60 HIKES
WITHIN 60 MILES
6th Edition

PORTLAND

**Including the Coast, Mount Hood,
Mount St. Helens, and the Santiam River**

D1056448

Paul Gerald

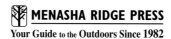

MENASHA RIDGE PRESS
Your Guide to the Outdoors Since 1982

60 Hikes Within 60 Miles: Portland

Printed in China
Published by Menasha Ridge Press
Distributed by Publishers Group West
Sixth edition, second printing 2018

Project editor: Kate Johnson
Cover and interior design: Jonathan Norberg
Cartography: Scott McGrew and Tim Kissel
Cover photos: (front) Vista Ridge; (back, clockwise from top) Ape Canyon, Triple Falls, Silver Star Mountain: Ed's Trail, and Lava Canyon, all by Paul Gerald
Interior photos: Paul Gerald, except those noted on page and the following: page 24: Tyler Hulett/Shutterstock; page 63: Marc Hallquist/Flickr; page 94: Chris Christian/Flickr; page 98: Gary Gilardi/Shutterstock; page 188: courtesy of Oregon's Mt. Hood Territory/public domain; and page 209: William Cushman/Shutterstock.
Proofreader: Susan Roberts McWilliams
Indexer: Rich Carlson

Library of Congress Cataloging-in-Publication Data

Names: Gerald, Paul, 1966- author.
Title: 60 hikes within 60 miles Portland / Paul Gerald.
Other titles: Sixty hikes within sixty miles Portland
Description: Sixth edition. | Birmingham, Ala. : Menasha Ridge Press, 2018. | Includes index.
Identifiers: LCCN 2018000286 | ISBN 9781634040846 (pbk.) | ISBN 9781634040853 (ebook)
Subjects: LCSH: Hiking—Oregon—Portland Region—Guidebooks. | Trails—Oregon—Portland Region—
    Guidebooks. | Portland Region (Or.)—Guidebooks.
Classification: LCC GV199.42.O72 P6738 2018 | DDC 796.5109795/49—dc23
LC record available at https://lccn.loc.gov/2018000286

MENASHA RIDGE PRESS
An imprint of AdventureKEEN
2204 First Ave. S, Ste. 102
Birmingham, AL 35233

Visit menasharidge.com for a complete listing of our books and for ordering information. Contact us at our website, at facebook.com/menasharidge, or at twitter.com/menasharidge with questions or comments. To find out more about who we are and what we're doing, visit blog.menasharidge.com.

DISCLAIMER This book is meant only as a guide to select trails in the Portland, Oregon, area and does not guarantee hiker safety—you hike at your own risk. Neither Menasha Ridge Press nor Paul Gerald is liable for property loss or damage, personal injury, or death that may result from accessing or hiking the trails described in this guide. Be especially cautious when walking in potentially hazardous terrains with, for example, steep inclines or drop-offs. Do not attempt to explore terrain that may be beyond your abilities. Please read carefully the introduction to this book, as well as safety information from other sources. Familiarize yourself with current weather reports and maps of the area you plan to visit (in addition to the maps provided in this guidebook). Be cognizant of park regulations, and always follow them. While every effort has been made to ensure the accuracy of the information in this guidebook, land and road conditions, phone numbers and websites, and other information can change from year to year.

Dedication

With immense gratitude and respect, I dedicate this book to the people who build and maintain the trails.

60 Hikes Within 60 Miles: Portland

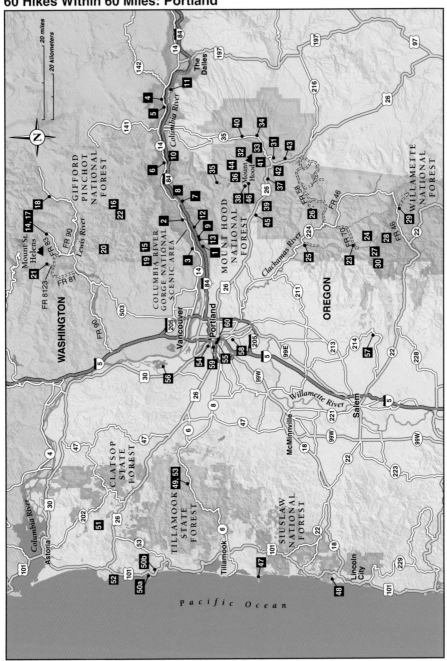

TABLE OF CONTENTS

At some point, the task of thanking everyone associated with this book just becomes too much. The whole idea that I am the one who writes it even starts to blur a little; I get so much help, information, support, and companionship—and so many of you read and use this work—that it seems more like ours than mine. Whenever I meet somebody out on the trail who is using this book (and assuming they aren't lost or injured), I get a powerful sense that we, together, are enjoying these places and benefiting from our work. So thank you, most of all.

Of course, there are dozens of people behind the scenes who make this happen, starting with all the people at Menasha Ridge Press—none of whom I've even had the chance to meet in person! First and foremost is Molly Merkle, who for years has patiently answered all my tedious questions and tolerated my somewhat adversarial relationship with deadlines. For this edition, it's mainly been project editor Kate Johnson putting up with me. Then there are the people who turn my Word files, photos, and GPS tracks into the book you're holding: Annie Long, Scott McGrew, and Tim Kissel. Thanks to Allison Brown for patiently explaining my royalties reports—many times—and to Tanya Twerdowsky and Liliane Opsomer for letting the world know the book exists.

I processed a lot of information for this book, much of which came from the U.S. Forest Service, Oregon State Parks, oregonhikers.org, the Columbia Gorge Visitors Center, Washington State Parks, the Mazamas, Friends of the Columbia Gorge, and the amazing book *Oregon Geographical Names* from the Oregon Historical Society Press. (I am proud to own a signed copy of the seventh edition, revised and updated by Lewis L. McArthur, and I recommend it highly.)

Once I put all the information together, I needed somebody to make sure I wasn't completely out of touch with reality. Enter a small army of patient employees of various federal, state, and private agencies who interrupted their busy schedule to review all the text. My humble thanks to them all: Stephen Anderson, Tom Atiyeh, Lynn Barlow, J. W. Cleveland, Jane Dooley, Susan Freston, Brandon Haraughty, Greg Hawley, Karen Houston, Lorie Hutton, Robin Jensen, Breanne Jordan, Heather Latham, Mark Marshall, Pete Marvin, Gary McDaniel, Jacquelyn Oakes, Randy Peterson, Erik Plunkett, Dean Robertson, Tom Robinson, Kevin Strandberg, Bob Stillson, Rick Swart, and Gary Walker. Special thanks also to Tom Kloster for his Wy'East Blog and that thing he and his friends did up at Mount Hood. Ryan Ojerio with the Washington Trails Association was fantastic with Coyote Wall and Cape Horn. And thanks to Becky Schreiber for helping out so much with the trails in Hoyt Arboretum—and for loaning me Buddy the beagle on occasion.

Of course, a hike is a lonely experience without good friends to share it with. Special mention here has to go to Kelly Podshadley for being my most frequent hiking buddy and my hiking safety check-in partner. May you finish all 60 soon! And here is a list of the folks who made "researching" this sixth edition such an enjoyable experience: Mehdi Akhavein, Debbie Bauer, Sherry Bourdin, Jennifer Brown, Peter Carew, Jim Chase, Tom Eggers, Gwen Farnham, Laura Foster, Andrew Franklin, Craig Frerichs, Jane Garbisch, Steve Gilbert, Regis Krug, Ann Johnson, Bob Malone, Lorin Moentenich, Avis Newell, Judy Olivier, West Post, Pam Probst, Martin Schwartz, Maria Shindler, Margaret Smith, Kathy Stefan, Sue Stonecliffe, Jim Van Lente, Norma Vincent, Eric Wheeler, and Leslie Woods-Eggers. I've done a horrendous job of keeping notes on who accompanied me along the way, and I absolutely left people out. I apologize in advance. I also literally copied and pasted those last two sentences from the fifth edition!

And finally, a lifetime of love and thanks to my family back east: Marjorie and Barry Gerald; Lee, Lela, and Jack Gerald and Max Simpson; and Lucy, Becky, David, Jeff, and Charlie Cook.

—*Paul Gerald*

Welcome to Menasha Ridge Press's *60 Hikes Within 60 Miles,* a series designed to provide hikers with the information they need to find and hike the best trails surrounding metropolitan areas.

Our strategy is simple: First, find a hiker who knows the area and loves to hike. Second, ask that person to spend a year researching the most popular and best trails around. And third, have that person describe each trail in terms of difficulty, scenery, condition, elevation change, and other categories that are important to most hikers. "Pretend you've just completed a hike and met up with other hikers at the trailhead," we told each author. "Imagine their questions, and be clear in your answers."

An experienced hiker and writer, Paul Gerald has selected 60 of the best hikes in and around the Portland, Oregon, metropolitan area. This sixth edition includes new hikes, as well as additional sections and new routes for some of the existing hikes. Gerald provides hikers (and walkers) with a great variety of hikes—all within roughly 60 miles of Portland—from urban strolls on city sidewalks to aerobic outings at Mount Hood or the coast.

You'll get more out of this book if you take a moment to read the Introduction, which explains how to read the trail listings. The "Maps" section will help you understand how useful topos are on a hike and will also tell you where to get them. And though this is a where-to, not a how-to, guide, readers who haven't hiked extensively will find the Introduction of particular value.

As much for the opportunity to free the spirit as to free the body, let these hikes elevate you above the urban hurry.

All the best,
The Editors at Menasha Ridge Press

Here's a funny admission from the author of a hiking book: There comes a time, almost every time I go hiking, when I kind of hate it.

Sometimes it's the weather, of course—I'm pretty much a fair-weather hiker. Sometimes it's the big uphills. Sometimes it's the big downhills. Sometimes it's the tedious drive back home (in particular, the stretch of I-84 between Troutdale and I-205). Sometimes it's the early start, or the late return, or all the chatter on the trail.

Maybe I'm just getting old. My 47-year-old legs and back complain a good bit more than their 25-year-old versions did. Maybe it's the pounds I put on while writing a breakfast guidebook. And maybe I fell into the trap of letting my favorite pastime become part of my job; slogging up a viewless hill in the rain because "I have to do it for my book" hardly screams "glamorous life of a writer."

So why do it? For the little moments in between.

Take Multnomah Falls, for example. You drive there, you see the falls, you fight the crowds, and maybe you drag yourself up the paved trail to the top of the falls for a look around. (And yes, I am being a horribly jaded Oregonian, but there's an element of "been there, done that.")

Ah, but if you keep going, there's a place just a little farther up, right past the old bridge over the creek, where the pavement ends, the crowds turn around, and it turns into a trail leading into the woods, bound for miles away. And every time I go there, there's a little moment waiting for me, like a present I'm always getting for the first time. It's the moving on, the letting go, the opening up, the knowing that behind me are town, life, work, money, cars, computers . . . and ahead of me are only more trails, trees, creeks, birds, cliffs, and mountains.

My brain knows that I can walk from that spot, using only forest trails, to Mount Hood, to countless other quiet, wild places—and that's a part of it. But it's my heart where the little moment happens: a kind of release and relaxation, a simple knowing that from here on, it's just me, or us, and the woods, and I can go wherever I feel, because I have everything I need right here with me.

Mountains have stirred my heart since I was a kid, and it's because they are filled with those little moments: walking over a ridge to see a great view, coming around a corner to surprise a deer on the path, catching a glimpse of an eagle or a big fish, or just sitting down for some peace next to a stream. Of course, it doesn't have to be in the mountains; much of Portland's magic lies in places like Macleay Park, where you leave "the city," in the metaphorical sense, and enter "the woods," where trout swim in the creek, massive trees grow all around, and a bird sanctuary lies just up the hill. It's there in the wooded ravine around Marquam Trail, which was at one time to be filled with apartments but instead remains a quiet, shady way to reach the highest place in the city.

My original, superficial reason for writing this book, way back in 2000, was so I could walk into Powell's, buy a latte, point at a book on the shelf, and say, "I wrote that." In other words, it was mostly ego. (Believe me, it wasn't the money.) There was something deeper, though. I have always wanted to visit interesting places, meet interesting people, and do interesting things, then tell people about them. Part of that is still ego, sure, but a bigger part is that I just think life is cool, and I want to share that coolness with people. I think hiking is particularly cool, even when I hate it, because, after all, don't you feel a little more satisfaction walking to the top of, say, Larch Mountain than driving up there? Especially if you start by the banks of the Columbia and walk to the top of a Cascades peak? The work, if you can do it, enhances the payoff. You get a connection with the whole mountain.

Over the years, the deeper reason for writing this book has really come to the surface. Tens of thousands of people have bought it, which amazes and humbles me, and more than a few have told me they like it. Ego again, sure, but also something else: they (you) are having those little moments, too! To think I drove all the ridiculous way to Whetstone Mountain to that somewhat boring hike—ah, but to get that mind-boggling view—and then somebody else read about it, made the same drive, and got the same view, well, it makes me feel warm and fuzzy. People often thank me for writing the book, and all I can think to say is, "Thanks for enjoying it."

And that's when they ask me The Question: "What's your favorite hike?" (Everybody asks it, and if you do too, it's not a problem.) And I, being a wordy writer (have you noticed?), always say, "Well, that depends." It depends, in my case, almost entirely on what month it is. I often think of Catherine Creek (page 35) and Coyote Wall and The Labyrinth (page 40), hikes that in April and May are awash in flowery, sunny, breezy, birdsong-y little moments and that in July or August would probably kill you with heat and boredom.

My "favorite" also depends on what mood I'm in. Sometimes I want a big adventure like Trapper Creek Wilderness (page 114), maybe even an overnight, and sometimes I just want to stroll along the Salmon River (page 196) for a couple of miles, to gaze at the big trees and look for salmon.

I have written this book, six times now, with one intention: to help my fellow humans get out to some cool spots so they can experience those little moments. I wrote the book as if you're actually going to carry it along with you, so I can point stuff out along the way and give you some things to think about while you're doing the dull stuff. I'll tell you why Ramona Falls (page 192) is called that (it's a sweet story), where the Throne of the Forest King sits (page 248), and why there are cables around stumps high above the Clackamas River (page 133). I assume you want to know these things.

What I also assume is that, like most people I talk to, you may want to know what my favorite hike is. Like I said, that depends, so here, by way of introduction to the book, is my personal hiking calendar. I don't stick to this—or anything else in life—very strictly, but I bet that if you follow it you'll have a fine year of hiking, and there's a decent chance we'll bump into each other.

I get through winter the way most outdoorsy Portlanders do: I'll go up the Macleay Trail (page 268) or Marquam Trail (page 272) to stretch my legs, to Tryon Creek (page 285) to look for trillium, and maybe out to Angels Rest (page 21) for a sunset. Otherwise it's snowshoes, coffee, and planning for better weather. For this edition, I've even included a list of good snowshoeing hikes.

What I really look for, usually on oregonhikers.org, is the first picture of a grass widow. What's a grass widow? Well, objectively speaking, it's a small, unassuming, mostly purple flower, barely 6 inches tall. But to the local hiker's heart, it's The Beginning of It All, the first spring wildflower that blooms where such flowers bloom. Most often, the grass widow is first seen in March at Catherine Creek (page 35), and its appearance means that we can now leave rainy old Portland, drive an hour east, and listen to the meadowlarks while we look for the hundreds of types of flowers that will soon drape the slopes at Coyote Wall (page 40) and Tom McCall Preserve (page 67).

That show goes until May, and in the meantime, the few dry days offer a chance to go to Silver Falls State Park (page 281), where you can walk 7 miles, see 10 full-tilt waterfalls, and sip a hot drink by a fireplace before or after you go. It's also time to start getting into shape, and for that there is Hamilton Mountain in Beacon Rock State Park (page 26), itself a flowery scene by April, when flowers on the Oregon side of the Gorge have yet to bloom but the Washington side is catching rays. I also use, as a conditioner and a reminder of why I live here, the loop from Wahkeena Falls over to Multnomah Falls (page 75). You might like it as well, if you're into stuff like creeks, waterfalls, springs, views, and soft-serve ice cream. And now, you get to be amazed how nature recovers from a fire.

Other April favorites? The plunging waters of Eagle Creek (page 48) or Falls Creek (page 90) and the irises out at the end of Cape Falcon (page 50).

By May, in theory, I'm getting in pretty good shape, and the sun is starting to win its annual battle against the clouds. Barely. But May means one big thing in my hiking life: Dog Mountain (page 44). It's physically big but psychologically bigger. The flower show there from mid-May to mid-June wipes me out every year, and whenever I tell people the balsamroot is a "sea of yellow," it's an understatement. Really, if you do one hike this year, go up Dog Mountain in late May or so. Well, first do some other hikes to prepare.

By June the bloom is spreading and the clouds are clearing. June can be maddening, though; you want to get up high, but most years the snow still blankets those trails. June is about transition and midelevation: too late for spring flowers, too early for Mount Hood, just right for being around 2,000–3,000 feet for the first blast of summer. My June favorites are Silver Star Mountain (page 19) for the flowers, Bull of the Woods (page 126) for the rhododendrons, Kings and Elk Mountains (page 49) to see what shape I'm really in, or Saddle Mountain (page 253) for both the flowers and a meal at Camp 18.

In July I play two little games called Beat the Heat and Follow the Mosquitoes. See, for the first month after the snow melts, the mosquitoes will make you hate life. And July tends to be pretty warm. So I wait for word that the little varmints are gone from various shady forests, and then I move in to hike. This leads me to lower-elevation places like Breitenbush (page 148), Opal Creek (page 152), and Lewis River (page 98), or the ever-cool coast, where July means the big bloom at Cascade Head (page 238), and July 16, the opening of the upper trailhead there.

August is what it's all about around here. The snow and mosquitoes are gone, and my hiker's life is all about getting as high up as possible. For me, this means it's Mount Hood time: McNeil Point barely edges out Vista Ridge, Paradise Park, and Lookout Mountain as a favorite, but anything in the "Around Mount Hood" section (page 158) will be a day well spent. And now we get to watch Vista Ridge recover from a tremendous fire as well.

For a lot of hikers, September is the best month. The weather is cooling, the crowds are gone, and there will just start to be some fall colors somewhere. I like Cooper Spur (page 164) this time of year, because at about 8,000 feet you can just barely sense winter coming over the ridge. September is also your last shot at the high stuff, so it's a good time to hit Bull of the Woods (page 126) for that big view as well.

For this hiker, October is the grand finale. You're in shape, you've got your hiking crowd of friends, you can still do any hike in the book, and there's a sweet sadness as the season closes, plus a sense of rush to get it all in before the snow blows. For highlights, it's all about two things: salmon and fall colors. October is when the ocean-run fish make it into the Salmon River (page 196) and the Wilson River (page 261), and when the vine maples at Trapper Creek (page 114) or Ape Canyon (page 82) will blow your mind.

After a year like that, frankly, I'm more interested in watching college football or English soccer for November and December than I am in hiking. And I know that I just listed at least a third of the book as a favorite, but what can I say? The whole book is favorites! I've done well over 100 different hikes around here, and these are the 60 I believe anyone will enjoy.

So please do enjoy them, and take care of them. And remember: If you have one of those moments when you hate hiking, just keep truckin', and you'll soon get to one of those other little, but glorious, moments in between.

Weisendanger Falls on the Larch Mountain Trail (Hike 9, page 58)

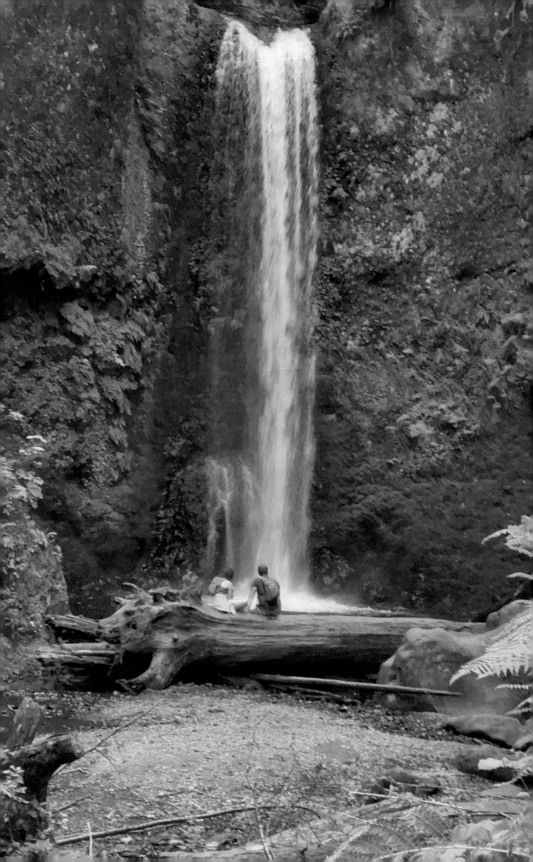

REGION Hike Number/Hike Name		Page #	Mileage	Difficulty	Months Open	Best Time	Kid Friendly	Backpacking	Running
IN THE COLUMBIA RIVER GORGE									
1	Angels Rest and Devils Rest	21	4.6/8.6	M–S	all	clear days	sort of		
2	Beacon Rock State Park	26	1.8/8	E–S	all	4–5	✓		
3	Cape Horn	31	4–6.3	E–M	all	4–5/10	✓		
4	Catherine Creek	35	Up to 4.1	E–M	all	3–6	✓		
5	Coyote Wall and The Labyrinth	40	4.6/5.2	M	all	4–5			✓
6	Dog Mountain	44	6.9	S	all	5–6			✓
7	Eagle Creek	48	4/12	E–M	all	3–5/9–10	sort of	✓	✓
8	Herman Creek	53	6–20	E–S	all	4–5/10	✓	✓	
9	Larch Mountain	58	6.8–18	M–S	all	8			
10	Mount Defiance	63	3–11.6	E–S	all	4/9	sort of		
11	Tom McCall Preserve	67	2.5–6	E–M	all	4–5	✓		
12	Triple Falls	71	4.5	M	all	4/10	✓		
13	Wahkeena Falls to Multnomah Falls	75	4.9	M	all	anytime			
AROUND MOUNT ST. HELENS									
14	Ape Canyon	82	11.6	M	6–10	9–10			✓
15	Bluff Mountain Trail	86	13.2	S	6–10	7/10			
16	Falls Creek Falls	90	3.4/6.1	E–M	5–11	5–6	✓	✓	
17	Lava Canyon	94	1.3–6	E–S	6–10	6/10			
18	Lewis River	98	5.2	E	4–11	6/10	✓		✓
19	Silver Star Mountain: Ed's Trail	102	4.8	M	6–10	7/10	✓		
20	Siouxon Creek	106	Up to 10.8	E–S	3–11	6/10	✓	✓	✓
21	South Fork Toutle River	110	11.2	S	6–10	8–9		✓	
22	Trapper Creek Wilderness	114	Up to 14.5	E–S	5–11	9–10		✓	
UP THE CLACKAMAS RIVER									
23	Bagby Hot Springs	122	3–3.6	E	3–11	4–10	✓	✓	✓
24	Bull of the Woods	126	2.2/7	E–S	6–10	8–9	✓	✓	
25	Clackamas River	130	8.2/8	M	all	5/10	✓	✓	✓
26	Roaring River Wilderness	134	1.4–12.6	E–S	7–10	8–9	✓	✓	
27	Whetstone Mountain	138	4.8	M	6–10	6/10			
UP THE SANTIAM RIVER									
28	Battle Ax Mountain	144	5.1/6.5	S	6–10	8–9		✓	
29	Breitenbush Hot Springs Area	148	1–8	E–S	4–11	9–10	✓	✓	
30	Opal Creek Wilderness	152	7–13	E–M	4–11	7–10	✓	✓	✓
AROUND MOUNT HOOD									
31	Barlow Pass	160	5–10	M	7–10	8–9		✓	
32	Cooper Spur	164	6.8	S	7–10	8–9		✓	
33	Elk Meadows	169	2–12	M–S	7–10	8–9	✓	✓	

REGION Hike Number/Hike Name	Page #	Mileage	Difficulty	Months Open	Best Time	Kid Friendly	Backpacking	Running
34 Lookout Mountain	174	3/9.6	E–S	7–10	8–9	✓		
35 Lost Lake	179	3.3–16	E–S	6–10	8–9	✓	✓	✓
36 McNeil Point	184	12	E–S	7–10	8–9		✓	
37 Mirror Lake	188	2.8/6	E–S	6–10	8–9	✓		
38 Ramona Falls	192	7.1/16	E	5–10	7–9	✓	✓	✓
39 Salmon River	196	5.2/6.6	E–S	all	10	✓	✓	✓
40 Tamanawas Falls	200	3.4	E	6–11	7–9	✓		
41 Timberline Lodge	204	1–13	E–S	7–10	8–9	✓	✓	
42 Trillium Lake	209	1.9	E	6–10	8–9	✓		✓
43 Twin Lakes	213	9.4	M	6–10	8–9	✓	✓	✓
44 Vista Ridge	218	4–11	M	7–10	8–9		✓	
45 Wildwood Recreation Site	223	1.75/10.6	E–S	all	8–10	✓		
46 Zigzag Mountain	227	4.6/6.8/9.4	E–S	6–10	8–9	✓	✓	✓
THE COAST AND COAST RANGE								
47 Cape Lookout State Park	234	3.6–4.8	M	all	3–4/7–9	✓		
48 Cascade Head	238	2.5–5.4	M	all/7–12	7–9			
49 Kings Mountain and Elk Mountain	243	5.2–13.4	M–S	all	5–6			
50 Oswald West State Park	248	2.5–9	E–S	all	clear days	✓		
51 Saddle Mountain	253	5.2	S	all	6–7			
52 Tillamook Head	257	3–12	E–M	all	3–4	✓	✓	
53 Wilson River	261	Up to 20.6	E–S	all	3–4/10	✓		✓
PORTLAND AND THE WILLAMETTE VALLEY								
54 Macleay Trail	268	2.26/4.5	E–M	all	clear days	✓		✓
55 Marquam Trail to Council Crest	272	3.7	E–M	all	clear days	✓		
56 Sauvie Island	276	3/7	E	all/4–9	4–5/10	✓		✓
57 Silver Falls State Park	281	Up to 7	E–M	all	3–4/9–10	✓		
58 Tryon Creek State Natural Area	285	3	E	all	4	✓		✓
59 Washington Park and Hoyt Arboretum	289	4	E	all	3/10	✓		✓
60 Willamette River Greenway	293	Up to 12.2	E–M	all	anytime	✓		✓

DIFFICULTY RATINGS		
E = Easy	M = Moderate	S = Strenuous

MONTHS OPEN

Numbers correspond to months (3 = March, etc.).

See paulgerald.com/hike-list *for an online version of this chart.*

MORE HIKE CATEGORIES

REGION Hike Number/Hike Name	Page #	Wheelchair/ Stroller Friendly	Big Views	Waterfalls	Snowshoeing	Swimming	Good for Shuttles	Camping at Trailhead
IN THE COLUMBIA RIVER GORGE								
1 Angels Rest and Devils Rest	21		✓	✓			✓	
2 Beacon Rock State Park	26	✓	✓	✓				✓
3 Cape Horn	31		✓					
4 Catherine Creek	35	✓	✓					
5 Coyote Wall and The Labyrinth	40	✓	✓					
6 Dog Mountain	44		✓					
7 Eagle Creek	48			✓			✓	✓
8 Herman Creek	53		✓	✓			✓	✓
9 Larch Mountain	58	✓	✓	✓			✓	
10 Mount Defiance	63	✓	✓	✓				
11 Tom McCall Preserve	67		✓					
12 Triple Falls	71			✓				
13 Wahkeena Falls to Multnomah Falls	75	✓		✓				
AROUND MOUNT ST. HELENS								
14 Ape Canyon	82		✓				✓	
15 Bluff Mountain Trail	86		✓					
16 Falls Creek Falls	90			✓		✓		
17 Lava Canyon	94	✓		✓				
18 Lewis River	98			✓		✓		✓
19 Silver Star Mountain: Ed's Trail	102		✓					
20 Siouxon Creek	106			✓		✓		
21 South Fork Toutle River	110		✓					
22 Trapper Creek Wilderness	114		✓		✓			
UP THE CLACKAMAS RIVER								
23 Bagby Hot Springs	122					✓		
24 Bull of the Woods	126		✓			✓		
25 Clackamas River	130			✓		✓	✓	✓
26 Roaring River Wilderness	134					✓		✓
27 Whetstone Mountain	138		✓					
UP THE SANTIAM RIVER								
28 Battle Ax Mountain	144		✓					✓
29 Breitenbush Hot Springs Area	148				✓		✓	✓
30 Opal Creek Wilderness	152					✓		

REGION Hike Number/Hike Name	Page #	Wheelchair/Stroller Friendly	Big Views	Waterfalls	Snowshoeing	Swimming	Good for Shuttles	Camping at Trailhead
AROUND MOUNT HOOD								
31 Barlow Pass	160		✓		✓		✓	
32 Cooper Spur	164		✓		✓			✓
33 Elk Meadows	169		✓		✓			
34 Lookout Mountain	174		✓					
35 Lost Lake	179	✓	✓			✓		✓
36 McNeil Point	184		✓					
37 Mirror Lake	188		✓		✓	✓		
38 Ramona Falls	192			✓				
39 Salmon River	196				✓	✓		✓
40 Tamanawas Falls	200			✓	✓			
41 Timberline Lodge	204	✓	✓		✓			✓
42 Trillium Lake	209	✓			✓	✓		✓
43 Twin Lakes	213				✓	✓		✓
44 Vista Ridge	218		✓					
45 Wildwood Recreation Site	223	✓			✓	✓		
46 Zigzag Mountain	227		✓			✓		
THE COAST AND COAST RANGE								
47 Cape Lookout State Park	234		✓				✓	✓
48 Cascade Head	238		✓				✓	
49 Kings Mountain and Elk Mountain	243		✓			✓	✓	✓
50 Oswald West State Park	248		✓				✓	
51 Saddle Mountain	253		✓					✓
52 Tillamook Head	257		✓				✓	
53 Wilson River	261					✓	✓	✓
PORTLAND AND THE WILLAMETTE VALLEY								
54 Macleay Trail	268	✓						
55 Marquam Trail to Council Crest	272		✓					
56 Sauvie Island	276					✓		
57 Silver Falls State Park	281			✓				✓
58 Tryon Creek State Natural Area	285	✓						
59 Washington Park and Hoyt Arboretum	289	✓						
60 Willamette River Greenway	293	✓					✓	

See paulgerald.com/hike-list for an online version of this chart.

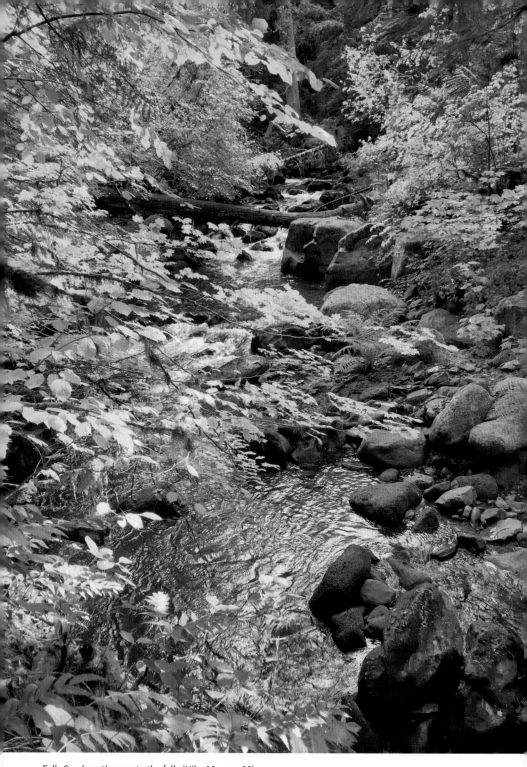

Falls Creek on the way to the falls (Hike 16, page 90)

Welcome to *60 Hikes Within 60 Miles: Portland*! If you're new to hiking or even if you're a seasoned trekker, take a few minutes to read the following introduction. We'll explain how this book is organized and how to get the best use of it.

About This Book

I suppose there's one thing I should get out of the way right up front: yes, many of these hikes are more than 60 driving miles from Portland. When the idea was first proposed, that was the suggested range, but driving 60 miles from the middle of Portland doesn't get you to most trailheads on Mount Hood, or any on the coast. And I didn't want to write that book. So I changed it to 60 miles as the crow flies from the edge of the metro area. And even then, some are beyond it. But virtually all are within a two-hour drive of Pioneer Courthouse Square. Here is a quick rundown of the geographical areas covered:

IN THE COLUMBIA RIVER GORGE goes as far east as just past Mosier. This means an amazing territory that goes from waterfalls, moss, and ferns to oak savannas and wildflower meadows. It also goes up from the river to subalpine ridges, thousands of feet above.

AROUND MOUNT ST. HELENS is only on the south side, including up onto the peak itself. Hikes here also explore the wooded mountains between the Columbia and the mountain, and some of the effects the mountain has had on the environment.

UP THE CLACKAMAS RIVER means trails that are all accessed by driving up OR 224 past Estacada. This is mainly forest and lake country, with a lot of wilderness, and it goes all the way up to high lookouts in the Cascades.

UP THE SANTIAM RIVER means up OR 22 east of Salem. This is similar to the Clackamas area and neighbors it, creating a great swath of forest, hills, and solitude between Mounts Hood and Jefferson.

AROUND MOUNT HOOD means literally that: hikes basically in a circle around the mountain. Here you will go from creekside strolls to rocky ridges next to glaciers.

THE COAST AND COAST RANGE means west of Forest Grove and from Cape Lookout near Tillamook up to Seaside. The Coast Range offers younger forest but great hiking variety, and at the coast you can find sweeping views of the ocean, sandy beaches, and tremendously large trees.

PORTLAND AND THE WILLAMETTE VALLEY really means the Portland area plus Silver Falls State Park. This can mean sidewalks or city parks, farm country or waterfall heaven.

Within each of those areas, I have tried to offer a good selection and variety of hikes. For example, in each area you should be able to find easy walks for the whole family, river walks, lake visits, scenic viewpoints, challenging treks, and connections to larger areas with more options like backpacking trips. I wrote the book with the whole range of hikers in mind; some of you are just starting out or want to take it easy, and some of you want to go really big. I tried to accommodate everyone.

How to Use This Guidebook

The following information walks you through this guidebook's organization to make it easy and convenient to plan great hikes.

OVERVIEW MAP AND MAP LEGEND

Use the overview map on page iv to assess the general location of each hike's primary trailhead. Each hike's number appears on the overview map and in the table of contents. As you flip through the book, a hike's full profile is easy to locate by watching for the hike number at the top of each page. The book is organized by region, as indicated in the table of contents. A map legend that details the symbols found on trail maps appears on page 17.

REGIONAL MAPS

The book is divided into regions, and prefacing each regional section is an overview map. The regional maps provide more detail than the overview map, bringing you closer to the hikes.

TRAIL MAPS

A detailed map of each hike's route appears with its profile. On each of these maps, symbols indicate the trailhead, the complete route, significant features, facilities, and topographic landmarks such as creeks, overlooks, and peaks.

To produce the highly accurate maps in this book, the author used a handheld GPS unit to gather data while hiking each route, and then sent that data to the publisher's expert cartographers. However, your GPS is not really a substitute for sound, sensible navigation that takes into account the conditions that you observe while hiking.

Further, despite the high quality of the maps in this guidebook, the publisher and author strongly recommend that you always carry an additional map, such as the ones noted in each entry's listing for "Maps."

ELEVATION PROFILES (DIAGRAM)

For trails with any significant elevation changes, the hike description *will* include this profile graph. Entries for fairly flat routes, such as a lake loop, *will not* display an elevation profile.

For hike descriptions where the elevation profile is included, this diagram represents the rises and falls of the trail as viewed from the side, over the complete distance (in miles) of that trail. On the diagram's vertical axis, or height scale, the number of feet indicated between each tick mark lets you visualize the climb. To avoid making flat hikes look steep and steep hikes appear flat, varying height scales provide an accurate image of each hike's climbing challenge.

THE HIKE PROFILE

Each hike contains a brief overview of the trail, a description of the route from start to finish, key at-a-glance information—from the trail's distance and configuration to contacts for local information—GPS trailhead coordinates, and directions for driving to the trailhead area. Each profile also includes a map (see "Trail Maps," previous page) and elevation profile (if the elevation gain is 100 feet or more). Many hike profiles also include notes on nearby activities.

KEY INFORMATION

The information in this box gives you a quick idea of the statistics and specifics of each hike.

DISTANCE & CONFIGURATION Distance notes the length of the hike round-trip, from start to finish. If the hike description includes options to shorten or extend the hike, those round-trip distances will also be factored here. Configuration defines the trail as a loop, an out-and-back (taking you in and out via the same route), a figure eight, or a balloon.

DIFFICULTY The degree of effort that a typical hiker should expect on a given route. For simplicity, the trails are rated as easy, moderate, or strenuous.

SCENERY A short summary of the attractions offered by the hike and what to expect in terms of plant life, wildlife, natural wonders, and historical features.

EXPOSURE A quick check of how much sun you can expect on your shoulders during the hike.

TRAFFIC Indicates how busy the trail might be on an average day. Trail traffic, of course, varies from day to day and season to season. Weekend days typically see the most visitors. Other trail users that may be encountered on the trail are also noted here.

TRAIL SURFACE Indicates whether the trail surface is paved, rocky, gravel, dirt, boardwalk, or a mixture of elements.

HIKING TIME How long it took me to hike the trail. I like to dawdle, and I can easily fritter away time eating or admiring wildflowers. On average, I cover 2 miles an hour (more hiking downhill, fewer on steady ascents, particularly during hot weather). If you're an experienced hiker in great shape, you'll finish the hikes with time to spare, but if you're a beginner or you like to stop to take in the views, allow for a little extra.

ELEVATION CHANGE Lists the cumulative elevation change along the trail.

SEASON The time of year when a particular hike is accessible. In most cases, the determining factor is snow. Except where specific hours are noted, hikes are accessible daily, sunrise–sunset.

BEST TIME If you want to save a hike for when it's at its best, this is the time to shoot for.

BACKPACKING OPTIONS Feel like spending the night out? Here's a quick glance; more details can be found in the text.

DRIVING DISTANCE How far each hike is from Pioneer Courthouse Square in downtown Portland. Not that you'd want to start from here necessarily, but the numbers should give you a good estimate of travel times to the trailheads from where you live. Driving times are provided as well.

ACCESS Fees or permits required to hike the trail are detailed here—and noted if there are none. Trail-access hours are also shown. A number of trailheads in this book require a Northwest Forest Pass. All of the outdoors shops listed in Appendixes A and B sell the pass, which costs $5 for one day and $30 for one year; you can also buy it at discovernw.org/store.

Other passes, such as the Interagency Senior Pass and various national passes, are available, so make sure to get the one that best meets your needs. Visit tinyurl .com/usfsregion6passesandpermits for more information.

MAPS Resources for maps, in addition to those in this guidebook, are listed here. (As previously noted, the publisher and author recommend that you carry more than one map—and that you consult those maps before heading out on the trail to resolve any confusion or discrepancy.)

WHEELCHAIR ACCESS At a glance, you'll see if there are paved sections or other areas for safely using a wheelchair.

FACILITIES This item alerts you to restrooms, water, picnic tables, and other basics at or near the trailhead.

CONTACT Listed here are phone numbers and websites for checking trail conditions and gleaning other day-to-day information.

LOCATION The address for the trail.

COMMENTS Here you will find assorted nuggets of information, such as whether or not dogs are allowed on the trails.

IN BRIEF

Think of this section as a taste of the trail, a snapshot focused on the historical landmarks, beautiful vistas, and other sights you may encounter on the hike.

DESCRIPTION

The heart of each hike. Here, the author provides a summary of the trail's essence and highlights any special traits the hike has to offer. The route is clearly outlined, including landmarks, side trips, and possible alternate routes along the way. Ultimately, the hike description will help you choose which hikes are best for you.

NEARBY ACTIVITIES

Look here for information on things to do or points of interest, such as nearby parks, museums, and restaurants. Note that not every hike has a listing.

DIRECTIONS

Used in conjunction with the GPS coordinates, the driving directions will help you locate each trailhead. Once at the trailhead, park only in designated areas.

GPS TRAILHEAD COORDINATES

As noted in "Trail Maps," page 2, the author used a handheld GPS unit to obtain geographic data and sent the information to the publisher's cartographers. The coordinates included with each hike profile—the intersection of the latitude (north) and longitude (west)—will direct you to the trailhead for that hike. In some cases, you can drive within viewing distance of a trailhead. Other hiking routes require a short walk to the trailhead from a parking area. You will also note that this guidebook uses the degree–decimal minute format for presenting the GPS coordinates:

N45° 33.613' W122° 10.365'

The latitude and longitude grid system is likely quite familiar to you, but here is a refresher, pertinent to visualizing the GPS coordinates:

Imaginary lines of latitude—called parallels and approximately 69 miles apart from each other—run horizontally around the globe. The equator is established to be 0°, and each parallel is indicated by degrees from the equator: up to 90°N at the North Pole, and down to 90°S at the South Pole.

Imaginary lines of longitude—called meridians—run perpendicular to latitude lines. Longitude lines are likewise indicated by degrees. Starting from 0° at the Prime Meridian in Greenwich, England, they continue to the east and west until they meet 180° later at the International Date Line in the Pacific Ocean. At the equator, longitude lines are approximately 69 miles apart, but that distance narrows as the meridians converge toward the North and South Poles.

To convert GPS coordinates given in degrees, minutes, and seconds to degree–decimal minute format, divide the seconds by 60. For more on GPS technology, visit usgs.gov.

TOPOGRAPHIC MAPS

The maps in this book have been produced with great care and, used with the hike text, will direct you to the trail and help you stay on course. However, you'll find superior detail and valuable information in the U.S. Geological Survey's 7.5-minute-series topographic maps. At mytopo.com, for example, you can view and print free USGS topos of the entire United States. Online services such as Trails.com charge annual fees for additional features such as shaded relief, which makes the topography stand out more. If you expect to print out many topo maps each year, it might be worth paying for such extras. The downside to USGS maps is that most are outdated, having been created 20–30 years ago; nevertheless, they provide excellent topographic detail. Of course, Google Earth (earth.google.com) does away with topo maps and their inaccuracies, replacing them with satellite imagery and its inaccuracies. Regardless, what one lacks, the other augments. Google Earth is an excellent tool whether you have difficulty with topos or not.

The author used the Gaia app on his iPhone for this edition and found it quite a bargain for $20. It works particularly well if you download maps of the area you're hiking ahead of time, and remember that it works in airplane mode, as well. This saves on battery power immensely.

If you're new to hiking, you might be wondering, "What's a topo map?" In short, it indicates not only linear distance but also elevation, using contour lines. These lines spread across the map like dozens of intricate spiderwebs. Each line represents a particular elevation, and at the base of each topo a contour's interval designation is given. If, for example, the interval is 20 feet, then the distance between each contour line is 20 feet. Follow five contour lines up on the same map, and the elevation has increased by 100 feet. In addition to the sources listed previously and in Appendix B, you'll find topos at major universities, outdoors shops, and some public libraries, as well as online at nationalmap.gov and store.usgs.gov.

Weather

For most folks, the hiking season around Portland starts in March or April, when flowers bloom and temperatures start to rise. Unfortunately, that's the least stable season, weather-wise. Forecasts are notoriously off the mark during spring, so if you aren't absolutely, positively sure it will be clear, plan for 50-something degrees and drizzling into June.

Snow is a different matter: The higher-elevation hikes in this book generally won't be completely clear until July. Also note that in the Columbia River Gorge, wind is a near-constant reality, so even on a sunny June day, a hike such as the one to Dog Mountain (Hike 6, page 44) can have you reaching for a hat and gloves. By mid- to late June, and all the way into October, you'll see mostly sunny skies, mild temperatures, and happy hikers. Then winter comes, and for all intents and purposes it rains until spring. We try to think of it as "waterfall loading."

The following chart lists average temperatures and precipitation by month for the Portland area. For each month, "Hi Temp" is the average daytime high, "Lo Temp" is the average nighttime low, and "Rain or Snow" is the average precipitation. And remember, this is for the city: subtract degrees across the board as you go higher up into the mountains.

	January	February	March	April	May	June
HI TEMP	47°F	51°F	57°F	61°F	68°F	74°F
LO TEMP	36°F	36°F	40°F	43°F	49°F	54°F
RAIN or SNOW	4.88"	3.66"	3.66"	2.72"	2.48"	1.69"
	July	August	September	October	November	December
HI TEMP	81°F	81°F	76°F	64°F	53°F	46°F
LO TEMP	58°F	58°F	53°F	46°F	40°F	35°F
RAIN or SNOW	.67"	.67"	1.46"	2.99"	5.63"	5.47"
Source: usclimatedata.com						

Water

How much is enough? Well, one simple physiological fact should convince you to err on the side of excess when deciding how much water to pack: a hiker walking steadily in 90° heat needs approximately 10 quarts of fluid per day. That's 2.5 gallons. A good rule of thumb is to hydrate prior to your hike, carry (and drink)

6 ounces of water for every mile you plan to hike, and hydrate again after the hike. For most people, the pleasures of hiking make carrying water a relatively minor price to pay to remain safe and healthy. So pack more than you anticipate needing, even for short hikes.

If you are tempted to drink "found" water, do so with extreme caution. Many ponds and lakes encountered by hikers are fairly stagnant, and the water tastes terrible. Drinking such water presents inherent risks for thirsty trekkers. Giardia parasites contaminate many water sources and cause the dreaded intestinal giardiasis that can last for weeks after ingestion. For information, visit The Centers for Disease Control website at cdc.gov/parasites/giardia.

For that reason, effective treatment is essential before using any water source found along the trail. Boiling water for 2–3 minutes is always a safe measure for camping, but day hikers can consider iodine tablets, approved chemical mixes, filtration units rated for giardia, and UV filtration. Some of these methods (for example, filtration with an added carbon filter) remove bad tastes typical in stagnant water, while others add their own taste. As a precaution, carry a means of water purification to help in a pinch, if you realize you have underestimated your consumption needs.

Clothing

Weather, unexpected trail conditions, fatigue, extended hiking duration, and wrong turns can individually or collectively turn a great outing into a very uncomfortable one at best—and a life-threatening one at worst. Thus, proper attire plays a key role in staying comfortable and, sometimes, in staying alive. Here are some helpful guidelines:

Choose silk, wool, or synthetics for maximum comfort in all of your hiking attire—from hats to socks and in between. Cotton is fine if the weather remains dry and stable, but you won't be happy if that material gets wet.

Always wear a hat, or at least tuck one into your day pack or hitch it to your belt. Hats offer all-weather sun and wind protection as well as warmth if it turns cold.

Be ready to layer up or down as the day progresses and the mercury rises or falls. Today's outdoor wear makes layering easy, with such designs as jackets that convert to vests and zip-off or button-up legs.

Wear hiking boots or sturdy hiking sandals with toe protection. Flip-flopping along a paved urban greenway is one thing, but never hike a trail in open sandals or casual sneakers. Your bones and arches need support, and your skin needs protection.

Pair that footwear with good socks. If you prefer not to sheathe your feet when wearing hiking sandals, tuck the socks into your day pack; you may need them if the weather plummets or if you hit rocky turf and pebbles begin to irritate your feet. And, in an emergency, if you have lost your gloves, you can use the socks as mittens.

Don't leave rainwear behind, even if the day dawns clear and sunny. Tuck into your day pack, or tie around your waist, a jacket that is breathable and either water-resistant or waterproof. Investigate different choices at your local outdoors retailer. If you are a frequent hiker, ideally you'll have more than one rainwear weight, material, and style in your closet to protect you in all seasons in your regional climate and hiking microclimates.

Essential Gear

Today you can buy outdoor vests that have up to 20 pockets shaped and sized to carry everything from toothpicks to binoculars. Or, if you don't aspire to feel like a burro, you can neatly stow all of these items in your day pack or backpack. The following list showcases never-hike-without-them items, in alphabetical order, as all are important:

- **Extra clothes:** raingear, warm hat, gloves, and change of socks and shirt
- **Extra food:** trail mix, granola bars, or other high-energy foods
- **Flashlight or headlamp** with extra bulb and batteries
- **Insect repellent.** For some areas and seasons, this is vital.
- **Maps and a high-quality compass.** Even if you know the terrain from previous hikes, don't leave home without these tools. And, as previously noted, bring maps in addition to those in this guidebook, and consult your maps prior to the hike. If you are versed in GPS usage, bring that device too, but don't rely on it as your sole navigational tool, as battery life can dwindle or die, and be sure to compare its guidance with that of your maps.
- **Pocketknife and/or multitool**
- **Sunscreen** Note the expiration date on the tube or bottle; it's usually embossed on the top.
- **Water** As emphasized more than once in this book, bring more than you think you will drink. Depending on your destination, you may want to bring a container and iodine or a filter for purifying water in case you run out.
- **Whistle** This little gadget will be your best friend in an emergency.
- **Windproof matches and/or a lighter,** as well as a fire starter

FIRST AID KIT

In addition to the aforementioned items, those below may appear overwhelming for a day hike. But any paramedic will tell you that the products listed here—in alphabetical order, because all are important—are just the basics. The reality of hiking is that you can be out for a week of backpacking and acquire only a mosquito bite. Or you can hike for an hour, slip, and suffer a bleeding abrasion or broken bone.

Fortunately, these listed items will collapse into a very small space. You can also purchase convenient, prepackaged kits at your pharmacy or online.

➤ Adhesive bandages

➤ Antibiotic ointment (Neosporin or the generic equivalent)

➤ Athletic tape

➤ Benadryl or the generic equivalent, diphenhydramine (for allergic reactions)

➤ Blister kit (such as Moleskin/Spenco 2nd Skin)

➤ Butterfly-closure bandages

➤ Elastic bandages or joint wraps

➤ Epinephrine in a prefilled syringe typically by prescription only, for people known to have severe allergic reactions to hiking occurrences such as bee stings

➤ Gauze one roll and a half dozen 4-by-4-inch pads

➤ Hydrogen peroxide or iodine

➤ Ibuprofen or acetaminophen

Note: Consider your intended terrain and the number of hikers in your party before you exclude any article cited above. A botanical garden stroll may not inspire you to carry a complete kit, but anything beyond that warrants precaution. When hiking alone, you should always be prepared for a medical need. And if you are a twosome or with a group, one or more people in your party should be equipped with first aid material.

General Safety

The following tips may have the familiar ring of your mother's voice as you take note of them.

➤ Always let someone know where you will be hiking and how long you expect to be gone. It's a good idea to give that person a copy of your route, particularly if you are headed into any isolated area. Let them know when you return. I always text a friend with my exact route and the instructions to call the sheriff if she doesn't hear from me by a certain time.

➤ Always sign in and out of any trail registers provided. Don't hesitate to comment on the trail condition if space is provided; that's your opportunity to alert others to any problems you encounter.

➤ Do not count on a cell phone for your safety. Reception may be spotty or nonexistent on the trail, even on an urban walk—especially if it is embraced by towering trees.

➤ Always carry food and water, even for a short hike. And bring more water than you think you will need. (That cannot be said often enough.)

- ➤ **Ask questions.** State forest and park employees are there to help. It's a lot easier to solicit advice before a problem occurs, and it will help you avoid a mishap away from civilization when it's too late to amend an error.

- ➤ **Stay on designated trails.** Even on the most clearly marked trails, there is usually a point where you have to stop and consider which way to go. If you become disoriented, don't panic. As soon as you think you may be off track, stop, assess your current direction, and then retrace your steps to the point where you went astray. Using a map, a compass, and this book, and keeping in mind what you have passed thus far, reorient yourself, and trust your judgment. If you become absolutely unsure of how to continue, return to your vehicle the way you came in. Should you become completely lost and have no idea how to find the trailhead, remaining in place along the trail and waiting for help is most often the best option for adults and always the best option for children.

- ➤ **Always carry a whistle,** another precaution that cannot be overemphasized. It may be a lifesaver if you do become lost or sustain an injury.

- ➤ **Be especially careful when crossing streams.** Whether you are fording the stream or crossing on a log, make every step count. If you have any doubt about maintaining your balance on a log, ford the stream instead: use a trekking pole or stout stick for balance *and face upstream as you cross.* If a stream seems too deep to ford, turn back. Whatever is on the other side is not worth risking your life.

- ➤ **Be careful at overlooks.** While these areas may provide spectacular views, they are potentially hazardous. Stay back from the edge of outcrops, and make absolutely sure of your footing; a misstep can mean a nasty and possibly fatal fall.

- ➤ **Standing dead trees and storm-damaged living trees pose a significant hazard to hikers.** These trees may have loose or broken limbs that could fall at any time. While walking beneath trees, and when choosing a spot to rest or enjoy your snack, look up.

- ➤ **Know the symptoms of subnormal body temperature, known as hypothermia.** Shivering and forgetfulness are the two most common indicators of this stealthy killer. Hypothermia can occur at any elevation, even in the summer, especially when the hiker is wearing lightweight cotton clothing. If symptoms present themselves, get to shelter, hot liquids, and dry clothes as soon as possible.

- ➤ **Know the symptoms of heat exhaustion (hyperthermia).** Light-headedness and loss of energy are the first two indicators. If you feel these symptoms, find some shade, drink your water, remove as many layers of clothing as practical, and stay put until you cool down. Marching through heat exhaustion leads to heatstroke, which can be fatal. If you should be sweating and you're not, that's the signature warning sign. Your hike is over at that point—heatstroke is a life-threatening condition that can cause seizures, convulsions, and eventually death. If you or a companion reaches that point, do whatever can be done to cool the victim down, and seek medical attention immediately.

➤ **Most important of all, take along your brain.** A cool, calculating mind is the most important asset on the trail. It allows you to think before you act.

In summary: Plan ahead. Watch your step. Avoid accidents before they happen. Enjoy a rewarding and relaxing hike.

Watchwords for Flora and Fauna

Be aware of the following concerns regarding plants and wildlife.

BLACK BEARS In my 20-plus years of hiking around Portland and Oregon, I have seen black bears exactly five times; three of those were running away before I spotted them, one never saw me, and one was so engrossed in huckleberries that it didn't care about me at all. Though attacks by black bears are uncommon, the sight or approach of a bear can give anyone a start. If you encounter a bear while hiking, remain calm and avoid running in any direction. Make loud noises to scare off the bear, and back away slowly. In primitive and remote areas, assume bears are present; in more-developed sites, check on the current bear situation prior to hiking. Most encounters are food related, as bears have an exceptional sense of smell and not particularly discriminating tastes. While this is of greater concern to backpackers and campers, on a day hike, you may plan a lunchtime picnic or munch on an energy bar or other snack from time to time. So remain aware and alert.

BLACK FLIES Though certainly a pest and maddening annoyance, the worst a black fly will cause is an itchy welt. In this area, they are most active in the Cascades just after the snow melts, in June and July, during the day, and especially before thunderstorms, as well as during the morning and evening hours. Insect repellent has some effect, though the only way to keep out of their swarming midst is to keep moving.

MOSQUITOES Mosquitoes will mainly enter your hiking experience up in the Cascades in June and July, just after the snow melts. Ward off these pests with insect repellent and/or repellent-impregnated clothing. In some areas, mosquitoes are known to carry the West Nile virus, but in Oregon they are quite rare. The year 2016, for example, saw just four human cases. Still, all due caution should be taken to avoid their bites.

POISON OAK When using this book, your chances of encountering poison oak are greatest in the Columbia River Gorge, with the odds going up as you travel east. It likes dry country, so while you probably won't see it at Multnomah Falls, you will see great stands of it at Catherine Creek. It also grows almost exclusively below 3,000 feet elevation, so on some hikes you will eventually get above it. Most people encounter poison oak while bushwhacking or traveling off-trail, so stay on established trails whenever possible.

Recognizing and avoiding poison oak is the most effective way to prevent the painful, itchy rash associated with it. The plant occurs as either a vine or a shrub, with three leaflets. It's easiest to spot in summer and early autumn, when the leaves flush bright red. Beware of unknown bare-branched shrubs and vines in winter—the entire plant can cause a rash, no matter what the season.

Urushiol, the oil in the sap of the plant, is responsible for the rash. Within about 14 hours of exposure, raised lines and/or blisters will appear on the affected area, accompanied

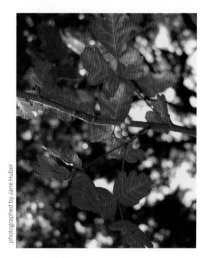

photographed by Jane Huber

Poison oak

by a terrible itch. If you do happen to touch the plant, you must remove the oil within 15–20 minutes to avoid a reaction. Rinsing it off with cool water—hot water spreads it—is impractical on the trail, but some commercial products, such as Tecnu, are effective in removing it from your skin without the use of water.

Refrain from scratching because bacteria under your fingernails can cause an infection. As soon as possible, wash and dry the affected area thoroughly, applying a calamine lotion to help dry out the rash. If itching or blistering is severe, seek medical attention. To keep from spreading the misery to someone else, wash not only any exposed parts of your body but also any oil-contaminated clothes, hiking gear, and pets.

SNAKES In the region described in this book, you will very often encounter non-venomous and nondangerous garter snakes; in the eastern Columbia Gorge, you might see a rattlesnake, although I never have. The best rule is to leave all snakes alone, give them a wide berth as you hike past, and make sure any hiking companions (including dogs) do the same.

The following is good advice for rattlesnake country, which again is really just the hikes east of Hood River. When hiking, stick to well-used trails, and wear over-the-ankle boots and loose-fitting pants. Do not step or put your hands beyond your range of detailed visibility, and avoid wandering around in the dark. Step *onto* logs and rocks, never *over* them, and be especially careful when climbing rocks. Always avoid walking through dense brush or willow thickets.

Should you encounter a rattlesnake, its body language will reveal its mood. A coiled rattler is primed for a strike, while a relaxed rattler is more sanguine. If the snake is within striking distance, stand motionless and wait for it to calm down and move on. Taking small, slow steps backward is another smart strategy. If you're out of immediate range, you can either skirt the snake or wait for it to move. Some people believe tapping the ground with a stick—from a safe distance, rather than in the snake's face—will encourage the snake to move on.

TICKS Ticks are often found on brush and tall grass, where they seem to be waiting to hitch a ride on a warm-blooded passerby. Adult ticks are most active April–May and again October–November. Among the varieties of ticks, the black-legged tick, commonly called the deer tick, is the primary carrier of Lyme disease. But Lyme disease is rare in Oregon, averaging 35–45 cases statewide per year. In 2016 Multnomah County had four reported cases.

Still, getting a tick is a hassle, so a few tips are in order. Use insect repellent that contains DEET. Wear light-colored clothing to make it easier for you to spot ticks before they migrate to your skin. At the end of the hike, visually check your hair, the back of your neck, your armpits, and your socks. During your posthike shower, take a moment to do a more complete body check. For ticks that are already embedded, removal with tweezers is best. Grasp the tick close to your skin, and remove it by pulling straight out firmly. Do your best to remove the head, but do not twist. Use disinfectant solution on the wound.

These arachnids like to hang out in the brush that grows along trails. I've noticed ticks mostly in the eastern Columbia River Gorge, but you should be tick-aware throughout the spring, summer, and fall. Ticks are ectoparasites, meaning they need a host for most of their life cycle in order to reproduce. The ticks that alight onto you while hiking will be very small, sometimes so tiny that you won't be able to spot them. All ticks need to attach for several hours before they can transmit disease.

Hunting

Separate rules, regulations, and licenses govern the various hunting types and related seasons. Though there are generally no problems, hikers may wish to forgo their trips during the big-game seasons, when the woods suddenly seem filled with orange and camouflage. In our part of the world, this basically means the autumn, whether it's deer, elk, or game birds. The only times I have ever encountered hunters on a hike around here were on Sauvie Island in late October and way up in the Cascades in mid-October. And that's a total of three times.

REGULATIONS

The only regulations we need to concern ourselves with have to do with parking, registration, and the size of our groups.

For parking, if you have a Northwest Forest Pass, Oregon State Parks Pass, and a Washington State Parks Discovery Pass, you will have access to almost every trail in this book. A few have their own parking costs, and those will be mentioned in the text.

In designated wilderness areas, two more regulations come into play. One is that you will be required to fill out a free permit when entering the wilderness. The other is that, within wilderness areas, groups size is limited to 12 people.

Trail Etiquette

Always treat the trail, wildlife, and fellow hikers with respect. Here are some reminders.

➤ **Plan ahead in order to be self-sufficient at all times.** For example, carry necessary supplies for changes in weather or other conditions. A well-planned trip brings satisfaction to you and to others.

➤ **Hike on open trails only.** In seasons or construction areas where road or trail closures may be a possibility, use the websites or phone numbers shown in the "Contacts" line for each hike to check conditions prior to heading out. And do not attempt to circumvent such closures.

➤ **Avoid trespassing on private land,** and obtain all permits and authorization as required. Also, leave gates as you found them or as directed by signage.

➤ **Be courteous** to other hikers, bikers, and equestrians you encounter on the trails.

➤ **Never spook wild animals or pets.** An unannounced approach, a sudden movement, or a loud noise startles most critters, and a surprised animal can be dangerous to you, to others, and to itself. Give animals plenty of space.

➤ **Observe the yield signs** around the region's trailheads and backcountry. Typically they advise hikers to yield to horses, and bikers to yield to both horses and hikers. By common courtesy on hills, hikers and bikers should yield to any uphill traffic. When encountering mounted riders or horsepackers, hikers can courteously step off the trail, on the downhill side if possible. So that the horse can see and hear you, calmly greet the riders before they reach you and do not dart behind trees. Also resist the urge to pet horses unless you are invited to do so.

➤ **Stay on the existing trail** and do not blaze any new trails. Don't cut short the switchbacks!

➤ **Be sure to pack out what you pack in,** leaving only your footprints. No one likes to see the trash someone else has left behind. And yes, this includes bags of dog poop.

15

Tips on Enjoying Hiking Around Portland

It would be hard to have a bad time hiking around Portland, but there are degrees of enjoyment. Here are my tips to help you make the most of your day.

➤ **Try to avoid the crowds.** I know it's hard for many people to get out during the week, but understand that if you hike in the Gorge or at Mount Hood on weekends, it may be a madhouse. Go early in the morning. Or go after work (and bring a headlamp). Or go somewhere else! For the Gorge, in particular, I have offered a less crowded alternative for some of the most popular hikes.

➤ **Try hiking at different times of day.** I love hitting a crowded trail in mid-afternoon, when the morning shift has left and the midday crowd is clearing out. Go nuts sometime and hike for the sunrise or sunset.

➤ **Bring food you actually like.** Sounds silly, I know, but if you don't like energy bars, don't bring them. Bring something you want to eat. I also carry a couple of freezer packs on many hikes to keep my sandwich or fruit fresh.

➤ **Potluck it.** Plan on a group meal along the way.

➤ **Have a hot meal or beverage.** Who says you can't bring your camp stove on a day hike? Pasta for lunch in a flowery meadow works pretty well.

➤ **Bring group snacks.** People like people with snacks.

➤ **Carpool, and pitch in for gas.**

➤ **Bring fresh socks and sandals** or other comfortable footwear for the trip home. Kicking off those hiking shoes and filthy socks is the best!

➤ **Bring a bag to stash your dirty hike gear in** for the drive home—especially if you're a passenger.

➤ **Pack a cooler and posthike snacks in the car.** Nothing beats finishing up the hike, kicking off your shoes, tearing into a bag of salty goodness, and washing it down with some liquid sugar. Or a beer, if you're not driving. Or fruit, if that's your thing.

➤ **Seriously consider shuttles and key swaps.** I mention them where they make sense, but a key swap is a blast. Get two groups of people, swap cars on the way to the hike, park at either end, hand off keys when you meet, and then you're hiking to your own car for the trip out. Or do the swap posthike over coffee or food. Bringing a spare for your ride is a good idea, too.

➤ **Make it an overnighter.** Whether camping near the trailhead or spending a night in a hotel, why not make it two days in a row? I love spending a couple of nights every spring in Hood River, exploring the town and only doing that tedious drive home once. Same thing for the coast.

➤ **Get a cushion to sit on.** Every time I whip out my little foam sit pad, people gawk and say they have to get one. Best $12 I ever spent.

➤ **Get a bladder for your water.** It's nice to take a sip without taking off your pack.

← → Directional arrows	Featured trail	Alternate trail
Freeway	Highway with bridge	Minor road
Boardwalk	Unpaved road	
Railroad	Boundary line	Power line
Park/forest	Water body	River/creek/ intermittent stream

⛏ Bicycle trail	❓ Information/kiosk	🚽 Pit toilet/outhouse
Boat launch	Lighthouse	Radio tower
🚌 Bus stop	△ Overlook	Restroom
△ Campground	Marsh/bog	Scenic view
Drinking water	✕ Mine/quarry	Shelter
Fishing	Monument	Spring
✕ Footbridge	P Parking	Trailhead
✳ Garden	▲ Peak/hill	Viewing platform
Gate	Picnic area	// Waterfall/cascades
● General point of interest		

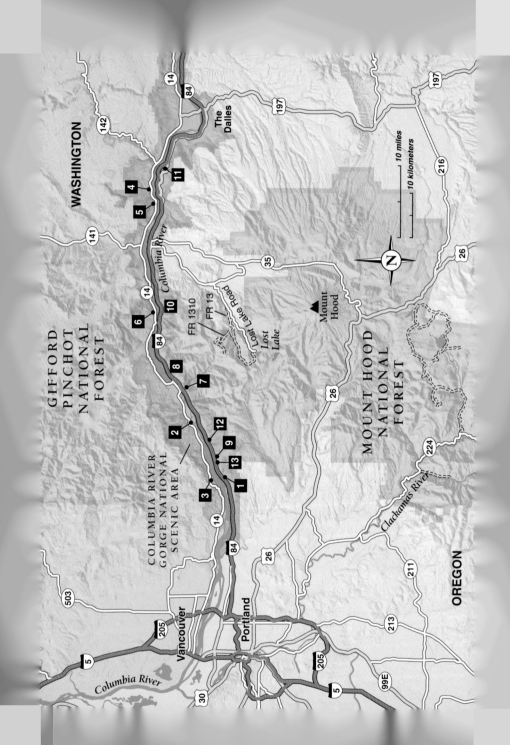

IN THE COLUMBIA RIVER GORGE

CHAPTER FOREWORD:
A Special Statement on the Columbia Gorge Trails

The Eagle Creek Fire of 2017 had an enormous impact on the Oregon side of the Columbia River Gorge. Unfortunately, as this edition was being written, very little was known about that impact, when (or if) all the trails would reopen, or what they would look like. The affected hikes in this book are Angels Rest, Eagle Creek, Herman Creek, Larch Mountain, Mount Defiance, Triple Falls, and Wahkeena Falls to Multnomah Falls.

Even the Historic Columbia River Highway through "waterfall alley" wasn't expected to open until the summer of 2018. In fact, as we went to press, massive changes to traffic and parking patterns on that road were also being considered.

What I have done here—all I can do—is offer a description of what everything was like before that fire. For the affected hikes here, and until we can update this book, you will have to check with OregonHikers.org, the Forest Service, and Friends of the Gorge (gorgefriends.org) for the latest conditions and openings. I will also keep updates on my website at paulgerald.com/eaglecreekfire. It may be years before these trails are back as we knew them prefire, and some may not return. Then again, more may be built.

To support and perhaps help with construction and maintenance, check with Trailkeepers of Oregon at trailkeepersoforegon.org.

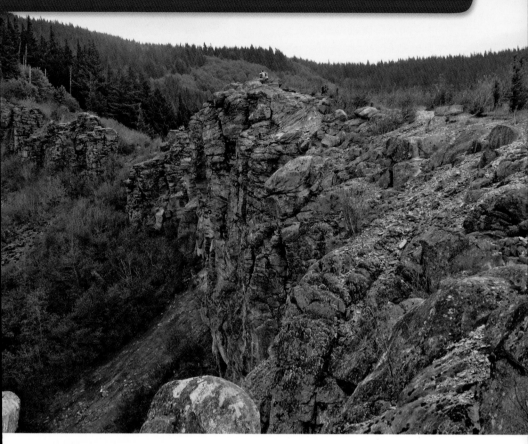

The ridge leading out to Angels Rest

THIS TRAIL IS one of the more accessible hikes in the region, with a gentle grade to a spectacular lookout point above the Columbia River. And that's why it has become so overcrowded. Try to go in spring, during the week, or after work—or check the Nearby Activities (page 25) for another option entirely. It also connects with Wahkeena Trail, making longer loops or one-way hikes with shuttles possible.

DESCRIPTION

As you drive out I-84, you can actually see Angels Rest, a flat-topped rock outcropping sticking out over the road at the end of a ridge. What looks like a building on top is in fact a clump of trees. You should also be able to make out the effects of the 2017 Eagle Creek Fire, much of which burned the same area as a 1991 fire near the summit.

Angels Rest Trail #415 starts off easy enough, then hits a rocky climb that's steep only for a few moments, leading to an early reward: a rare view from above a

DISTANCE: 4.6-mile out-and-back to Angels Rest, 8.6 miles point-to-point to Devils Rest

DIFFICULTY: Moderate to Angels Rest because of altitude gain and a little rock-scrambling at top; tougher to Devils Rest because of length and elevation

SCENERY: Forest, waterfall, creek crossing, panorama from Angels Rest

EXPOSURE: Mostly shady; one section at the top lies along a narrow, rocky ridge with steep drops.

TRAFFIC: Heavy year-round and utterly insane on nice-weather weekends. Do all you can to avoid these.

TRAIL SURFACE: Packed dirt with some roots; rocks

HIKING TIME: 2.5 hours to Angels Rest, 5 hours to Devils Rest

ELEVATION CHANGE: 1,450' to Angels Rest, 2,250' to Devil's Rest

SEASON: Year-round, but often gets snow in winter

BEST TIME: Any clear day when the whole world isn't hiking there

BACKPACKING OPTIONS: One decent campsite just past Angels Rest

DRIVING DISTANCE: 28 miles (30 minutes) from Pioneer Courthouse Square

ACCESS: No fees or permits required as of 2017

MAPS: Green Trails *Map 428 (Bridal Veil)* or *Map 428S (Columbia River Gorge–West)*

WHEELCHAIR ACCESS: No, but nearby Bridal Veil Falls State Park (503-695-2261, tinyurl.com /bridalveilfallssp) has some accessible trails.

FACILITIES: Restrooms and water 0.5 mile west at Bridal Veil Falls State Park

CONTACT: Columbia River Gorge National Scenic Area, 541-308-1700, www.fs.usda.gov/crgnsa

LOCATION: Angels Rest Trailhead at the intersection of E Bridal Veil Road and the Historic Columbia River Highway in Bridal Veil, Oregon.

COMMENTS: Dogs must be on a leash not exceeding 6 feet. Also, see the note at the start of this section (page 20) about the 2017 Eagle Creek Fire.

waterfall, in this case the 100-foot Coopey Falls, named for Charles Coopey, a Portland tailor who owned land here. A short way past this, the trail crosses a wooden bridge over Coopey Creek; just below this bridge, you can take a side trail down to see 35-foot Upper Coopey Falls. Beyond the bridge, the trail starts climbing again.

After about a mile, you'll start switchbacking through an area that burned in 1991; note the blackened trunks of some of the bigger trees. Mostly just the underbrush and smaller trees burned, which opened up the forest floor to the sun and let wildflowers come in to take your mind off the climb. (On the other hand, much of this area appears to have also burned in 2017.) Follow a series of small switchbacks into more-open (perhaps charred) country, getting a view of the rocky face of Angels Rest as you go. When the trail traverses 100 yards of rockslide, you're almost done.

Just past the slide, the trail reenters the woods briefly, and then you turn left out onto the final ridge. This last stretch of the trail might make you think twice about bringing small children: it gets a little narrow, with cliffs to the east falling away a few hundred feet, and in one spot you'll have to scramble up about 10 feet of rock. When the trail to Devils Rest goes back and to the right on the ridgetop, continue straight another 0.2 mile.

The reward for your effort is a view to rival any other in the Gorge, especially for the relative ease with which you got here. To the east you can see Beacon Rock

Angels Rest and Devils Rest

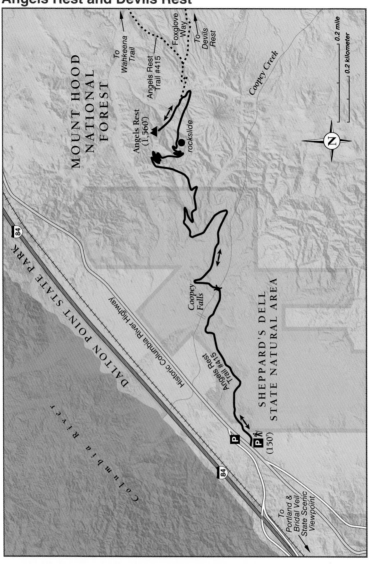

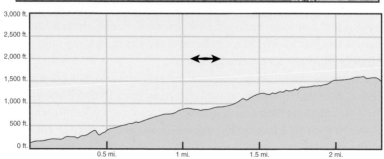

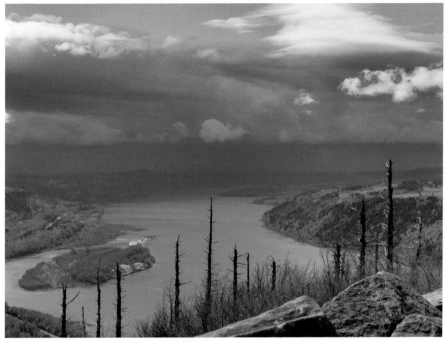

Looking west down the Columbia from Angels Rest, with trees showing fire damage

and the high walls on either side of the river. To the west you can see Vista House (built in 1916 as a pioneer memorial and rest stop for travelers, now an interpretive center, museum, and gift shop) and the hills falling away toward Portland and the Willamette Valley. The Columbia River, right below you, seems close enough that if you got a running start you could jump into it. You might see some windsurfers out there; on one trip, I watched a floatplane practicing touch-and-go landings on this stretch of the river.

You can also see three other hikes from this book: right next to Beacon Rock is the step-shaped Hamilton Mountain in Beacon Rock State Park (see next hike), and farther west on the Washington side are the bare peaks of Silver Star Mountain (Hikes 15 and 19). There's even a nice bench to sit on out here. Around to the left of the summit, a notch in some rocks offers shelter from frequently high winds. All in all, it's hard to imagine a better place to have lunch. The sunsets are rather amazing, as well—just bring a light for the trip back down.

If you're up for more hiking, you can turn this into a longer out-and-back or do a one-way hike with another car parked farther east. To do either, as you walk back down the ridge, veer left (east) at the junction instead of continuing straight, which is where you came from. After a few minutes you'll come to another junction. For the campsite, stay left 0.6 mile. For Devils Rest, follow the Foxglove Way

Trail uphill a mile to its junction, in an area that's often a bit marshy, with Foxglove Trail. Follow that 0.4 mile to Devils Rest, which oddly is some 800 feet higher than Angels Rest. Anyway, the official summit has neither a view nor a sign. The view up here is 0.2 mile farther along, on a side path left just after the trail starts down the hill on the other side.

You can go back the same way, or if you have a car at Wahkeena Falls or even Multnomah Falls, connect with that loop hike (page 75) by continuing past the viewpoint 1.4 miles to a big junction and heading for wherever your car is. This junction is 5.9 miles from the Angels Rest trailhead. From there, it's 1.9 miles to the Wahkeena Falls trailhead (making a total of 7.8 miles one-way) and 2.7 miles to Multnomah Falls trailhead (for a total of 8.6 miles).

NEARBY ACTIVITIES

Instead of a nearby activity for this and other supercrowded Gorge hikes, I am going to suggest another hike for those days when Angels Rest is a zoo. For a shorter but steeper hike to another amazing Gorge view, check out Mitchell Point. Take I-84 to Exit 58 and follow the trail up 1,300 feet in 1.3 miles. It gets sketchy and exposed at times, and you will want poles, but plans are afoot to rebuild the trail into something more user-friendly. Be sure to take the side trail to Mitchell Spur, as well. Check the field guide at oregonhikers.org for details.

• •

GPS TRAILHEAD COORDINATES
Angels Rest Trailhead N45° 33.613' W122° 10.365'
Devils Rest Trailhead N45° 33.734' W122° 7.704'

DIRECTIONS Take I-84 from Portland, driving 21 miles east of I-205 to Exit 28 (Bridal Veil). Bearing right off the exit, drive less than a mile, and park in the parking area at the intersection with the Historic Columbia River Highway; a second parking lot is down the road, to the right. The signed trailhead is on the old highway, across from the entrance to the lower lot.

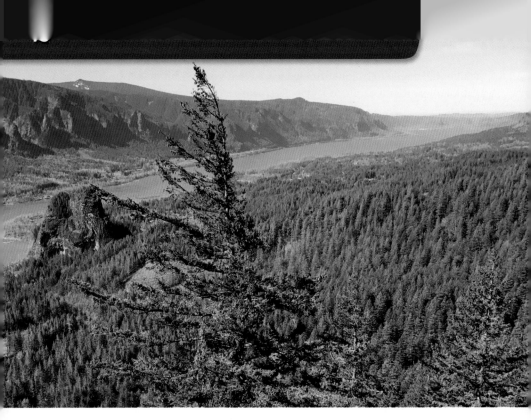

The Columbia River from Little Hamilton Mountain

ONE OF THE most recognized symbols of the Columbia River Gorge, Beacon Rock is also a fascinating, if short, hiking experience—and it's not even all this Washington state park has to offer. There's also a rigorous climb to scenic Hamilton Mountain, with a couple of amazing waterfalls along the way, and two supereasy nature loops.

DESCRIPTION

Beacon Rock

Beacon Rock got its name on Halloween 1805, when William Clark described it in his journal. It was originally called Beaten Rock because of the weather, but apparently something got crossed up in transcription. For the Corps of Discovery and the people who then lived along the Columbia River, Beacon Rock meant two important things: the last of the rapids on the Columbia River and the beginning of tidal influence on the river. Today, it means a unique hiking experience to its summit, and the state park around it means a chance to take in more nice views of the Columbia.

To climb Beacon Rock, which ascends 680 feet in less than a mile, start at a sign on the south side of WA 14, and give thanks to Henry J. Biddle. It was he who bought the rock (which is what's left of the inside of an ancient volcano) in 1914 to save it

DISTANCE & CONFIGURATION: 1.8-mile out-and-back to top of Beacon Rock, 8-mile loop to Hamilton Mountain

DIFFICULTY: Easy–moderate for Beacon Rock, strenuous for Hamilton Mountain

SCENERY: Overlooks of the Columbia, waterfalls, and spring wildflowers

EXPOSURE: Hamilton Mountain is mostly shady, with one rocky section near clifftops; Beacon Rock is on the side of a cliff but has handrails.

TRAFFIC: Heavy on weekends, moderate otherwise

TRAIL SURFACE: Packed dirt with rocks, some pavement

HIKING TIME: 1 hour for Beacon Rock, 4.5 hours for Hamilton Mountain

ELEVATION CHANGE: 680' to Beacon Rock, 2,100' to Hamilton Mountain

SEASON: Year-round, daily, 8 a.m.–sunset; call for trail conditions in winter.

BEST TIME: April and May

BACKPACKING OPTIONS: None

DRIVING DISTANCE: 51 miles (1 hour) from Pioneer Courthouse Square

ACCESS: A Washington State Discover Pass ($10/day, $30/year) is required and can be bought at the park or online at discoverpass .wa.gov.

MAPS: Green Trails *Map 428 (Bridal Veil)* or *Map 432S (Columbia River Gorge–West)*; free map at park headquarters and at website below

WHEELCHAIR ACCESS: Nearby on Hadley Trail; 1-mile loop at the Doetsch Day Use Area

FACILITIES: Water and restrooms at both trailheads

CONTACT: Beacon Rock State Park, 509-427-8265, parks.state.wa.us/474/beacon-rock

LOCATION: 34841 WA 14, Skamania, WA

COMMENTS: Dogs must be on a leash not exceeding 8 feet.

from being blasted to pieces for jetty material. He said his purpose was simply to build the trail you're about to hike, which he did with Italian stonemasons who had worked on the Columbia River Highway. Eventually, his family donated the land to the state. Though Biddle never charged hikers a penny, it remains the only trail I know of with a gate on it; it's open daily from 8 a.m. to dusk.

The trail is something of an engineering wonder: 4,500 feet long and 4 feet wide, it includes 52 switchbacks, 100 concrete slabs, and, originally, 22 wooden bridges. Some of the original work remains, such as wrought-iron handrails at some switchbacks and steel eyebolts in the rock wall.

To get to the top, just persevere and, if heights bother you, don't look down. Past the gate, it's virtually all rails and bridges and platforms until you're just below the summit, where you'll have a view east to Bonneville Dam, north to Hamilton Mountain, and straight down the other side to the boat docks of the state park.

Hamilton Mountain

For a more challenging and rewarding hike, drive—or walk, if the gate is closed—up the road across WA 14 to the Hamilton Mountain Trailhead. From here, you'll climb gently through forest until you reach a bench to take a break; the power lines you're under here aren't all that scenic, but you do get a view ahead to the summit of Hamilton Mountain. At 0.5 mile, continue straight at a trail leading left to the campground

Beacon Rock State Park

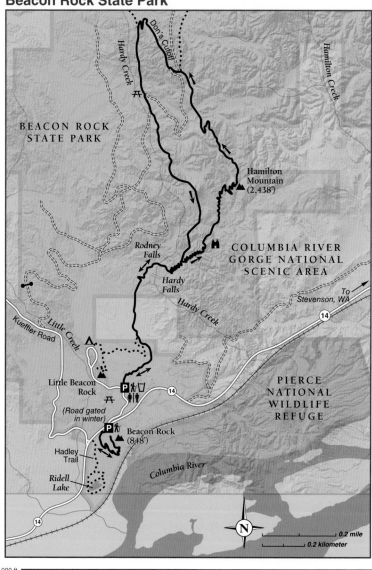

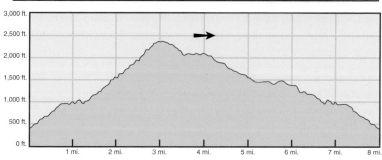

and a rock formation called Little Beacon Rock; 0.4 mile later, you'll come to a trail leading down and to the right 100 yards to two viewpoints overlooking Hardy Falls. A minute past that on the main trail, you'll see a sign that reads HAMILTON MOUNTAIN; oddly enough, it points downhill.

For a sight to remember, and perhaps a soak to cool you down, walk 100 yards left and check out Pool of the Winds at the top of Rodney Falls. Here the creek almost explodes out of a bowl in the rock face before tumbling down into the falls. You can get right in its spray, but in winter and spring you will be essentially wading the last part of the trail.

If you don't feel like climbing anymore, turn back here—it gets tougher quickly. To get to Hamilton Mountain, follow the signed trail as it descends to, then crosses, Hardy Creek and then heads up the hill. After 0.2 mile of climbing, you'll come to a junction with Hardy Creek Trail coming in from the left. This is the return portion of my suggested loop hike, so keep right on Hamilton Mountain Trail, and after 0.7 mile of sturdy climbing you'll reach the spectacular lookout at Little Hamilton Mountain. There's nothing wrong with turning back here, but be careful as you walk around on these rocks—in some spots it's more than 200 feet straight down.

If you want the real views, keep climbing. You'll see side trails on the right leading to meadows on top of the ridge. (You can take one of the side trails to get a view of the river.) Along the main trail, you'll pass two viewpoints of the mountain's rocky face while gaining 700 feet in just over a mile, bringing you to a mountain-top junction. The view from the summit of Hamilton Mountain, just to your right, is somewhat blocked by brush, but you can see Table Mountain to the northeast, Mount Adams just east of that, and Mount St. Helens to the northwest. You should also be able to make out Dog and Wind Mountains up the river, Eagle Creek and the Benson Plateau across it, and the town of Cascade Locks.

To add some new scenery and make your hike a loop, continue 0.9 mile north along the dramatic north ridge of Hamilton, which actually has better views than the summit. Turn left onto an old road, and go 100 yards to take Don's Cutoff Trail. This scenic but uneventful side trip—named for Don Cannard, cofounder of the Chinook Trails Association—leads down to Hardy Creek Trail, which at this point looks like a road. Turn left, follow the trail downhill past a picnic table, make another left to get back on a proper trail, and after another mile you'll be back at the junction mentioned above, just east of Rodney Falls. Turn right and you'll reach the Hamilton Mountain Trailhead in 1.6 miles.

Four More Easy Walks

Elsewhere in this park you can find the 1.2-mile, flat Doetsch Walking Path around a large meadow; the 1.5-mile River to Rock Trail, which gains 272 feet and goes through a 100-year-old filbert orchard; and two trails from the campground—0.5 mile to Little Beacon Rock and 1.2 miles on the ADA-accessible Hadley Trail.

NEARBY ACTIVITIES

The Columbia Gorge Interpretive Center Museum (990 SW Rock Creek Drive, Stevenson, WA; 800-991-2338 or 509-427-8211; columbiagorge.org), 10 miles east of the park on WA 14, features historical displays ranging from the geological (descriptions of the formation of the gorge) to the mechanical (examples of steam engines used on railroads a bit more recently).

. . . .

GPS TRAILHEAD COORDINATES
Beacon Rock Trailhead N45° 37.723' W122° 1.297'
Hamilton Mountain Trailhead N45° 37.929' W122° 1.207'

DIRECTIONS Take I-84 from Portland, driving 37 miles east of I-205 to Exit 44 (Cascade Locks). As soon as you enter the town, take your first right to get on Bridge of the Gods, following a sign for Stevenson. Pay a $2 toll on the bridge and, at the far end, turn left (west) on WA 14. Proceed 6.9 miles to Beacon Rock State Park. To hike up Beacon Rock, park on the left; to go toward Hamilton Mountain, turn right on the campground access road and drive 0.4 mile to the trailhead. The gate to the upper trailhead is closed in winter, but the trail is open; you'll just have to park on the south side of WA 14 and walk up the access road.

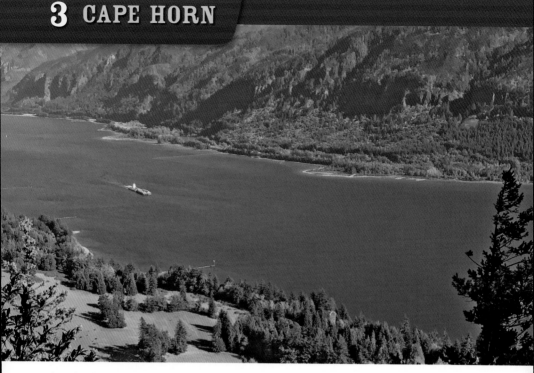

The Columbia River and the burned face of Angels Rest from Cape Horn Trail

THIS IS ONE of the newest trails in the Columbia River Gorge, and it's easy to see why it has become so popular. You can enjoy spectacular views of the Columbia from high up on the hill or just 200 feet above a riverside railroad, and in between you have a pleasant walk through forest and rolling-hill countryside reminiscent of a stroll in Europe.

DESCRIPTION

This trail has been sort of emerging for years: from off-limits private property to conservation struggle to informal trails to finally full-on U.S. Forest Service–approved design and maintenance. (You can get all the history at gorgefriends .org.) Now that it's official, with tunnels under the highway and everything, it's really two hikes put together: an upper section of 2.6 miles to viewpoints high above the river, and a lower section of about 4 miles that skirts the edge of cliffs just above the river and visits a waterfall—but is closed February 1–July 15 every year to protect nesting peregrine falcons.

When the lower portion is open, you can hike the whole loop in 6.3 miles. I should point out, if only for fun, that opinions vary wildly on how long this loop actually is: The Forest Service says 6 miles, the Cape Horn Conservancy says 7.7 miles, the Portland Hikers Field Guide says 7.1 miles, and Friends of the Columbia Gorge says 8.3 miles. My GPS said 6.3 miles, and my internal measuring device agreed.

DISTANCE & CONFIGURATION: 5.2-mile out-and-back for upper section, 4-mile out-and-back for lower section, 6.3-mile loop (when open)

DIFFICULTY: Easy–moderate

SCENERY: Forest, countryside, waterfall, clifftop viewpoints of Columbia River

EXPOSURE: Shaded, with several points on clifftops with railings

TRAFFIC: Moderate on spring and summer weekends

TRAIL SURFACE: Packed dirt, gravel, rocks

HIKING TIME: 2 hours for either section, 3.5 hours for whole loop

ELEVATION CHANGE: 1,350'

SEASON: Upper loop open year-round, with possible snow and ice in winter; lower loop closed February 1–July 15

BEST TIME: April and May for wildflowers, October for fall colors

BACKPACKING OPTIONS: None

DRIVING DISTANCE: 33 miles (40 minutes) from Pioneer Courthouse Square

ACCESS: No fees or permits required

MAPS: Green Trails *Map 428S (Columbia River Gorge–West)*; online map at capehorn conservancy.org

WHEELCHAIR ACCESS: No

FACILITIES: Outhouse at trailhead

CONTACT: Friends of the Columbia Gorge, gorgefriends.org; Columbia River Gorge National Scenic Area, 541-308-1700, www.fs.usda.gov /crgnsa; Cape Horn conservancy, capehorn conservancy.org

LOCATION: Cape Horn Trail at the intersection of Salmon Falls Road and Canyon Creek Road, east of Washougal, WA

COMMENTS: For the best photos of gorge views, do this hike in the afternoon, when the sun is behind you. Also, Friends of the Columbia Gorge hopes to purchase a 90-acre parcel to extend this trail, so check online to see if that has happened.

The trail starts right across the road from the trailhead and follows a wide gravel path in a thick forest, which in October has great fall colors, mainly from big-leaf maples. The first mile crosses several massive trees and a small creek and then gains 650 feet in a series of mellow switchbacks with not much to see, though it's interesting to look for the old sections of volunteer-built trail, now blocked with logs and branches. At 0.9 mile ignore a trail leading to the right, and at 1.1 miles you'll pass almost under a set of power lines.

At 1.2 miles you come to a funny sign offering a choice between VIEWPOINT and HORSES. Turns out it's because the viewpoint is on a narrow, rocky ledge that's unsafe for our four-legged friends. Don't be a horse: go left and check out the view of the gorge. This is Pioneer Point, with a view mostly east; a couple of minutes later you'll see another side trail leading to Fallen Tree Viewpoint, with a view mostly west. Both of these offer a good, if sad, view of the burned face of Angels Rest (page 21) across the way.

At this point you've gone 1.3 miles with 800 feet of elevation gain, and you're done climbing for now. The trail crosses the viewless summit, drops for just over 0.5 mile, briefly joins an old road in the woods, and then at 2.1 miles crosses paved Strunk Road. The next 0.5 mile or so reminds me of walking in England or Italy: rambling along country lanes past fields, houses, and horses, with wooded hillsides in the background.

Cape Horn

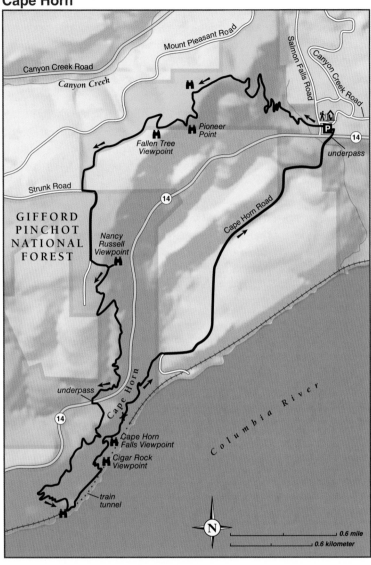

Mount Pleasant Road

Canyon Creek Road

Canyon Creek

Salmon Falls Road

Canyon Creek Road

Pioneer Point

Fallen Tree Viewpoint

underpass

Strunk Road

14

GIFFORD PINCHOT NATIONAL FOREST

Nancy Russell Viewpoint

Cape Horn Road

underpass

14

Cape Horn

Columbia River

Cape Horn Falls Viewpoint

Cigar Rock Viewpoint

train tunnel

N

0.6 mile

0.6 kilometer

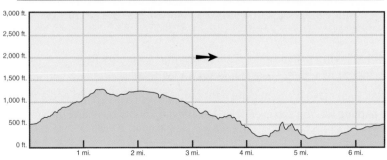

Now walking along a gravel road, look for the trail heading left, just as you reach the second clump of trees. The next big highlight is a new viewpoint built to honor Nancy Russell, founder of Friends of the Columbia Gorge, the group that did much of the work to save this place from development. In fact, the first time I hiked Cape Horn years ago, a big house stood near here. The Friends bought the land and tore the house down.

The Nancy Russell Viewpoint is at the 2.6-mile mark, so when the lower trail is closed, you might as well turn around here; that's the 5.2-mile option. But when you can do the whole loop, keep on truckin'. The trail now drops a few hundred feet in 0.5 mile to a new tunnel under WA 14—so much better than the death-defying dash of the old days.

Just past the tunnel, a new section of trail was clearly hacked out of a wall of blackberries. At the bottom of the hill, now at the 4.2-mile mark, an unsigned junction turns out to be another horse-versus-viewpoint decision. Again, don't be a horse: go right and follow the trail to a series of viewpoints recently made safer with retaining walls. You're actually above a long railroad tunnel here, and the Columbia River shipping channel is close to this bank, so you might get to see some cool machinery moving around.

After a final viewpoint that features tall, skinny Cigar Rock, you'll climb up a rocky slope (look for waterfalls up above), and then the trail crosses a bridge in front of Cape Horn Falls. In the old days, this trail went behind the falls, which was fun in the spring and summer, not so much in the winter.

Another steep (and occasionally rugged) drop brings you, after 0.4 mile, to the only semi-unfortunate aspect of this hike, which is that the last 1.3 miles are on a paved road. Nothing to be done, as both sides are private property and there's no room for another trailhead. So just enjoy the country-road rambling and watch out for cars. Right before the end, you'll use another tunnel to cross under WA 14, putting you back where you started.

If you just want to do the lower section when it's open, simply start at the trailhead and do these last few paragraphs in reverse, back to the Nancy Russell Viewpoint.

· ·

GPS TRAILHEAD COORDINATES N45° 35.359' W122° 10.711'

DIRECTIONS From Portland take I-205 across the Columbia River into Washington, and take Exit 27 (WA 14/Camas). Follow WA 14 for 20 miles and turn left onto Salmon Falls Road; then make an immediate right onto Canyon Creek Road and another right into the parking lot. You can even take a Skamania County bus here; the stop is called Salmon Falls, and the schedule is at tinyurl.com/hikebybus.

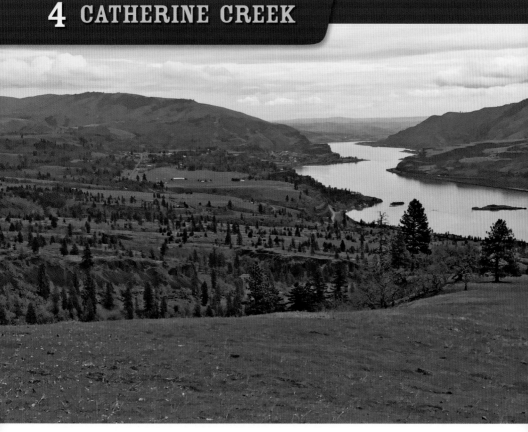

View east of the Columbia River from the Catherine Creek high country

FOR NINE MONTHS of the year there's really no reason to go to Catherine Creek, but from March to May there's no better place to be, for at that time it is wildflower heaven, with close to 100 species blooming at some point.

DESCRIPTION

There isn't much to this hike, physically speaking. In fact, you could knock out the paved and wheelchair-accessible section below the road in about 15 minutes. It's really all about the flowers and the wide-open vistas uncommon elsewhere in our local hiking world. Just try to avoid weekends if you can, or start early or late; crowds here have gotten nuts in the last few years.

From the road, walk through a gate and choose a path to the right, toward a small canyon just up the hill. If you're like me, you'll stop within a few feet and start admiring flowers. One enthusiast has counted as many as 82 species in bloom here on an April day, with such fantastic names as chocolate lily, common bastard toadflax, least hop clover, poet's shooting star, rigid fiddle-neck, great hound's-tongue, slender popcorn flower, small-flowered blue-eyed Mary, and chickweed monkey flower.

DISTANCE & CONFIGURATION: Loop of up to 4.1 miles

DIFFICULTY: Easy–moderate

SCENERY: Wide-open vistas; a geological curiosity; and (in spring) flowers, flowers everywhere!

EXPOSURE: Out in the open most of the way; optional trips to a clifftop

TRAFFIC: Heavy on weekends in late spring and early summer, moderate otherwise

TRAIL SURFACE: Dirt and some rock, plus a small paved section

HIKING TIME: 30 minutes–4 hours

ELEVATION CHANGE: 200'–1,040'

SEASON: Year-round

BEST TIME: Late March–early June

BACKPACKING OPTIONS: None

DRIVING DISTANCE: 72 miles (1 hour, 30 minutes) from Pioneer Courthouse Square

ACCESS: No fees or permits required

MAPS: Green Trails *Map 432S (Columbia River Gorge-East)*

WHEELCHAIR ACCESS: A series of loops below the parking area offers access to flowers, birds, views of the Columbia River, and a waterfall on Catherine Creek.

FACILITIES: Portable restroom at the trailhead February–May; no drinkable water

CONTACT: Columbia River Gorge National Scenic Area, 541-308-1700, www.fs.usda.gov/crgnsa

LOCATION: Catherine Creek Day Use Area/Trailhead on Old Highway 8, 5 miles west of Lyle, WA

COMMENTS: Dogs must be leashed.

Follow a gravel road into the canyon and up the creek. Watch out for poison oak; it's everywhere—beware an "old growth" stand of it on the right as you near the creek. After 0.25 mile, you could follow County Road Trail up the hill to the left if you want some exercise or you're connecting over to Coyote Wall (see below), but for now, cross the creek on a bouncy plank bridge and, 100 yards later, arrive at an old homestead. Above you now is a geological curiosity: a natural arch we'll see the top of later.

Past the homestead, stay right and ascend a slight rise into a meadow. Just after you pass the power lines, a total of 0.9 mile from your car, you come to a junction where you have three options: a lower loop, an upper loop, and a trip to the high country. For the lower loop, follow a trail to the right and then along the top of a little ridge, and your hike will be 2 miles. I'll describe that section in a bit, because you really should do at least part of the upper loop—and I will add that trails in this area have been in a state of flux for years. They were not, when I wrote this, completely official, but you should be able to follow along here. The best map (other than mine, of course) is the Green Trails *Map 432S, Columbia River Gorge-East*.

For the upper loop, follow Trail CA3 left and up the draw until you see a faint, signed road headed right and up the hill; follow it up into the meadows, then either head down toward the lower loop or find a trail east and across the meadows to eventually reach an overlook of Major Creek. (Some of this area burned in 2013, so you can see how it's coming back.)

For the high country, from this second junction keep heading up the draw until the trail climbs into the meadows, then go down and back toward the car or follow

Catherine Creek

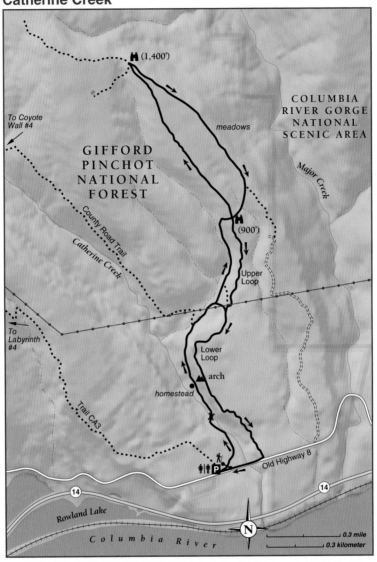

Ħ (1,400')

To Coyote
Wall #4

COLUMBIA
RIVER GORGE
NATIONAL
SCENIC AREA

meadows

Major Creek

GIFFORD
PINCHOT
NATIONAL
FOREST

County Road Trail

Catherine Creek

Ħ (900')

Upper
Loop

To
Labyrinth
#4

Lower
Loop

▲ arch

homestead

Trail CA3

Old Highway 8

P

14

14

Rowland Lake

C o l u m b i a   R i v e r

N

0.3 mile
0.3 kilometer

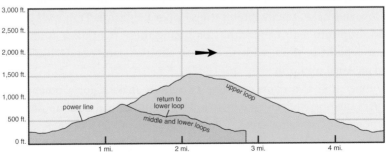

3,000 ft.
2,500 ft.
2,000 ft.
1,500 ft.
1,000 ft.
500 ft.
0 ft.

power line

return to
lower loop

upper loop

middle and lower loops

1 mi.   2 mi.   3 mi.   4 mi.

Trail CA3 up to the treeline, where there's a lovely picnic spot among magnificent oak trees. From here turn east and follow a trail over to viewpoints of Major Creek, then circle back to the Lower Loop for a roughly 4-mile day. Or look for a trail that goes west, crosses another line of trees, and enters yet another huge meadow. Above and to the right you'll see a clump of trees that shelters a tiny spring. Just below that a berm gathers the spring water into a surprising pond. And on that berm you could have quite a fine picnic, with the Columbia River laid out at your feet, flowers all around, and Mount Hood across the way.

Now for the lower loop, which is also the way down from the upper loop, or high country. Wherever you're starting, follow a trail that eventually hugs the top of the ridge above Catherine Creek. You'll get a view into the canyon where the homestead is, and then you'll walk along a fence at the top of the arch.

Keep descending the hill, and you'll cross a little draw filled with purple camas (in April), with creek access on your right, and a few minutes later you'll be at the road—and probably as close to power lines as you'll ever be in your life. Turn right and a little rock scramble will put you on the road's shoulder. Cross the creek again and see the parking lot, just up the hill.

Connection to Coyote Wall

But wait—there's more. Catherine Creek has a neighboring hike to the west called Coyote Wall (Hike 5, page 40), with a neat area called The Labyrinth in between. An entire system of official trails—with signs and everything—has been constructed in here, which makes for less adventure but more clarity.

From the Catherine Creek trailhead, go left on Trail CA2, Rowland Ridge Trail; it climbs gently through marshy areas and over small hills, and after 0.25 mile arrives at an uphill turn back to the right, near the top of a cliff. CA2 goes uphill here, but I suggest going left, where a small trail heads down along the face of the cliff, then hugs a steep, rocky hillside for a short time before dropping into a grassy bowl. Here, it intersects yet another old road (officially Labyrinth Trail CO7) heading steeply uphill. Follow this trail as it swings left and passes a series of rock pits that American Indians used as vision-quest sites—please don't disturb them.

The path, still CO7, eventually leads through several meadows some 700 feet above Rowland Lake, finally intersecting Upper Labyrinth Trail #4424. Stay left here and drop into The Labyrinth. Combining these two hikes as an out-and-back or as a point-to-point with an easy car shuttle is one of my absolute favorites, and an April tradition.

An upper trail also connects these two areas, making for a potentially epic loop. That's the one you can take by following County Road Trail up the hill from the junction near Catherine Creek. Climb that trail for 1,000 feet of elevation, then follow Atwood Road Trail to the west until you intersect the upper reaches of the

Coyote Wall hike. You could come back down CO8 and return to your car that way or connect all the way over to Coyote Wall. Options galore!

NEARBY ACTIVITIES

Crowds at Catherine Creek got you down, but you still want some flowers and views? Head over to gorgefriends.org and search for the Mosier Plateau Trail, a 3.5-mile loop that starts and ends in the town of Mosier. It has a waterfall, river views, flowers, and a town.

• •

GPS TRAILHEAD COORDINATES N45° 42.630' W121° 21.727'

DIRECTIONS Take I-84 from Portland, driving 56 miles east of I-205 to Exit 64, the third exit for Hood River. Turn left at the end of the ramp, following the signs for White Salmon. Pay a $1 toll (as of 2017) to cross the Columbia River, then turn right on WA 14. Travel 5.9 miles and turn left onto Old Highway 8. The parking area is 1.5 miles ahead, on the left.

The "yellow wall" near the Catherine Creek trailhead

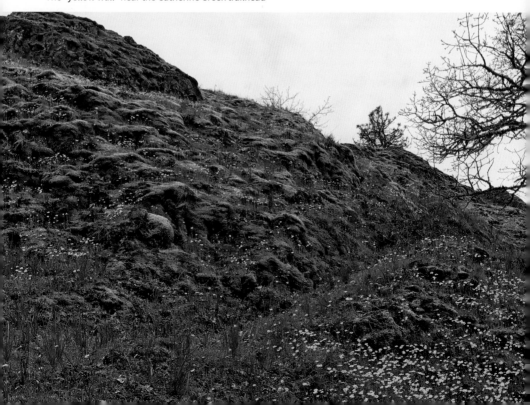

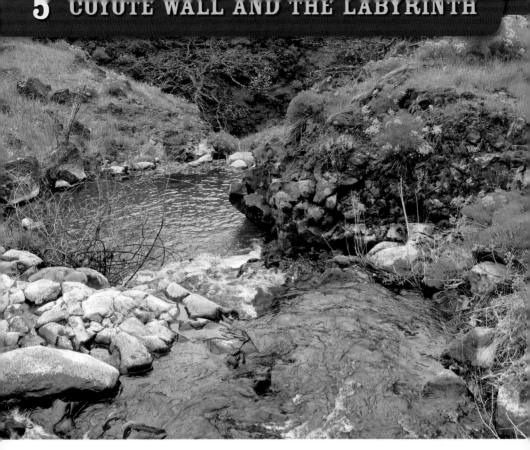

The Labyrinth is filled with creeks and flowers.

SAY IT'S SPRINGTIME, at least according to the calendar, but Portland is socked in and wet. Go east, fair hiker!—to the high and dry lands of the Columbia River Gorge, where flowers bloom, birds croon, and Coyote Wall looms.

DESCRIPTION

Standing at the trailhead, looking up at Coyote Wall, you might feel a bit intimidated. Fear not, for the way is gradual and the work rewarding. Just walk around the gate, and follow the old road along Locke Lake and eventually around the base of the wall itself. Turn left onto Trail #4426 and immediately you're faced with numerous trails. Mountain bikers zip through here in every direction, but our path is always the one to the left and uphill. Follow #4426 until, just under a mile out, it runs into Little Moab Trail #4429. Take #4429 and follow it to, and then up and along, the top of the wall. Just less than a mile up from the junction with #4426, the trail leaves the wall and you reach a junction where the #4426 comes back in. Here, you have a choice to make: high, medium, or low.

DISTANCE: 4.6-mile loop to the top of the wall; 5.2-mile loop to include The Labyrinth; a number of other possibilities, including connecting to Catherine Creek (Hike 4, page 35)

DIFFICULTY: Moderate

SCENERY: Clifftop vistas, wide-open country, spring wildflowers

EXPOSURE: Along a cliff at times, and out in the open almost the whole way

TRAFFIC: Heavy on spring weekends, moderate otherwise

TRAIL SURFACE: Dirt; can be slick when wet

HIKING TIME: 3–5 hours

ELEVATION CHANGE: 915'–1,790'

SEASON: Year-round

BEST TIME: April and May

BACKPACKING OPTIONS: None

DRIVING DISTANCE: 69 miles (1 hour, 15 minutes) from Pioneer Courthouse Square

ACCESS: No fees or permits required

MAPS: Green Trails *Map 432S (Columbia River Gorge–East)*

WHEELCHAIR ACCESS: First 0.5 mile on an old paved road that extends beyond the trail

FACILITIES: Restroom at the trailhead

CONTACT: Columbia River Gorge National Scenic Area, 541-308-1700, www.fs.usda.gov/crgnsa

LOCATION: Coyote Wall on Old Highway 8, 3 miles east of Bingen, WA

COMMENTS: Dogs must be leashed January–June. The trails here are somewhat in flux as land ownership shifts and more planning takes place. Call ahead or check the website above or wta.org to get the latest information.

High Route to the Top of Coyote Wall

If you're going up, stay left and follow Trail #4428 along the top of Coyote Wall. Just past a set of power lines, you'll see a trail off to the right, which you can take to cut some elevation, but I say keep going. After 1.3 miles of steep and steady climbing, through a sea of springtime flowers with views behind you to the Columbia and Mount Hood and down the face of Coyote Wall, you'll reach a forested junction with the Atwood Road Trail. Stick with #4428 as it loops back down to the right, paralleling the trail you came up, and after 0.6 mile reaches that junction you saw below. Head east from here, away from the wall, another 0.7 mile to, once again, Old Ranch Road #4426. At this junction, you can head down that for a mile until you see Little Maui Trail #4425—which will be after Little Moab—and follow that down and through The Labyrinth. Or you can head east and follow the middle path, described below.

Middle Route on #4426

At the Old Ranch Road decision point above, go uphill on #4426; it climbs to a three-way junction after nearly a mile. Turn right onto Atwood Road Trail, and soon you'll pass between two giant oak trees to a viewpoint at what looks like the site of an old house. (In fact, you'll be able to see a house off to your left—don't go over there.)

Stick with Atwood Road headed east, and in 0.6 mile you'll see Upper Labyrinth Trail #4424 on the right. This one wanders down and around, with great views down to Rowland Lake and the Columbia, and after 0.7 mile it comes to Labyrinth Trail.

Coyote Wall and The Labyrinth

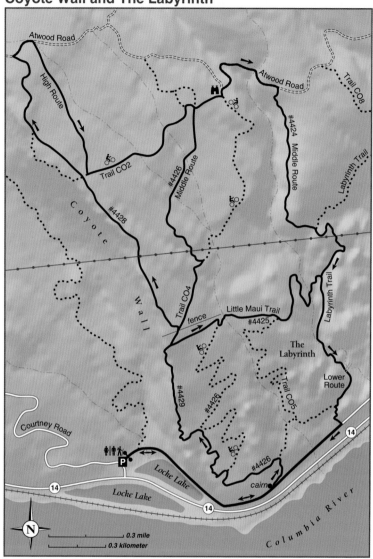

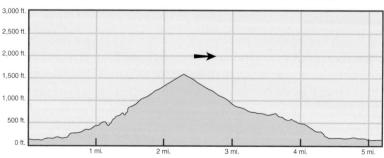

Go straight ahead at this junction, now on Labyrinth Trail and headed back to the west toward The Labyrinth, which you can see spread out below you.

Lower Route to The Labyrinth

Back at that decision spot, if you just stick with the lower, flatter #4426 (instead of the #4429 up the wall or #4426 going uphill), you will hit Little Maui Trail in less than half a mile. From here, just follow Little Maui into The Labyrinth.

Whichever way you get there, The Labyrinth is filled with hidden wonders: waterfalls, a small cave, small buttes to climb, and hidden meadows filled with flowers and surrounded by oak trees. So take your time, stick with Little Maui, look out for mountain bikers, and enjoy yourself. When in doubt, head downhill, and you will eventually pop out at the paved road you started on; turn right to get back to your car.

I know this is some confusing stuff; I'm doing my best! There are a lot of trails, and the bottom line for me is, it's a cool area, but obey the signs and don't trespass. Green Trails maps have one set of numbers; the signs have another, but trust my map and yourself, and just have a good time.

NEARBY ACTIVITIES

Sticking with my theme of offering alternatives for supercrowded Gorge trails, this time I will say look for the Memaloose Hills Hike, over in Oregon's Memaloose State Park. The unofficial but easy-to-follow 5.2-mile loop visits two flower-covered hillsides with terrific views. Look for it in the oregonhikers.org field guide.

• •

GPS TRAILHEAD COORDINATES N45° 41.998' W121° 24.202'

DIRECTIONS Take I-84 from Portland, driving 56 miles east of I-205 to Exit 64, the third exit for Hood River. Turn left at the end of the ramp, following the signs for White Salmon. Pay a $1 toll (as of 2017) to cross the Columbia River, then turn right on WA 14. Go 4.6 miles and turn left onto Courtney Road; the parking lot is on the right.

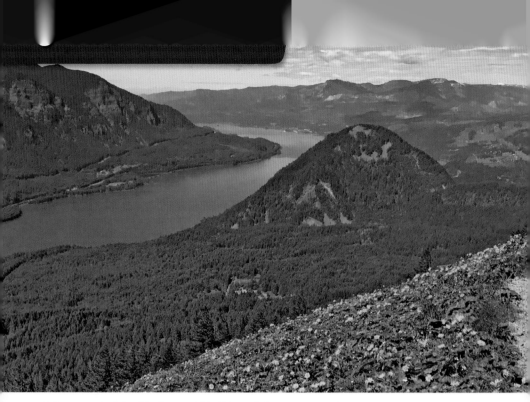

Balsamroot, the Columbia River, and Wind Mountain from Dog Mountain

THIS IS PROBABLY the most popular of the real hiking trails in the Columbia River Gorge—"real" meaning it requires some real effort. But with an easy-access trailhead, great views of the river, and sunshine and wildflowers at a time when it's usually still raining in Portland, it's no wonder everybody on Earth comes here.

DESCRIPTION

It seems that every hiker around Portland has been up Dog Mountain or at least heard about it. Climbers use it as an early-season conditioner. Wildflower enthusiasts flock to it in early summer. In spring, when it's still raining in Portland, it's often sunny here. And while staggering up the hill is tedious enough, it can be even more so when 500 people are coming back down toward you.

So I have an idea: let's make this thing a one-way loop. Seriously. If we all go the same way, which I think is a superior loop anyway, we don't have to run into each other so much. Follow along, try it, and see what you think. We'll go up the super-steep way and come down the normal-steep way.

From the parking lot, take the trail to the right, past the picnic table, and up to the restroom. Then follow the Dog Mountain Trail up a bunch of switchbacks 0.7 mile to a junction. Stay right, and after another 1.2 miles of climbing, you'll come

DISTANCE & CONFIGURATION: 6.9-mile loop

DIFFICULTY: Strenuous

SCENERY: Second-growth forest, wildflowers, panoramic view of the Columbia River Gorge

EXPOSURE: Alternately shady and open

TRAFFIC: Berserk on weekends, especially in early summer; very heavy otherwise. Not so bad outside the months of April–June.

TRAIL SURFACE: Packed dirt with rocks, some gravel

HIKING TIME: 4 hours

ELEVATION CHANGE: 2,800'

SEASON: Year-round, but occasional snow and ice on top

BEST TIME: Mid-May–early June

BACKPACKING OPTIONS: None

DRIVING DISTANCE: 56 miles (1 hour, 30 minutes) from Pioneer Courthouse Square

ACCESS: Northwest Forest Pass (see page 14); $5/vehicle/day without pass

MAPS: Green Trails *Map 430 (Hood River)* or *Map 428S (Columbia River Gorge–West)*

WHEELCHAIR ACCESS: No

FACILITIES: Restrooms at trailhead; no water

CONTACT: Columbia River Gorge National Scenic Area, 541-308-1700, www.fs.usda.gov/crgnsa

LOCATION: Dog Mountain Trailhead on WA 14, 4 miles east of Home Valley, WA

COMMENTS: Crowds here are so ridiculous in flower season, even during the week, that there is now a shuttle bus from the town of Stevenson. Please consider taking it, or carpooling, or coming during the week, or going for sunrise or sunset, or *something*. Long-term plans for a new and bigger trailhead are in the works, as well. For info on the shuttle, call 509-427-3990 or go to tinyurl.com/dogmtbus.

to the first viewpoint that combines river and flowers. Get used to this. There is even a little bench here to rest on.

After this, it gets really steep. (Sorry if you thought it was bad so far.) The next mile gains 900 feet, bringing you well and truly out in the open and to a former fire lookout spot called Puppy Point. Halfway along, when the other trail rejoins from the left, there's a small bench to rest on again. At Puppy Point, you will have a choice of trails, one of which heads off toward the woods and away from, if it's April to early June, one of the most amazing wildflower displays you've ever seen. Take the one that heads for the flowers.

In May and June, the open slopes of Dog Mountain are awash in flowers, especially big yellow balsamroot, purple lupine, and red paintbrush. But year-round, the views here of the river and other mountains—including Mount Hood, which peeks over the far side—are sublime. You'll climb in the open, stopping to catch your breath and say "wow" over and over, 0.4 mile to a junction. This is where you leave Dog Mountain Trail and head up 0.1 mile to the summit, but remember this spot: we're going the other way down from here.

I once counted 72 people on this summit. It's not hard to understand why, as arriving at this magical place is an annual ritual for many of us, as well as a sought-after goal for many others. The view here stretches from the high desert of central Oregon to Beacon Rock in the west—look how small it is! Way to the right is Mount St. Helens. Directly opposite is the 4,960-foot Mount Defiance, the one with the

Dog Mountain

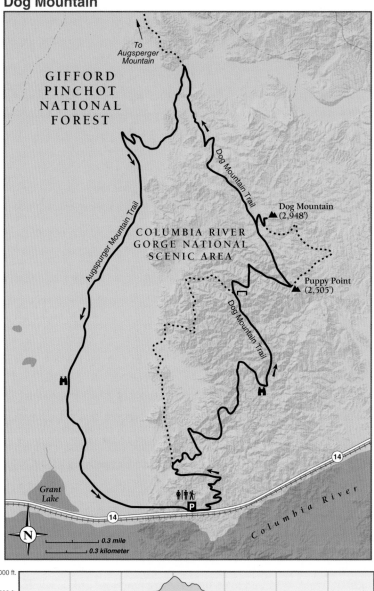

GIFFORD PINCHOT NATIONAL FOREST

To Augsperger Mountain

Dog Mountain Trail

Dog Mountain (2,948')

Puppy Point (2,505')

Augspurger Mountain Trail

COLUMBIA RIVER GORGE NATIONAL SCENIC AREA

Dog Mountain Trail

14

Grant Lake

14

P

Columbia River

N

0.3 mile
0.3 kilometer

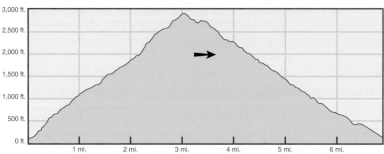

radio towers on top. The highest point in the gorge, it seems to taunt, "Yeah, right, you've climbed barely half of me." That would be Hike 10 (page 63), if you're feeling up for it.

I'd like to take a moment to explain why Dog Mountain is called Dog Mountain. It's neither because of all the dogs on the trail, nor because the hike is a real bitch. It's because some pioneers in the area were forced to eat dog meat to avoid starvation. The town of Hood River was in fact first called Dog River, but the name was changed because nobody liked it. Imagine that.

For the return loop, turn right at the aforementioned junction, following a sign for Augspurger Mountain. Aside from the one-way-loop advantages I propose, this route is also 0.6 mile longer than the way you came up, and hence less steep and easier on the knees and ankles. And the first part is an amazing section of trail that most people don't hike. You'll stroll along through more of the meadows, past pockets of evergreens, with immense views all around, 0.9 mile before dropping back into the woods and intersecting the Augspurger Mountain Trail.

If you're feeling particularly badass, turn right and add Augspurger to your day, a combination known among certain nutjobs as the Dogspurger Loop. All it adds is 5.9 miles and 2,000 feet of elevation to your day—oh, and another great, flowery viewpoint. Assuming you're not a nutjob, though, turn left and enjoy a casual, mostly shady descent back to the trailhead, passing viewpoints of Wind Mountain and Grant Lake by WA 14 down below. When you see the lake, you're 0.5 mile from home.

NEARBY ACTIVITIES

As with most of these Gorge hikes, I am going to recommend a somewhat similar, and almost certainly less crowded, option. It's beyond the range of this book, but go check out the hike at Dalles Mountain Ranch in Washington's Columbia Hills State Park. It's 4 miles out-and-back on an old road, but the flowers are everything Dog Mountain offers, with only 1,150' of elevation gain. Details are at gorgefriends.org and the oregonhikers.org field guide.

· ·

GPS TRAILHEAD COORDINATES N45° 41.960' W121° 42.477'

DIRECTIONS Take I-84 from Portland, driving 37 miles east of I-205 to Exit 44 (Cascade Locks). As soon as you enter the town, take your first right to get on Bridge of the Gods, following a sign for Stevenson. Pay a $2 toll on the bridge and, at the far end, turn right (east) onto WA 14. Proceed 12 miles to the trailhead, on the left. And don't forget the shuttle bus option, above.

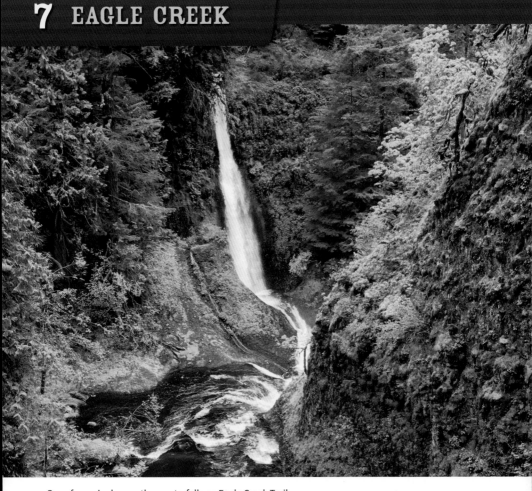

One of seemingly countless waterfalls on Eagle Creek Trail

EAGLE CREEK IS easily one of the classic and most popular hikes in Oregon. It's easy to get to, is easy to hike, and traverses a deep, forested canyon filled with waterfalls. With that in mind, start early, or go on a weekday, so you won't have to share the trail with the rest of Oregon. And, taking the 2017 fire into account, mourn the loss while admiring, for the rest of our lives, nature's recovery powers.

DESCRIPTION

The magic of this hike, at certain times of the year, begins before you even hit the trail itself. Eagle Creek has a small run of fall chinook salmon—fish that spend their adult lives in the ocean, come more than 70 miles up the Columbia, swim the fish ladder at Bonneville Dam, and then arrive here to spawn. A small dam blocks their

DISTANCE & CONFIGURATION: 4-mile out-and-back to Punchbowl Falls, 12-mile out-and-back to Tunnel Falls

DIFFICULTY: Easy–moderate depending on how far you go

SCENERY: Waterfalls, old-growth forest, spawning salmon in the fall, a forest recovering from fire

EXPOSURE: Several sections of trail follow the tops of ledges and cliffs—only sometimes with cables to hold on to.

TRAFFIC: Very heavy all summer, moderate in spring and fall

TRAIL SURFACE: Packed dirt and rocks

HIKING TIME: 2.5 hours to Punchbowl Falls, 6 hours to Tunnel Falls

ELEVATION CHANGE: 500'–1,640'

SEASON: Year-round, but muddy in winter and spring; you may also encounter snow and ice in winter.

BEST TIME: March–May for big water flows, September and October for fall colors and fish

BACKPACKING OPTIONS: Several sites starting a few miles up

DRIVING DISTANCE: 41 miles (50 minutes) from Pioneer Courthouse Square

ACCESS: Northwest Forest Pass required (see page 14)

MAPS: Green Trails *Map 428S (Columbia River Gorge–West)*

WHEELCHAIR ACCESS: A road along (and bridge over) Eagle Creek near trailhead

FACILITIES: Restrooms at trailhead; no water

CONTACT: Columbia River Gorge National Scenic Area, 541-308-1700, www.fs.usda.gov/crgnsa

LOCATION: Eagle Creek Trailhead on NE Eagle Creek Loop, 5 miles east of Warrendale, OR

COMMENTS: This isn't a good trail for dogs, and you shouldn't hike it if you're afraid of heights—people have died here. Also, be aware that hikers have had their cars broken into at the trailhead. And of course, since the 2017 fire started here and was named for Eagle Creek, there is just no telling when this trail will reopen or what it will look like. Contact the U.S. Forest Service or visit gorgefriends.org for the latest.

further progress up Eagle Creek, but in October and November they spawn in little round pools cleared by volunteers.

The trail was built in 1916 to coincide with the opening of the Columbia River Highway; the area around the fish hatchery was also the site of the first National Forest Service campground. The construction of the Eagle Creek Trail was a heroic feat. Trail builders chipped the path into cliff faces, built High Bridge over a deep gorge, and blasted a tunnel behind a waterfall 6 miles up. It's work like this that inspired me to dedicate this book to the builders and maintainers of trails.

In the first mile, you'll get an idea of what you're in for: a deep canyon, waterfalls, and a lovely creek without too much elevation gain. At 1 mile, you come to the first of several places where you walk a ledge—in this case, but not all, with a cable to hang on to. The importance of being careful cannot be overstated: people have fallen to their deaths from this trail.

Just over a mile out, look ahead through the trees for a big gash on the left side of the canyon. This is where there used to be a viewpoint of Metlako Falls (named for an American Indian goddess of salmon). But in December 2016, a section of the canyon wall some 300–400 feet long fell 200 feet into the creek. In fact, workers at the hatchery

Eagle Creek

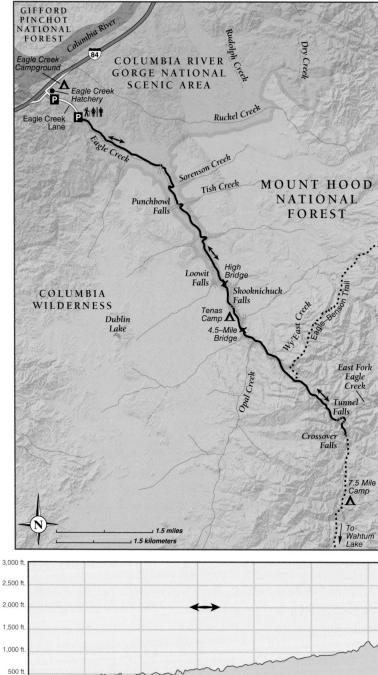

say Eagle Creek stopped flowing for about 45 minutes. The viewpoint is now gone for good, and sadly we can't see Metlako Falls anymore. Let's hope the U.S. Forest Service builds another one, and perhaps we could encourage them to do so.

Just past the former viewpoint, 1.5 miles out, is a bench. Another one is at 1.8 miles, and from here a side trail leads down to Punchbowl Falls, a must-see sight and the end of the line for a lot of people. Descend this trail 0.2 mile to reach Lower Punchbowl Falls; just above that is a large clearing that's often filled with swimmers and sunbathers. At the upstream end of the clearing is a lovely (and often photographed) view of the main Punchbowl Falls.

If you turn back here, you'll have hiked 4 miles, but it's not much more work to go at least as far as High Bridge, another 1.2 miles up. If you continue, you'll get a bird's-eye view of Punchbowl Falls just 0.3 mile ahead; then the gorge narrows considerably. One interesting site to look for is at 2.5 miles out, where the top of a concrete post sticks out of the trail at an odd angle. This is actually an old 3-mile marker (it says 11 on the other side, the distance to Wahtum Lake). A hiker and reader named Jerry King found at least two more of them: one at the (former) Metlako Falls viewpoint trail, and another just 0.5 mile from the trailhead. See if you can spot them on the way out.

Heading farther up, at 3.1 miles you'll see Loowit Falls on the right just before High Bridge, a spectacular sight at 120 feet above the river in a narrow gorge. It's above here that you're allowed to camp.

If you turn around at High Bridge, you'll have a 6.4-mile day. But before you turn back, put in another 0.3 mile to reach Tenas Camp, just 100 yards after a rare chance for creek access at the top of Skooknichuck Falls. Just past that are some very impressive Douglas-firs right on the trail.

Continuing up the trail, you'll soon cross what is officially known as 4.5 Mile Bridge. The map acknowledges that this is exactly 4 miles from the trailhead—what gives? Well, the fish hatchery back at the trailhead wasn't there when the trail was built, so the trailhead used to be 0.5 mile farther north, right by the highway. Same thing on those old mileage posts, which are probably from the 1930s.

Just past the bridge, look on the right for a double waterfall—that's Opal Creek, but don't confuse it with the world-famous Opal Creek described elsewhere in this book (Hike 30, page 152). About 0.5 mile above that waterfall, a sign explains that the area you're now entering was burned in a 1902 fire; you can still see some charred stumps around. So all the trees you'll see in this area are less than 100 years old (if there are any left from the 2017 blaze).

Hiking another 1.2 miles will bring you to a fascinating section of trail called the Potholes, where blasting for the trail created a section of crazily shaped rocks that are kind of tricky to walk on. Another 0.3 mile brings your total to 6 miles hiked, and you'll come into a deep gorge, where Tunnel Falls plunges 160 feet and the trail continues behind it through a 35-foot tunnel. Tunnel Falls is actually on East Fork Eagle Creek, which flows from Wahtum Lake. You could get to Wahtum Lake by hiking another 8 miles (and 2,500 feet) up this trail or by following the directions in the Herman Creek profile on page 53. (You can also drive there, but what fun is that?)

To return to Eagle Creek and see one final, dramatic falls, hike on about 0.2 mile. This falls doesn't have an official name, but it does have an interesting crisscross feature in its upper section, leading many people to call it Crisscross Falls or Crossover Falls.

If you're backpacking, you'll find good camping at 7.5 Mile Camp (again, 7 miles up) and at Wahtum Lake. Otherwise, if you head back at this point, you'll wind up having put in 12 miles.

NEARBY ACTIVITIES

Stop at Bonneville Dam Hatchery on your way home (70543 NE Herman Loop, Cascade Falls, OR; 541-374-8393; tinyurl.com/bonnevillehatchery). They have a fish ladder where you can often see fish swimming past the dam, and year-round ponds where you can view big trout and sturgeon. It's 1 mile west of Eagle Creek on I-84, and admission is free.

GPS TRAILHEAD COORDINATES N45° 38.205' W121° 55.182'

DIRECTIONS Take I-84 from Portland, driving 34 miles east of I-205 to Exit 41 (Eagle Creek). Go 0.2 mile, turn right, and drive 0.6 mile to the end of the road. If the parking area is crowded, you might have to park closer to the highway and hike that much farther.

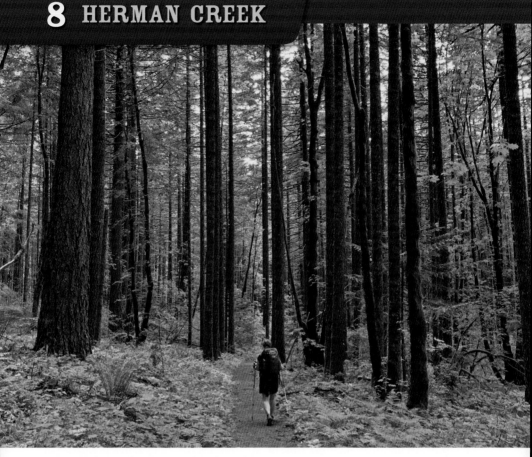

Forest grandeur on the Gorton Creek Trail just above Herman Camp

THE HIKING HUB at Herman Creek offers something for everyone: a midwinter riverside stroll, a spring get-in-shape workout, or a long summer backpack hike. The prize of the area, though, is Indian Point. That's the hike shown on the elevation profile; none of the others described here are nearly as steep as this one.

DESCRIPTION

Every spring, at some point, most of us trail hounds will wind up at the Herman Creek trailhead; whatever you're looking for, you can find it on these forested slopes. So, rather than one hike, here are a few options, from easiest to hardest, with enough variations that you may not know which to choose—and that's why so many of us return to Herman Creek time and time again.

All the hikes start at the same place, the Herman Creek trailhead, which until May 1 will mean a 0.5-mile walk from Forest Lane to the trailhead. From the trail sign, hike a short, steep section to some power lines, and follow the trail past them, for a total of 0.6 mile, to a junction. The options start here, as do the mileage counts.

DISTANCE & CONFIGURATION: 6–20 miles, out-and-back or loops

DIFFICULTY: Easy–strenuous

SCENERY: Old-growth forest, a clear stream, waterfalls, views of mountains and the gorge

EXPOSURE: Almost all shaded, with one optional bit of very exposed rock

TRAFFIC: Moderate on weekends, light otherwise

TRAIL SURFACE: Dirt, rocks

HIKING TIME: 2 hours–2 days

ELEVATION CHANGE: 1,000'–5,070'

SEASON: Year-round for the lower hikes, but snow possible; Nick Eaton Ridge likely snow-free April–November

BEST TIME: April–May, October

BACKPACKING OPTIONS: Fantastic

DRIVING DISTANCE: 46 miles (1 hour) from Pioneer Courthouse Square

ACCESS: Northwest Forest Pass required at summer trailhead only

MAPS: National Geographic *Columbia River Gorge,* Green Trails *Map 428S (Columbia River Gorge–West)*

WHEELCHAIR ACCESS: No

FACILITIES: Restroom and water at summer trailhead; water turns off when campground closes around Labor Day.

CONTACT: Columbia River Gorge National Scenic Area, 541-308-1700, www.fs.usda.gov/crgnsa

LOCATION: Herman Creek Trailhead on Herman Creek Road, 3 miles east of Cascade Locks, OR

COMMENTS: In winter and early spring, you'll have to park 0.5 mile down the access road at the gate; parking is free there, but it adds a mile to your day. Also, this is another area affected by the 2017 Eagle Creek Fire; check gorgefriends.org or oregonhikers.org for the latest conditions.

Pacific Crest Falls and the Pinnacles (4.1 miles, 1,000', easy)

From this junction, turn right and descend 0.4 mile to cross Herman Creek on a large metal bridge. This creek does get runs of anadromous fish (which live in the ocean and spawn in the rivers). Steelhead enter from June through October, and salmon are in from August to November. Perhaps you can spot one of these, or the large trout that inhabit the deeper pools.

Beyond the bridge, climb again 0.8 mile to reach an intersection with the Pacific Crest Trail (PCT). Turn right here, pass through a rockslide, and in 0.5 mile arrive at the two-tiered Pacific Crest Falls, which is much more impressive in winter and spring than in summer or fall.

Continue 0.2 mile and you'll catch a glimpse of the Herman Creek Pinnacles, basalt cones that can be tough to spot through summer brush.

To add a bit more, hike another 1.5 miles along the PCT to Dry Creek, which isn't dry. A side trail leads 0.2 mile to the equally wet Dry Creek Falls. You could even stash a car at Bridge of the Gods and make this a one-way hike.

Herman Creek Trail (up to 22.2 miles and 5,070', moderate–strenuous)

Herman Creek leads to several side trips, many nice places, and one spectacular destination. Best of all, the average elevation gain here is a paltry 350 feet per mile.

From the same junction referenced above, continue uphill and to the left, and you'll climb (briefly on a road) 0.7 mile to reach Herman Camp and a big trail intersection.

Herman Creek

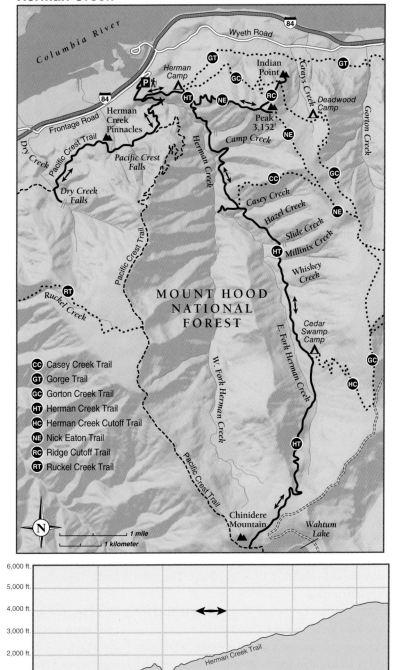

Legend:

CC Casey Creek Trail
GT Gorge Trail
GC Gorton Creek Trail
HT Herman Creek Trail
HC Herman Creek Cutoff Trail
NE Nick Eaton Trail
RC Ridge Cutoff Trail
RT Ruckel Creek Trail

From left to right, the trails are Gorge Trail, Gorton Creek Trail, and Herman Creek Trail. (If you're looking for a campsite, you can do a lot better than Herman Camp.)

Keep climbing Herman Creek Trail, which still looks like a road, and in 0.3 mile you'll pass the Nick Eaton Way junction (more on that later). After this, your trail begins a lazy climb in and out of small side canyons, though not yet near Herman Creek. Over the course of 2.4 miles, you'll pass a series of creeks and waterfalls until, at 4 miles total (3.4 since the first junction), you'll hit Casey Creek Camp and two trails.

For your first real view of Herman Creek on this hike, head down and to the right for a steep 0.3 mile to the confluence of Herman Creek's east and west forks. It's a fine place to have lunch and turn around for an 8-mile round-trip stroll.

For a major workout, go up Casey Creek Trail for 2.1 leg-killing miles that gain 2,540 feet. That gets you to Nick Eaton Trail; turn left and trace it back to the junction you just passed. That loop is only 11.3 miles with 4,035 feet of gain.

Farther along Herman Creek Trail, you'll pass more creeks and falls over the next 3.5 miles (notice a pattern?) and arrive at Cedar Swamp Camp, the first of three campsites in 0.5 mile. Things start to open up a bit here, and 3 more miles (a total of 11 since the car) put you at the PCT just below Chinidere Mountain and just above Wahtum Lake, where campsites and deep, blue water beckon. From Wahtum Lake, you could go back via Eagle Creek Trail for a spectacular two- or three-day backpack.

Nick Eaton Way to Indian Point (8 miles, 2,800', strenuous)

This is the pick of the area, at least for day hikers up for some "up." Nick Eaton Way (named for a pioneer-era farmer) is among the steeper paths around. I often use it to see what kind of shape I'm in by April; usually the answer is "not good."

From its start at Herman Creek Trail just above Herman Camp, Nick Eaton Way climbs 1,960 feet in 2 miles, making it steeper than Dog Mountain. But hey, it's only 2 miles, and along the way you'll traverse hanging meadows with flowers and great views. The meadow at 1 mile has a view down the Columbia to Bonneville Dam and Bridge of the Gods; another meadow, 0.2 mile on, has a rare view south—in this case, up Herman Creek's drainage.

After 2 miles of this, you'll enter Hatfield Wilderness and hit Ridge Cutoff Trail. Your path here is on the left, but if it's clear, it's worth staying on Nick Eaton Way 0.25 mile and looking for an unofficial but clear trail heading up to what's known simply as Peak 3,152 (its elevation). The view is better than the name, and it's a great lunch spot.

To continue the loop, take Ridge Cutoff Trail 0.6 mile to Gorton Creek Trail, where you have more choices. One option is to turn right and hike 6.5 miles, passing various camps and trails in a swing around to Wahtum Lake. The first campsite you encounter is Deadwood Camp, 0.8 mile along, which has a year-round stream.

If you're feeling slightly adventurous, your second option is to go about 50 yards right, then look for a seriously steep trail descending to the left. This path goes out toward Indian Point, a dramatic rock outcrop hundreds of feet above the Columbia. It's about 0.25 mile down to a flat spot at the base of the point; going any farther is enthusiastically discouraged if you have even the slightest fear of heights or lack of balance.

Back on Gorton Creek Trail, hike 2.6 mellow, lusciously green, big-tree-filled miles to Herman Camp, then turn right on Herman Creek Trail to return to the official trailhead after hiking another 1.3 uneventful miles.

NEARBY ACTIVITIES

Last I've seen, this trail wasn't getting too crowded, but if it is, here are a couple of options, both in the field guide at oregonhikers.org. If you want another forested river walk, check out Tanner Creek. If you want a big climb to a great view, head for Wauna Point. Also understand that all of those, like Herman Creek, were hit pretty hard by the fire in 2017.

• •

GPS TRAILHEAD COORDINATES N45° 40.92' W121° 50.52'

DIRECTIONS From Portland, take I-84, driving 37 miles east from I-205 to Exit 44 (Cascade Locks). Proceed through the town 3.2 miles, cross back under I-84, and stay straight onto Frontage Road. Go 1.7 miles and turn right onto Herman Creek Road, and follow that 0.3 mile to the trailhead. If the gate is closed down at Forest Lane, park there and walk up.

The Columbia River, Wind Mountain, and Dog Mountain from Indian Point

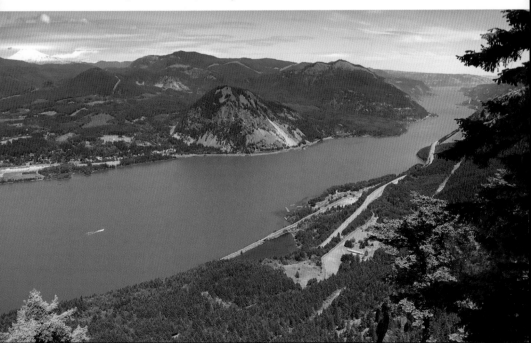

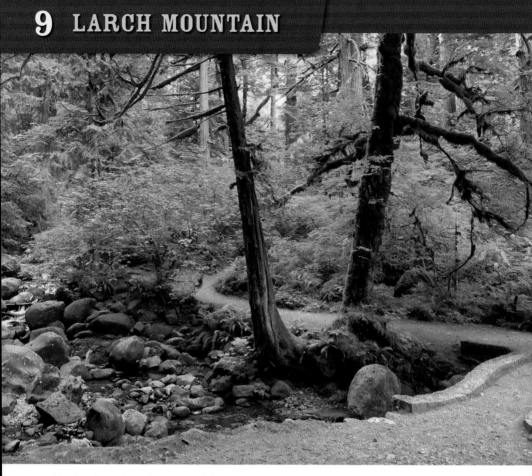

Bridge just above the trail to the top of Multnomah Falls

YOU CAN DRIVE to the top of Larch Mountain, but the trail between there and Multnomah Falls is one of the classic walks in Oregon—from the shores of the Columbia River to a high lookout in the Cascades, with old-growth forest on the way up and a view from the top that takes in everything from Portland to several volcanoes. A shorter loop hike encompasses the upper parts of the mountain only.

DESCRIPTION

Pick a clear day to get the best view, or think about timing your hike so that you arrive at the top at sunset—you'll get to see Mount Hood bathed in pink light, and the lights of Portland are spectacular from the summit. Consider doing this one in late August, when the upper parts of the hill are awash in huckleberries.

You can actually see Larch Mountain as you drive out I-84; it's just to the left of Mount Hood and has a notch in the top. The top of that notch is where you're headed.

DISTANCE & CONFIGURATION: 6.8-mile loop, with out-and-back and point-to-point options of up to 18 miles

DIFFICULTY: Moderate–strenuous

SCENERY: Waterfalls, creeks in wooded canyons, colossal trees, solitude, panoramic view

EXPOSURE: Mostly shady until summit

TRAFFIC: Always heavy on lower stretches and at the very top; low–moderate in between

TRAIL SURFACE: Pavement, packed dirt, some gravel

HIKING TIME: 5 hours one-way, 8 hours round-trip, 4 hours for upper loop

ELEVATION CHANGE: Options from 1,310' to 4,010'

SEASON: Year-round for lower parts; June–mid-October for upper

BEST TIME: Late August (for amazing huckleberries)

BACKPACKING OPTIONS: Poor

DRIVING DISTANCE: 31 miles (40 minutes) to lower trailhead or 36 miles (1 hour) to upper and middle trailheads from Pioneer Courthouse Square

ACCESS: No fees at Multnomah Falls or middle trailhead; Northwest Forest Pass (see page 14) or $5 daily pass required at upper trailhead

MAPS: National Geographic *Columbia River Gorge*, Green Trails *Map 428S (Columbia River Gorge–West)*

WHEELCHAIR ACCESS: First 0.2 mile to Benson Bridge and some trails from upper lot

FACILITIES: Full services at Multnomah Falls trailhead, restrooms atop Larch Mountain

CONTACT: Columbia River Gorge National Scenic Area, 541-308-1700, www.fs.usda.gov/crgnsa

LOCATION: 53000 Historic Columbia River Highway, 3 miles east of Bridal Veil, OR

COMMENTS: Here is another area greatly affected by the 2017 Eagle Creek Fire. Check with the Scenic Area or gorgefriends.org for the latest conditions.

As for the hike, you have several options, all quite worthwhile. You can start at the top or the bottom and put in 7.2 miles one-way, assuming you have a second car for a shuttle; you can do 14.4 miles round-trip; you can start in the middle and do a loop that takes in the view but with less work; or you can combine some of these.

Up from the Falls

Let's assume you put a second car at the top parking lot, and we'll start at the bottom then include the upper loop on the way. From Multnomah Falls Lodge, walk with the crowds up the paved trail that leads over Benson Bridge. This covers 1 mile (climbing 600 feet) to reach a junction with a side trail leading to the viewing platform at the top of the falls. Continuing past that junction, you'll leave 90% of your comrades behind so that, for the next several miles, you may well have Larch Mountain Trail #441 to yourself. You'll also enter one of the few areas of old-growth forest in the Columbia River Gorge (at least, before the Eagle Creek Fire).

The trail was built in 1916 to coincide with the opening of the Columbia River Highway. One thing we should get straight is that there are probably no larch trees on Larch Mountain. The name stuck after old-time settlers confused the noble fir with the larch, which grows only east of the Cascade Range (although a few grow at Hoyt Arboretum; Hike 59).

Larch Mountain

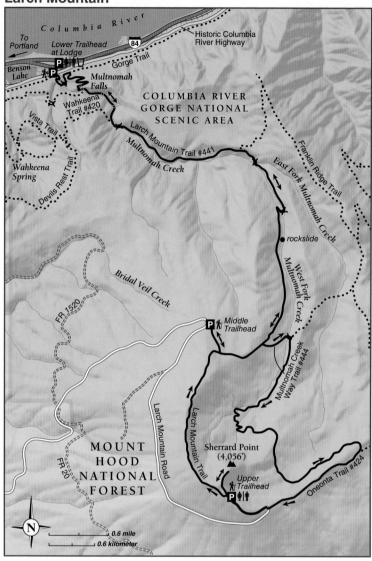

Columbia River

To Portland

Lower Trailhead at Lodge

Historic Columbia River Highway

84

Benson Lake

Gorge Trail

Multnomah Falls

Wahkeena Trail #420

COLUMBIA RIVER GORGE NATIONAL SCENIC AREA

Vista Trail

Larch Mountain Trail #441

Multnomah Creek

Wahkeena Spring

Devils Rest Trail

Franklin Ridge Trail

East Fork Multnomah Creek

rockslide

West Fork Multnomah Creek

Bridal Veil Creek

FR 1520

Middle Trailhead

Multnomah Creek Way Trail #444

FR 20

MOUNT HOOD NATIONAL FOREST

Larch Mountain Road

Larch Mountain Trail

Sherrard Point (4,056')

Upper Trailhead

Oneonta Trail #424

N

0.6 mile
0.6 kilometer

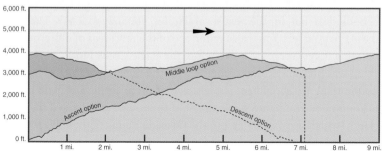

Middle loop option

Ascent option

Descent option

Staying on this trail, you'll cross Multnomah Creek and pass two lovely water-falls in a lush canyon. At 1.8 miles, ignore Wahkeena Trail #420, on the right. At 2 miles you'll cross Multnomah Creek again, and 0.5 mile past that you might have to take a diversion left onto the High Water Trail. At 3.2 miles, traverse East Fork Multnomah Creek. Just 0.5 mile later, you'll cross a one-log footbridge over West Fork Multnomah Creek.

At 3.9 miles you'll cross a rockslide and then start climbing through an old-growth forest of hemlock and Douglas-fir trees 6 feet or more in diameter and hundreds of years old. In late summer, this area abounds with huckleberries, and in autumn the red, yellow, and orange vine maple is astounding.

At 4.9 miles you'll come to a junction with Multnomah Creek Way Trail #444, and you'll have the option to simply stay on Larch Mountain Trail #441 (to reach the top in 2 somewhat boring miles) or to take Trail #444, to the left, a more scenic route to the top but one that's 1 mile longer.

Diversion onto Multnomah Creek Way Trail

If adding this loop sounds OK to you, follow Trail #444 0.2 mile, cross West Fork Multnomah Creek; turn right to follow Trail #444, and go 2.8 miles, past a marsh and up the ridge of Larch Mountain. The last bit of this is on the level bed of an old road, the remnant of decades of logging activity up here. Notice how the trees in that section aren't so big anymore?

When you come to Oneonta Trail #424 at the top of the ridge, turn right and follow it 0.9 mile slightly uphill to the shoulder of Larch Mountain Road. Walk up that 0.3 mile to the parking area, then take a signed, paved trail to Sherrard Point for the big view. Along the way you'll pass a picnic area with tables and grills. It's 0.7 mile from where you enter the road to Sherrard Point—a total of 7.7 miles from the trail-head at Multnomah Falls.

Any way you go, make sure to go have a look around from Sherrard Point—after you get over the aggravation of realizing, after all this work, you still have more than 100 steps to climb. It's named for Thomas H. Sherrard, who ran the Mount Hood National Forest from 1907 to 1934 and helped develop the Bull Run water preserve. If it's a clear day, you'll see Portland, Mount Hood, Mount Jefferson, Mount Adams, Mount St. Helens, and Mount Rainier. You'll also notice that you're at the top of a cliff on a semicircular ridge. That's because Larch Mountain is what remains of an ancient volcano, and what you're looking down into is the remnant of a crater.

The Upper Loop

As for your other hiking options on Larch Mountain, you can either start at the top and descend to Multnomah Falls, following Larch Mountain Trail all the way down or taking the Multnomah Creek Way Trail, or you can park at the middle trailhead (see Directions, next page). The middle trailhead accesses the upper part of Larch Mountain, saving you from climbing 3,000 feet from the Columbia.

From the middle trailhead, follow the gated gravel road 0.3 mile to intersect the Larch Mountain Trail, then either head right and walk 1.5 miles up to reach the top, or head left to descend 0.5 mile and take Multnomah Creek Way Trail #444 and the loop described above.

NEARBY ACTIVITIES

Check out the Portland Women's Forum State Scenic Viewpoint (39210 E Historic Columbia River Highway, Corbett, OR; 800-551-6949; oregonstateparks.org). Because it's a little farther west than the more famous Vista House, it's a less visited spot for viewing the Columbia River Gorge.

And if you want a less crowded, superlong hike to a mountain viewpoint, check out Table Mountain at oregonhikers.org. I used to have it in this book, but the best trailhead went away, making it a 15.5-mile, 4,320-foot extravaganza.

• •

GPS TRAILHEAD COORDINATES
Upper Trailhead N45° 31.776' W122° 5.303'
Middle Trailhead N45° 32.97' W122° 5.516'
Lower Trailhead N45° 34.659' W122° 7.032'

DIRECTIONS To start at the lower trailhead, take I-84 from Portland, driving 24 miles east of I-205 to Exit 31 (Multnomah Falls), the exit for the parking lot. Park and walk under the expressway to historic Multnomah Falls Lodge. For the middle and upper trailheads, take I-84, driving 15 miles east of I-205, and take Exit 22 (Corbett). At the exit, turn right onto NE Corbett Hill Road. After 1.5 miles, turn left onto E Historic Columbia River Highway. Drive 2 miles, then veer right onto Larch Mountain Road. The upper trailhead is in the parking lot at the end of the road, 14 miles up. The middle trailhead is 11.5 miles ahead, on the left, after Larch Mountain Road heads right and a gated gravel road takes off to the left.

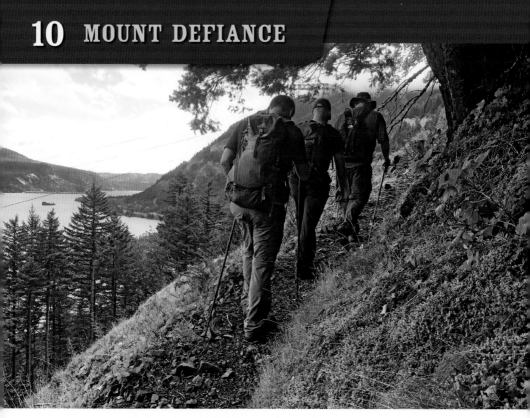

The journey is long and steep, but standing at the highest point in the gorge is worth the climb.

THERE'S A JOKE around here that one climbs Mount Hood to get in shape for Mount Defiance. That is a bit of an overstatement, but this climb to the gorge's highest point is relentless. I included it because a better hike to Table Mountain is now—thanks to the loss of a trailhead—15.5 miles long. The lower loop here is awfully nice as well, with four waterfalls in 3 miles.

DESCRIPTION

Whatever you're doing here, start by checking out Starvation Creek Falls, a minute's walk east of the parking area. It's a beautiful spot that, nearly every time I visit, I seem to have to myself. Now head back west on the Historic Columbia River Highway, on a section completed in 2016. After 0.3 mile you will come to a sign saying GORGE TRAIL 400 AND STARVATION RIDGE. This is where our paths diverge.

The Lower Loop

Head left up the Starvation Cutoff Trail. In the next 0.4 mile you might think I accidentally sent you up the big climb, as this stretch is amazingly steep and at times rocky. Stick with it; this is almost all the climbing you'll do on this loop. At the top you will intersect Starvation Ridge Trail #414. We're going to go right, but first walk 150 yards left to a viewpoint that includes the river and your car; look how

DISTANCE & CONFIGURATION: 3-mile loop or 11.6-mile loop

DIFFICULTY: Easy down low, strenuous up top

SCENERY: Forest, waterfalls, Columbia River views, highest point in the gorge

EXPOSURE: Mostly shady

TRAFFIC: Light–moderate

TRAIL SURFACE: Grass, packed dirt with rocks, rocky slopes; some loose rocks

HIKING TIME: 2–8 hours

ELEVATION CHANGE: 1,280' for lower loop, 4,940' for Defiance

SEASON: Year-round for lower loop, June–October for Defiance

BEST TIME: April for flowers down low, September for cool temperatures up high

BACKPACKING OPTIONS: A few sites at Warren Lake

DRIVING DISTANCE: 53 miles (1 hour) from Pioneer Courthouse Square

ACCESS: No fees or permits required

MAPS: Green Trails *Map 430 (Hood River)* or *Map 428S (Columbia River Gorge–West)*

WHEELCHAIR ACCESS: This trailhead is in the middle of a 1.6-mile paved section of the Historic Columbia River Highway.

FACILITIES: Restrooms at the trailhead

LOCATION: Starvation Creek State Park on Historic Columbia River Highway, 10 miles east of Cascade Locks, OR

CONTACT: Columbia River Gorge National Scenic Area, 541-308-1700, www.fs.usda.gov/crgnsa

high you've come! Return to the junction and continue west; in 0.1 mile you cross Cabin Creek. Climb again, sanely this time, 0.2 mile to another great river view under some power lines; the star of this view is Dog Mountain right across the way.

Now you'll descend 0.5 mile through meadows that will be bursting with color in the spring. You'll cross Warren Creek, which is lovely but could also be challenging in spring. After that it's slightly up again to yet another river view, this one featuring Wind Mountain, and then you drop down to a junction with Mount Defiance Trail #413. Before heading down that, walk west a minute to see Lancaster Falls, which spills almost right onto the trail.

Heading down the Mount Defiance Trail drops you down at Hole-in-the-Wall Falls, which has an interesting history. This is Warren Creek, but it's not the natural falls location; in 1938, workers blasted a hole through the rock to divert it away from the road. You can see the creek popping out of that hole at the top of the upper tier.

Now you just follow the paved old highway 0.6 mile back to your car, passing lovely Cabin Creek Falls on the way.

Mount Defiance

This journey is long and steep, there aren't many views for quite a while, and coming down will be worse. Sounds great, doesn't it? Well, standing at the highest point in the entire gorge is worth it, as is the sense of satisfaction from tackling this beast. And by the way, it got its name because it was always the last place around to lose its snow, thus defying the advent of spring. So off we go.

From the first junction mentioned above, stick with the pavement another 0.3 mile, passing Cabin Creek Falls and Hole-in-the-Wall Falls, then head up Mount

Mount Defiance

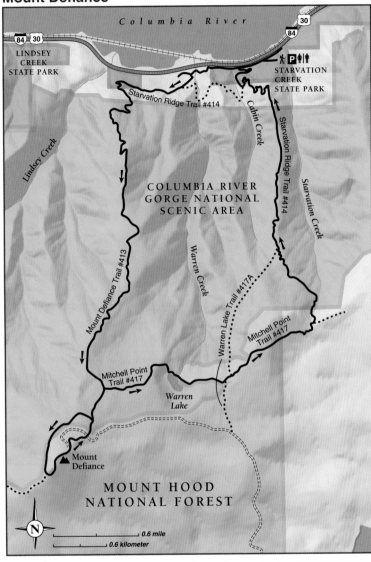

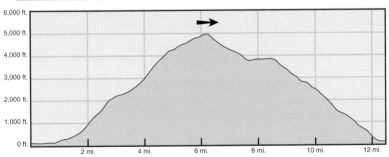

Defiance Trail #413. Stay right at a junction with Trail 414, pass Lancaster Falls, and very soon you will start up. Just put your head down and go for it, because over the next 2.7 miles you will gain 3,320 feet—considerably steeper than Dog Mountain, for reference—and really not have any views. When you get to the wilderness boundary, you've done 3.6 miles since the car, and your elevation is 3,600 feet.

During the next mile you will finally get a view from a rock slope at 4,100 feet—turn around and look *down* on Dog Mountain for some satisfaction—and then the environment opens up a bit, making it feel more like you're actually on a mountain. The grade also lets up, a little. At 5 miles and 4,280 feet you'll intersect Warren Lake Trail #417; keep going another 0.2 mile to another intersection, this with Defiance Cutoff Trail heading right. This is the beginning of a potential loop, with most of the great views to the right but also a boulder field to traverse.

If you're up for that, go right and traverse said boulder field, which has amazing views of the gorge, mountains everywhere, Bear Lake down to the right, and eventually Mount Hood peeking around the south side of the peak. Ignore a trail descending to the right. Soon you'll be at the top, where you will see a massive radio station, a bunch of trees, and one view of Mount Hood. You did it! You summited the gorge.

Now head northeast off the summit and look for Defiance Trail #413 heading back into the trees. After 0.5 mile, passing the Cutoff Trail again on the left, turn right for Warren Lake. This trail is easy for a bit before going steeply down to the shallow lake, where you will find the only water source and campsites on this whole trek. A total of 1.1 miles since leaving Defiance Trail, you'll intersect Starvation Ridge Trail, where you turn left. So begins the descent—as in 3,200 feet in around 2.5 miles. (By the way, you might want to start ibuprofen the day before this hike.). This puts you at an intersection with the Starvation Cutoff Trail, where you turn right for another 0.4 mile of entertainment that drops you out at the Historic Columbia River Highway. Kiss it if you'd like, then turn right and go 0.2 mile to your wonderful, padded car.

NEARBY ACTIVITIES

Full Sail Brewing Co. is in Hood River (506 Columbia St., 541-386-2247, fullsail brewing.com). How does a beer sound right now? Meanwhile, if this little trailhead is getting too crowded, you can do a climb of "only" 10.6 miles and 3,800 feet to Nesmith Point; see the oregonhikers.org field guide for details.

• •

GPS TRAILHEAD COORDINATES
Starvation Creek State Park N45° 41.314' W121° 41.425'

DIRECTIONS Take I-84 from Portland to Exit 55 (Starvation Creek Trailhead).

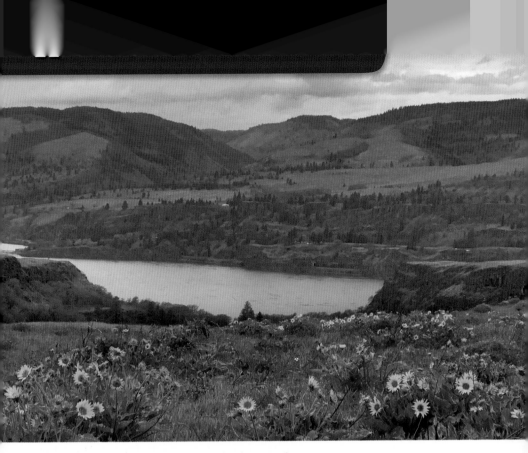

Balsamroot and the Columbia River from the Plateau Trail

THIS PLACE IS in a different world from most of the hikes in this book. It's a glimpse into central Oregon, a land of wide-open vistas, grass blowing in the nearly constant wind, and semiarid forests of oak and ponderosa pine. It also boasts panoramic vistas of the Columbia River and Mounts Adams and Hood, and more than 300 species of plants, some of them unique to the Columbia River Gorge.

DESCRIPTION

OK, so this one is more than 60 miles from Portland, even as the crow flies. But it's truly worth the extra bit of easy driving, especially in the spring and early summer. At those times of the year, there is a kind of rain shroud somewhere between Cascade Locks and Hood River; while it's still pouring in Portland, places like the McCall Preserve are bathed in sunlight and carpeted in a few dozen kinds of wildflowers all blooming at once.

Start with McCall Point Trail and get your exercise out of the way. The trail, which climbs just over 1,000 feet in 1.7 miles, starts out nearly flat and on an old

DISTANCE & CONFIGURATION: 3.5-mile out-and-back for McCall Point Trail, 2.5-mile balloon loop for Rowena Plateau

DIFFICULTY: Easy for Rowena Plateau Loop, moderate for McCall Point due to the climb

SCENERY: Wildflowers, the Columbia River below, two volcanoes, old oak trees

EXPOSURE: Wide open most of the time

TRAFFIC: Heavy on weekends when flowers are out, light otherwise

TRAIL SURFACE: Packed dirt

HIKING TIME: 1 hour for Rowena Plateau Loop, 2 hours to McCall Point

ELEVATION CHANGE: 1,070' to McCall Point, 100' for Rowena Plateau

SEASON: May–November for McCall Point, year-round for Rowena Plateau Loop

BEST TIME: April and May

BACKPACKING OPTIONS: No camping allowed

DRIVING DISTANCE: 76 miles (1 hour, 30 minutes) from Pioneer Courthouse Square

ACCESS: No fees or permits required

MAPS: Green Trails *Map 432S (Columbia River Gorge–East)*

WHEELCHAIR ACCESS: No

FACILITIES: None

CONTACT: Columbia River Gorge National Scenic Area, 541-308-1700, www.fs.usda.gov /crgnsa; The Nature Conservancy, 503-802-8100, tinyurl.com/tommccallpreserve

LOCATION: Rowena Crest Viewpoint on the Historic Columbia River Highway, 6 miles east of Mosier, OR

COMMENTS: Consider wearing long pants—ticks, poison oak, and rattlesnakes are all found in the area. Dogs are prohibited on both trails.

wagon road, winding through the kind of open space that is so rare in the western part of the state. The trees you eventually encounter are oaks, most of them Oregon white oak, and some as old as 800 years. After 0.5 mile, leave the road for a trail that ascends slightly when it gains the edge of the ridge, with ever-more-impressive views to the east. Keep an eye out for Mount Adams as its summit comes into view across the river.

The second half has had some serious work done in recent years, mostly to ease the grade and rebuild the tread so it isn't as slippery when wet. It also visits even more of the meadows than it used to, so it's a win all around. Keep an eye out for big stones laid in the trail as steps. Soon enough you'll come to McCall Point, an open hilltop with a sprawling view from Mount Hood to Mount Adams; you're actually about halfway between the two peaks, each of which is roughly 35 miles away. Looking west, you can see into the Columbia River Gorge; just to the left of it, the high peak with the towers on top is Mount Defiance, the highest point in the gorge.

You summit hounds out there might stand at McCall Point and notice there's more trail going south, through a notch, and then climbing again. I walked about a mile down (and then up) that trail, through some peaceful oak stands, but technically speaking, it didn't go anywhere special before it got pinched between a fence and the edge of a cliff. My advice is to have yourself a picnic at McCall Point and don't worry about that other trail.

Now for the Plateau Trail. Back at the trailhead, cross the highway and start on a wide path that actually drops 100 feet in elevation, traversing flower and grass

Tom McCall Preserve

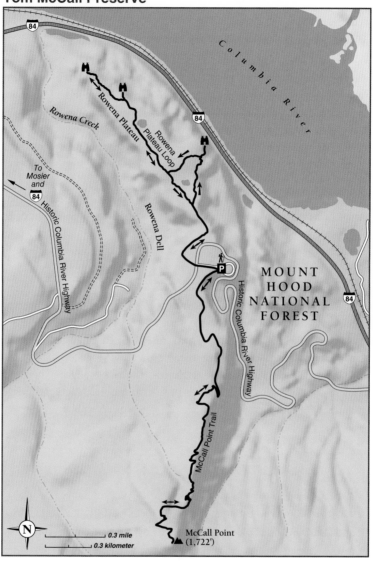

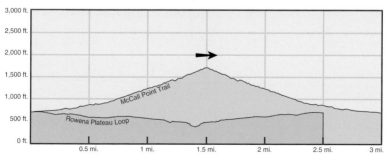

country to loop around a pond. Early in the year, there will be numerous other little ponds and wet areas, each supporting their own microhabitats. The small canyon below you on your left is called Rowena Dell.

There is officially one trail out here, which circles a pond and continues just over a mile out toward the river. In fact, there seem to be others around, including off to your right where you can visit the (not railed) top of a 500-foot cliff. The first, bigger pond has water lilies and frogs and birds, so rounding it is worthwhile. If you go all the way out, you can drop just below the plateau to a nice view of the river. The town across the river is Lyle, Washington, which lies on a gravel bar formed by catastrophic floods more than 10,000 years ago.

This trail isn't so much about the hiking or the points of interest; just plan to visit in April or May, try to avoid the crowds, and plan to spend a lot of time and take a lot of photos. For wildflowers and open vistas, it doesn't get any better than McCall Preserve in springtime.

NEARBY ACTIVITIES

As long as you're this far east, keep going to The Dalles to visit the Columbia Gorge Discovery Center (5000 Discovery Dr., The Dalles, OR; 541-296-8600, gorge discovery.org), where displays range from an exhibit about the Columbia River during the last ice age to an interactive installation about the Lewis and Clark expedition. And if this trail is too crowded, go across the river to Lyle Cherry Orchard, another flower spot owned by the Friends of the Columbia Gorge. See gorgefriends .org for details.

• •

GPS TRAILHEAD COORDINATES N45° 40.964' W121° 18.034'

DIRECTIONS Take I-84 from Portland, driving 62 miles east of I-205 to Exit 69 (Mosier). Turn right and follow Historic Columbia River Highway (US 30) 6.5 miles through Mosier to Rowena Crest Viewpoint. McCall Point Trail begins at a sign at the end of the stone wall. The Plateau Loop begins across the highway, where a set of steps leads over a fence.

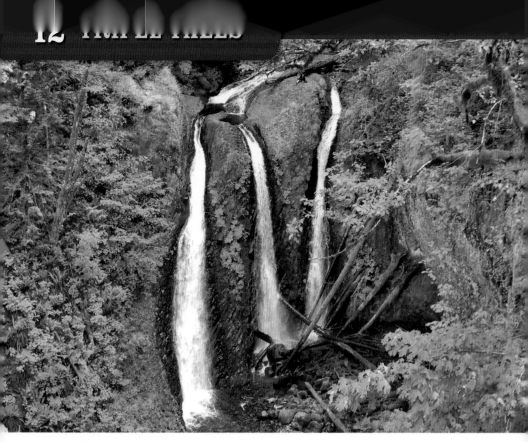

Triple Falls from the first viewpoint on the trail

A WATERFALL LIES at the end of this moderate hike, but you don't have to go that far to see some fine Columbia River Gorge scenery. You can, in fact, just drive by the trailhead and admire Horsetail Falls.

DESCRIPTION

If all you do is slow down while driving by Horsetail Falls, you'll be pleased. But at least cross the parking area to pick some blackberries over by the railroad tracks; they're ripe in late summer. The great thing about this trail is that the farther you go, the better it gets, and you never have to work very hard at all.

From Horsetail Falls, follow the gravel trail behind the sign describing some of the animals that live in the area. At 0.2 mile, stay right at a trail junction. A few hundred yards later, you'll come around a bend and see Upper Horsetail Falls, also known as Ponytail Falls. A popular turnaround spot because it's so near the car, these falls are also a hit with kids, who with supervision can go down by the water and catch some spray. The falls seem to shoot out of a basalt cliff face, and the area behind them is a grotto through which the trail passes. If you get under them, some

71

DISTANCE & CONFIGURATION: 4.5-mile out-and-back or loop

DIFFICULTY: Moderate

SCENERY: Four waterfalls, spectacular gorge, view of the Columbia River

EXPOSURE: In the forest all the way, with some sections very near steep hillsides

TRAFFIC: Heavy on summer weekends, moderate otherwise

TRAIL SURFACE: Gravel and packed dirt; roots, rocks

HIKING TIME: 3 hours

ELEVATION CHANGE: 610'

SEASON: Year-round but gets muddy in winter and spring

BEST TIME: April for water flow and flowers, October for fall colors

BACKPACKING OPTIONS: None

DRIVING DISTANCE: 35 miles (40 minutes) from Pioneer Courthouse Square

ACCESS: No fees or permits required

MAPS: Green Trails *Map 428 (Bridal Veil)* or *Map 428S (Columbia River Gorge–West)*

WHEELCHAIR ACCESS: No

FACILITIES: None at trailhead; water and restrooms 0.5 mile east at Ainsworth State Park (503-695-2261, tinyurl.com /ainsworthsp)

LOCATION: Horsetail Falls Trailhead on Historic Columbia River Highway, 2 miles west of Dodson, OR

CONTACT: Columbia River Gorge National Scenic Area, 541-308-1700, www.fs.usda.gov/crgnsa

smaller streams will trickle down onto your head. Just don't get directly under the main stream of water—even this relatively small waterfall is extremely powerful.

To keep going, simply follow the trail as it contours around the gorge wall. It soon comes to a brushy area on the right, through which several trails lead out to clifftop viewpoints over the Columbia River. You can make a side loop out there and work your way back to the main trail as it turns away from the river. A network of trails crisscrosses this tiny area, but they all lead to the same place. Just keep an eye on kids, as there is no rail on that clifftop; if you need a reminder, there is a memorial plaque for a 14-year-old boy who fell to his death near here in 1988.

A mile past Ponytail Falls, after you pass under a mossy "weeping" rock face, you'll descend to a bridge spanning the Oneonta Gorge. A geological and biological wonder, Oneonta alone is worth a visit; from here, you're looking down into it, with waterfalls above and below you. The one above you is Middle Oneonta Falls, and below is the upper lip of Lower Oneonta Falls. Just across the bridge, and after a little climbing, is another junction—here, you can go right to loop back to the highway (you'll have to walk nearly 0.5 mile along the road to get back to your car), or you can turn left and head up toward Triple Falls. The trail is rocky in places, and there's a little more elevation gain, but views of the narrow gorge will help keep you moving.

About a mile up you'll see Triple Falls. It's actually just one creek (Oneonta), but it splits just before it goes over the edge. Take your pictures from here, be careful at the viewpoint, then walk another minute or two to a wooden bridge across the wide stream just above the falls. Across it are some nice rocks for picnicking, and just upstream are pools the kids can jump into, if you've managed to get them this far. It

Triple Falls

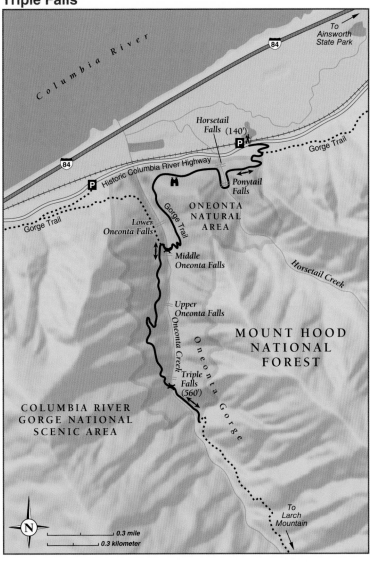

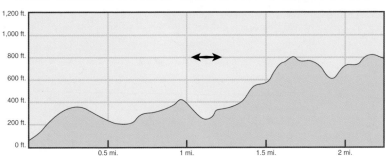

also appears the bridge was damaged by the fire, so check with the Forest Service to see its status.

And by the way, the next mile or so of trail above the falls sticks pretty close to the creek and is quite lovely, as well as less rarely hiked. If you're really feeling up for it, the top of Larch Mountain is 7 miles and 3,100 feet up, through an area that was definitely hit hard by the 2017 Eagle Creek Fire.

NEARBY ACTIVITIES

I used to recommend people check out Oneonta Gorge at this point but, honestly, it's just getting crushed by people. Give it a rest, literally, and instead go wander the newly developed waterfront in Hood River.

• •

GPS TRAILHEAD COORDINATES N45° 35.420' W122° 4.065'

DIRECTIONS Take I-84 from Portland to Exit 35 (Ainsworth). Turn right onto Frontage Road and then left onto Historic Columbia River Highway (following signs for Multnomah Falls). Continue 1.3 miles to the signed parking area at Horsetail Falls.

Ponytail Falls is a short way up the trail to Triple Falls.

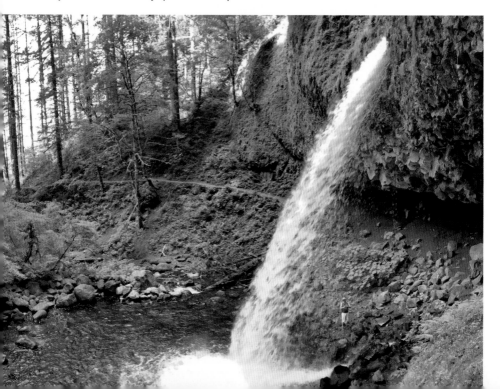

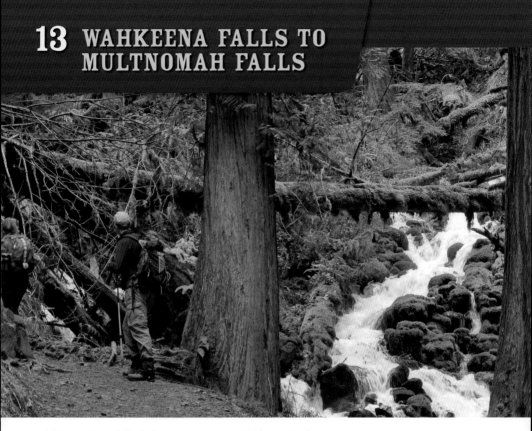

13 WAHKEENA FALLS TO MULTNOMAH FALLS

Hiking up through the lush, narrow canyon on Wahkeena Creek

JUST OFF I-84 and bookmarked by two waterfalls, this excursion is the ideal introduction to all the Columbia River Gorge has to offer, including great scenery, big crowds, waterfalls, and steep climbs. Word of warning: Parking is nearly impossible on summer weekends, so start very early if you can.

DESCRIPTION

When hiking friends come to visit Oregon, this is where I take them first. They get to see the scenic spectacle that is the Columbia River Gorge, they get to view the highest waterfall in Oregon, they get to see old-growth Douglas-firs, and they get their hearts pumping—from excitement and, at times, from effort.

You can hike either way on this trail and park at either falls; I prefer to park at Multnomah Falls and start the hike there. I'll tell you why in just a bit.

To do this, walk 100 yards down the historic highway west of Multnomah Falls Lodge, and take Return Trail #442, which parallels the road 0.6 mile to Wahkeena Falls. Along the way you'll pass under a giant boulder and be cooled by a mossy "weeping" rock wall.

DISTANCE & CONFIGURATION: 4.9-mile loop

DIFFICULTY: Moderate

SCENERY: Waterfalls, canyons, river views, flowers, a spring, big trees

EXPOSURE: In the forest all the way, a couple of sections of steep hillsides

TRAFFIC: Heavy, especially on weekends and around Multnomah Falls; moderate on weekdays

TRAIL SURFACE: Pavement, gravel, packed dirt with some rocky sections

HIKING TIME: 3 hours

ELEVATION CHANGE: 1,600'

SEASON: Year-round, but muddy and possibly icy in spots during winter and spring

BEST TIME: Whenever you can find parking

BACKPACKING OPTIONS: A couple of sites along the trail toward Angels Rest

DRIVING DISTANCE: 31 miles (35 minutes) from Pioneer Courthouse Square

ACCESS: No fees or permits required

MAPS: Green Trails *Map 428 (Bridal Veil)* or *Map 428S (Columbia River Gorge–West)*

WHEELCHAIR ACCESS: The first section of trail heading up from either falls is paved but kind of steep.

FACILITIES: Full services at Multnomah Falls Lodge

CONTACT: Columbia River Gorge National Scenic Area, 541-308-1700, www.fs.usda.gov/crgnra

LOCATION: 53000 Historic Columbia River Highway, 3 miles east of Bridal Veil, OR

COMMENTS: The upper parts of this trail probably saw some damage from the 2017 Eagle Creek Fire. Check the website above for the latest info.

Actually several falls in one, Wahkeena Falls encompasses everything from sheer drops to cascades to misty sprays. It is fed primarily by a spring up on the ridge that you'll see later. To start the loop, follow the paved trail across the creek and then 0.2 mile up to a footbridge at the base of the upper falls. Take a deep breath of that cool, refreshing air—your workout is about to begin.

In the next 0.4 mile of paved switchbacks, you'll gain about 400 feet; such quick climbs are the trademark of Gorge hikes. In the area around the bench set in the wall, see if you can find coins and other objects that workers stuck into the masonry of the walls. When you get to the top, turn right and walk a few minutes to Lemmon's Viewpoint, named for a firefighter who died in the area. This spot has a great lookout on the Columbia. Next, start back up past the junction, leaving the pavement. You can rest a few minutes later on a bench at the lovely Fairy Falls, sort of a miniature version of Ramona Falls (Hike 38, page 192). You still have some climbing to do; it's just that now it's more gradual and you have the creek and some lovely old forest to take your mind off it. Past fires took out smaller growth, blackened the trunks of bigger trees, and opened the forest floor for berries and wildflowers to move in. Just above Fairy Falls, you'll encounter Vista Point Trail—turn right here, staying on Wahkeena Trail #420. After another 0.4 mile, you'll come to an intersection with Angels Rest Trail #415. The sign here, also confusing, was helpfully edited: because it lacked the word *Trail* after *Vista Point, Devils Rest, and Larch Mountain*—the distances listed apply to those trails, not to the destinations—somebody came by and scratched *Trail* after each name. At any rate, you should at least take a 100-yard detour here on Angels

Wahkeena Falls to Multnomah Falls

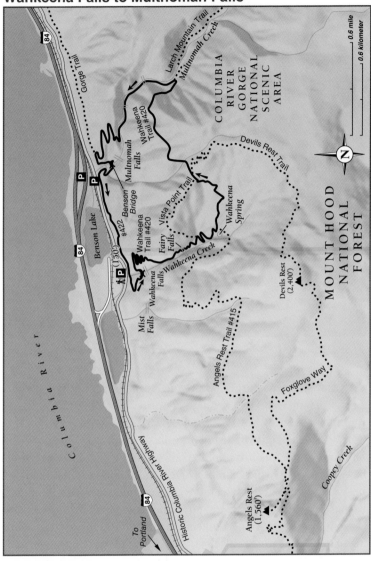

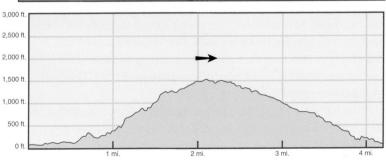

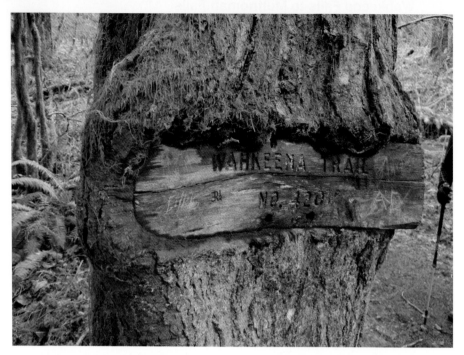

Tree versus sign on the Wahkeena Trail

Rest Trail to see Wahkeena Spring, where the creek emerges from the ground all at once in a magical (and tasty) scene. A few campsites sit a bit farther down this trail.

At the intersection of the Wahkeena and Angels Rest Trails, back near the spring, take Wahkeena Trail up the hill 0.4 mile to a four-way intersection. Ascending the hill from your left is Vista Point Trail—ignore it. Ascending the hill to your right is Devils Rest Trail, which climbs 820 feet in 1.6 miles to what, frankly, is a disappointing viewpoint. So unless you just want some more exercise, continue straight on Wahkeena Trail. Oh, and congratulations: no more climbing today!

This eastbound stretch on Wahkeena Trail soon descends and, in 0.9 mile, intersects Larch Mountain Trail #441, which connects Multnomah Falls with Larch Mountain (Hike 9, page 58). For our purposes, turn left and head 1 mile down the rock-filled Multnomah Creek along a truly magnificent section of trail. You'll pass several waterfalls: Ecola Falls and Weisendanger Falls, both 55 feet high; pass through Dutchman's Tunnel; and then pass three 10- to 15-foot falls known as Lower, Middle, and Upper Weisendanger Falls (Weisendanger was a U.S. Forest Service ranger).

After crossing what I consider a rather magical bridge over Multnomah Creek, you'll see a well-marked (and well-traveled) trail to the left leading 0.1 mile to the top of Multnomah Falls, where a wooden platform offers an ego-building view of the camera-toting throngs below. "Yeah," you can say later at the bottom, "I've been up there." This brings me to why I like to do the hike this way: From this point on, especially on a weekend, you'll be among hundreds of people. In my opinion, it's better (that is, faster) going downhill than uphill through such a mob. Multnomah Falls and Benson Bridge are just 1 mile on.

At 542 feet, Upper Multnomah Falls is the highest falls in Oregon. Be sure to stop at the information office at the lodge to see pictures of the various floods and a massive rockfall that have occurred there.

Now, for the final reason I like to start this hike at Wahkeena Falls but park at Multnomah Falls Lodge: when you're all done, you can get yourself an ice-cream cone or an espresso, or cruise the gift shop if you're into that, and your car is right there waiting for you.

NEARBY ACTIVITIES

The 1925 Multnomah Falls Lodge (503-695-2376, multnomahfallslodge.com) is well worth checking out, with its skylights and fireplace in the restaurant and its old-style stone-and-wood construction. The food isn't as good as the setting, but the Sunday brunch buffet is massive.

· ·

GPS TRAILHEAD COORDINATES
Wahkeena Falls Parking Area N45° 34.517' W122° 7.681',
Multnomah Falls Lodge N45° 31.776' W122° 5.303'

DIRECTIONS Take I-84 from Portland east 20 miles from I-205 to Exit 28 (Bridal Veil). Turn left onto Historic Columbia River Highway, and proceed 2 miles to the signed parking area at Wahkeena Falls or continue another 0.7 mile to Multnomah Falls Lodge. You can also stay on I-84 until Exit 31 for a larger parking area, then walk under the expressway to Multnomah Falls Lodge.

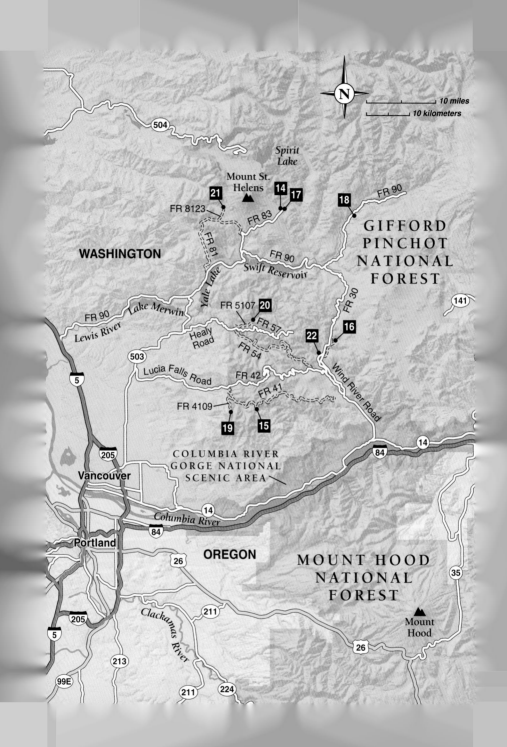

AROUND MOUNT ST. HELENS

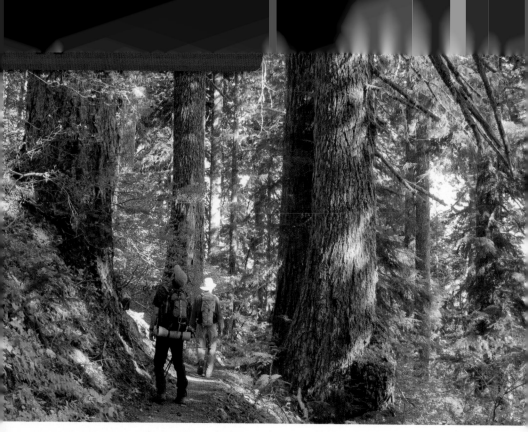

Big trees and fall colors on the Ape Canyon Trail

THIS TRAIL VISITS two worlds not often seen: the upper reaches of a volcano and the edge of what they call the "blast zone." Without too much climbing, you can stand in a wonderful old-growth forest and be mere feet from an area that was completely obliterated in 1980. At the top, you'll enjoy a sweeping view highlighted by an amazing geological oddity, right at the base of the volcano. And then you can go stand at the top of a waterfall with amazing views.

DESCRIPTION

As soon as you start walking, stay straight at an unsigned junction, and you'll get your first glimpse of the contrasts ahead when you've walked only 500 feet on this trail. At this point you'll be at the top of a little bluff, looking out over a wide area of rocks. Those rocks used to be on the upper slopes of Mount St. Helens, but on May 18, 1980, they tumbled down the hill at about 45 miles per hour, part of a lahar, or mudflow, triggered when the Shoestring Glacier melted moments after the volcano erupted. But the mudslide stayed generally within the boundaries of the Muddy River, so the forest you're standing in—even though it was within feet of the slide— was spared. You'll spend the next 5 miles climbing this ridge, but don't worry: you'll gain only around 1,500 net feet along the way.

DISTANCE & CONFIGURATION: 11.6-mile out-and-back

DIFFICULTY: Moderate

SCENERY: Old-growth forest, volcanic mudflow, narrow canyon, big-time views

EXPOSURE: Shady and open areas on the way up, then wide open at the top

TRAFFIC: Moderate on summer weekends, light otherwise

TRAIL SURFACE: Packed dirt with roots and rocks; rock at the top

HIKING TIME: 5.5 hours

ELEVATION CHANGE: 1,485'

SEASON: Late June–October

BEST TIME: July for water in the falls, September and October for fall colors

BACKPACKING OPTIONS: Poor (a few decent sites, but not much water available)

DRIVING DISTANCE: 75 miles (1 hour, 45 minutes) from Pioneer Courthouse Square

ACCESS: Northwest Forest Pass required (see page 14)

MAPS: USFS *Mount St. Helens National Volcanic Monument*

WHEELCHAIR ACCESS: No, but some of the nearby Lava Canyon Trail is accessible.

FACILITIES: None at trailhead; restrooms at Lava Canyon Trailhead

CONTACT: Mount St. Helens National Volcanic Monument, 360-449-7800, www.fs.usda.gov /mountsthelens

LOCATION: Ape Canyon Trailhead at the end of Forest Service Road (FR) 83, 18 miles east of Cougar, WA

COMMENTS: In June, check ahead to make sure FR 83 is open and snow-free.

Before you leave this viewpoint, look down. You're standing on several layers of rock, the result of a 1980 lahar that exposed the rock, giving scientists clues to the volcano's history of eruptions.

If you're on this trail in September or October, you'll be in the world of the vine maple; its red and orange explosion contrasts beautifully with the evergreen canopy. Keep an eye out for deer and elk as well. At 0.25 mile look for an island of trees on the edge of the mudflow and, after 0.5 mile enjoy your first view south (behind you) to Mount Hood. Ahead, on the slopes of Mount St. Helens, you can see the canyon left behind by Shoestring Glacier.

At 1.2 miles, you'll reach a little ridge, then soon after make a switchback to the right and climb a bit more; you'll also notice some social trails heading out to brushy viewpoints facing east to Mount Adams. You'll enter an impressive forest around 1.5 miles up; get your first view of Mount Adams at 1.7 miles; and at 2 miles start a series of switchbacks among old-growth hemlock and thick vine maple. Just past 3 miles, you'll actually lose some elevation before a viewpoint that takes in two-humped Mount Rainier off to your right. From here, you can also make out a large waterfall (mostly dry by late summer) on an eastern ridge of St. Helens—we'll be at the top of that soon.

At 4.4 miles, you'll be out in the open at the head of Ape Canyon proper—and in the "blast zone" itself. Up ahead, you'll see trees that were killed by the superheated gases produced when the mountain blew in 1980, and to the north (ahead of you) you'll see the utter desolation the eruption created. (The volcano exploded in that direction.)

Ape Canyon

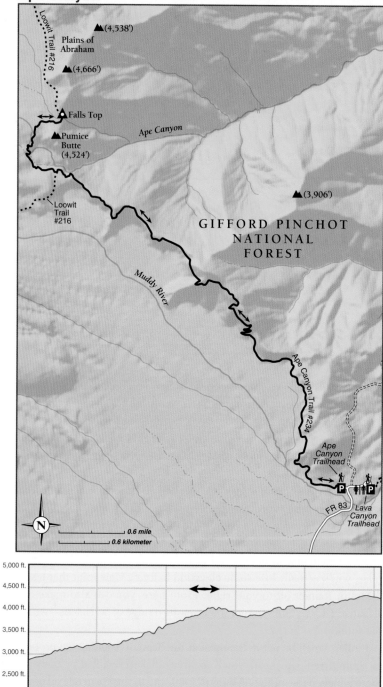

When you come to a lookout point on the right, you can scramble down a bit—be very careful—and look into the 300-foot slot at the head of Ape Canyon, which now stretches away to your right. It's also visible from a little farther up the trail, where, if you work it right, it makes a heck of a foreground for a picture of Mount Adams.

Just 0.2 mile farther up, Ape Canyon Trail #234 ends at an intersection with Loowit Trail #216, which goes all the way around Mount St. Helens. Walking up to a saddle on the left will get you a nice view south toward Mount Hood and the way you've come up, as well as a weather station and some rocks to sit on.

Back on the trail, stay to the right at the junction, now on Loowit Trail #216. Wind through another lahar as you go around Pumice Butte on your right, and 0.5 mile later you'll climb out of it to the east, where a series of rock cairns marks the trail's path onto the moonlike Plains of Abraham. When the trail dips to the cliff edge, you'll be at the top of that waterfall I told you about, with a sweeping view south. In early summer there should be some water in here; by autumn it's usually a trickle.

Turning around here gets you the 11-mile hike advertised, but it's more than worth it to continue a bit onto the Plains of Abraham, which were also created by the 1980 eruption. Look for trees on the nearby hilltops that are lying down and pointing away from the mountain; they were blasted down when the mountain blew. The Plains themselves are fantastic, especially when the weather is clear and the mountain looms over you. If you're up here in August, look for vast swaths of purple lupine on the slopes above.

If you're wondering about the name Ape Canyon, it recalls a 1920s incident in which an apelike "Bigfoot"—decades later found to be a kid playing a prank—threw rocks at some miners in the area. The only connection between Ape Canyon and Ape Cave is in the name: the Mount St. Helens Apes, a local Boy Scout troop that took its name from the Ape Canyon legend, first explored Ape Cave.

NEARBY ACTIVITIES

On the way back down FR 83, you'll pass a sign for Ape Cave, which is actually a long lava tube divided by an access ladder. Exploring the lower cave involves a 1.6-mile round-trip walk through a large cavern. Taking in the upper, 2.3-mile cave is trickier, requiring some rock scrambling here and there. Take two flashlights if you go.

• •

GPS TRAILHEAD COORDINATES   N46° 9.926' W122° 5.537'

DIRECTIONS Take I-5 from Portland to Exit 21. Turn right onto WA 503, which after 31 miles passes through Cougar and turns into FR 90. Continue 3.3 miles; turn left onto FR 83. The trailhead is 11.2 miles ahead on the left, just before the Lava Canyon trailhead.

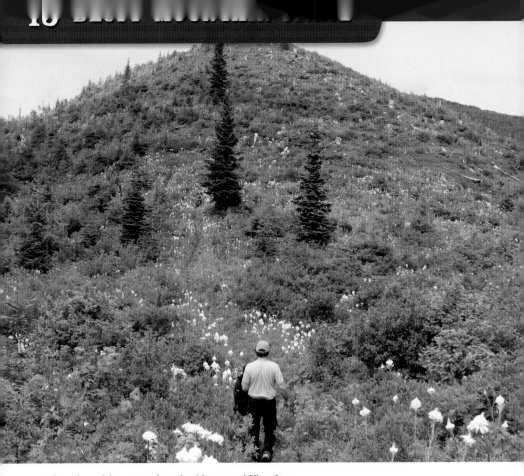

Hiking through beargrass along the ridge toward Silver Star

THERE ARE SEVERAL ways to reach the summit of Silver Star Mountain; this is the longest and toughest path to climb, and possibly the hardest to reach. But it is without question the most entertaining, offering excellent views, heaps of flowers, and few hikers, which gives it an almost expeditionary feel.

DESCRIPTION

Epic. That's the word that always comes to mind when I think of this hike. By the end of the (long, often hot) day, you'll feel like you've been on an adventure. And as you sit atop Silver Star, with all the slackers who came up one of the easy ways, you can tell 'em you ain't done nothin' if you ain't done Bluff Mountain Trail.

Speaking of those "easy" ways, one of them, Ed's Trail, is described in the Silver Star Mountain profile (Hike 19, page 102). Its access road is even worse, but the hike is easier than this one. The third option, via Grouse Vista (not in this book), has the advantage of good road access but the disadvantage of being dull and crowded.

DISTANCE & CONFIGURATION: 13.2-mile out-and-back

DIFFICULTY: Strenuous

SCENERY: Wide-open, flower-covered ridges; exposed mountainsides; waterfalls; panoramic vista

EXPOSURE: Open almost the whole way, occasionally on knife-edge ridges

TRAFFIC: Light

TRAIL SURFACE: Rocky

HIKING TIME: 7.5 hours

ELEVATION CHANGE: 1,660'

SEASON: Late June–October

BEST TIME: July for flowers, October for fall colors

BACKPACKING OPTIONS: Poor (a few decent sites, but not much water available)

DRIVING DISTANCE: 58 miles (2 hours) from Pioneer Courthouse Square

ACCESS: No fees or permits required

MAPS: Green Trails *Map 396 (Lookout Mountain)* and *Map 428 (Bridal Veil)*

WHEELCHAIR ACCESS: No

FACILITIES: None at the trailhead; restrooms and water at Sunset Falls Campground, on the way

CONTACT: Mount Adams Ranger District, 509-395-3400, www.fs.usda.gov/giffordpinchot

LOCATION: Bluff Mountain Trailhead on Forest Service Road (FR) 41, 20 miles southeast of Yacolt, WA

COMMENTS: FR 41, while passable, is rife with potholes and other problems—which have gotten worse over the years. Also, the last sections of the trail often retain snow well into July. Avoid this hike on a hot day, as you'll be in the open about 95% of the time.

From the trailhead, Bluff Mountain Trail #172 starts on an old jeep road along a ridge that looks and feels like it's way up in the alpine country of Mount Hood. That's because it's wide open and covered with flowers—but it's open because of a fire, not elevation. The 1902 Yacolt Burn was so intense that few trees have grown back, though the 1960s saw some terracing and replanting.

Wander along this ridge, with views of other peaks and ridges swept clean by the fire, for 2.5 sunbaked miles, then descend into a notch where the road ends. Here, look for the trail taking off for the right (west) side of the ridge and passing under a series of dramatic cliffs (the north side of Bluff Mountain), with views of Little Baldy off to the right. You'll probably have to skip over a couple of small creeks, which will be welcome sights on hot summer days.

At 3.5 miles, the trail climbs west into a patch of forest notable for thin but thickly packed trees that seem like clones of each other. Emerging from this forest at 3.8 miles, you'll be greeted by a big view of your destination, the two-humped Silver Star Mountain, ahead. Having come this far and climbed through a forest to be greeted by this view, don't you feel like you're on an expedition? Silver Star looks bigger and more dramatic than other peaks, as its generally treeless east face rises beyond an impressive foreground.

Back out in the sun, continue south along the east side of Little Baldy, and in just under 5 miles you'll have a view of a big waterfall on Silver Star's flanks. At 5.3 miles, continue straight through an intersection with Trail #175, and you'll

Bluff Mountain Trail

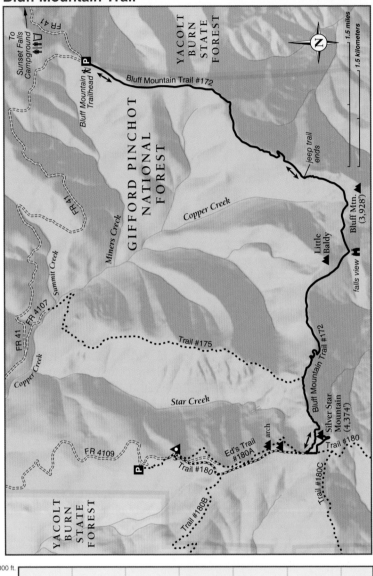

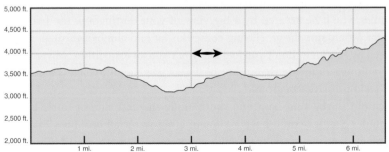

soon climb to the dramatic (perhaps nerve-wracking, for the acrophobic) ridges of Silver Star, which you wind along for almost a mile before descending into forest again just below the peak.

In these woods, your path intersects a road coming in from the right; this is the end of the Ed's Trail hike. Turn left on the road for a fairly steep climb—stay left again when the road splits—to a saddle between Silver Star's peaks. The higher one is on the left, and the view from here is as impressive as the one on the 6.6-mile hike you just did. On a clear day, you can see from the Three Sisters to Mount Rainier, and because you're on the highest peak in the immediate vicinity, there's a sense of being on a mountain throne.

The next rock to the south is Pyramid Rock. It's not impressive in and of itself, but in recent years there have been reports of at least one mountain goat hanging around there. So keep an eye out before returning the way you came.

• •

GPS TRAILHEAD COORDINATES N45° 46.803' W122° 10.010'

DIRECTIONS Take I-205 from Portland, driving 5 miles north of the Columbia River to take Exit 30B (Orchards). Turn right on WA 500 E, which turns into WA 503 in 0.9 mile (follow signs for Battle Ground). Continue 12.5 miles on WA 503, then turn right onto NE Rock Creek Road, which turns into Lucia Falls Road. Drive 8.5 miles on this road, then make a right onto NE Sunset Falls Road and follow it 7.4 miles to Sunset Falls Campground. Turn right to go through the campground and across a bridge over the East Fork Lewis River, and then leave the pavement, driving 9 bumpy miles on FR 41 to a big ridgetop parking area. The trailhead is on the right.

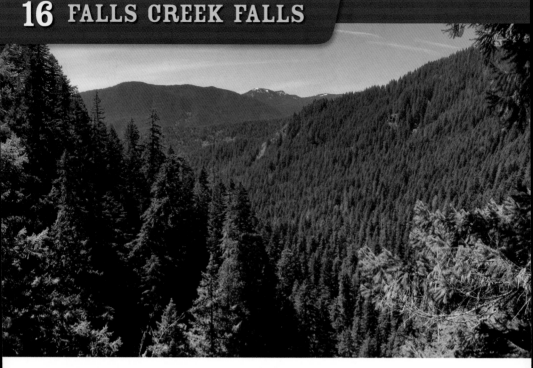

View down the valley from near the top of Falls Creek Falls

LOOKING FOR AN easy trail to a spectacular destination? This 1.7-mile ramble gains about 700 feet—which you will hardly notice on the way and will forget entirely when you reach one of the area's most impressive falls.

DESCRIPTION

The trail starts out flat through forest that's less than 60 years old, passing among huckleberry, Oregon grape, and Douglas-fir. Not much to see here, but at least you don't have to work hard. A hundred yards in, ignore Trail #152 on the left and continue up Trail #152A. (If you're doing the loop to the top of the falls, you'll see #152 later.)

After 0.5 mile, you'll traverse meadows with a view of an interesting rock formation to the left. In this area you will also find western larch, which normally grows east of the mountains. You won't notice this unless you visit in October, when its needles turn a dramatic gold. Soon after this, you'll cross Falls Creek on a suspension bridge over a narrow gorge; look for some cool round, water-formed rock faces.

At 0.6 mile, now in an older forest, you'll pass a couple of impressive root balls in an area that might get treacherous when wet. At 0.75 mile, you pass nearly under a big Douglas-fir; look for a dead one nearby with countless woodpecker holes.

After hiking 1 mile almost effortlessly, you'll reach a junction where the loop to the Upper Falls takes off, but for now stay on the path you've been hiking. It may sound odd, but on this creek, the Lower Falls is much more impressive than the Upper Falls.

DISTANCE & CONFIGURATION: 3.4-mile out-and-back for Lower Falls, 6.1-mile balloon if you also visit the Upper Falls

DIFFICULTY: Easy–moderate

SCENERY: Shady forest, serene stream, waterfall

EXPOSURE: Some cliff edges (easily avoided) at end of trail

TRAFFIC: Moderate on weekends, light otherwise

TRAIL SURFACE: Packed dirt

HIKING TIME: 2.5 hours to see the Lower Falls, 4 hours for whole loop

ELEVATION CHANGE: 700' to falls, 1,100' to top

SEASON: May–November; road gated December 1–March 31

BEST TIME: May and June

BACKPACKING OPTIONS: Decent site at Upper Falls

DRIVING DISTANCE: 66 miles (1 hour, 30 minutes) from Pioneer Courthouse Square

ACCESS: No fees or permits required

MAPS: Green Trails *Map 397 (Wind River)*

WHEELCHAIR ACCESS: No

FACILITIES: Outhouse at the trailhead

LOCATION: Falls Creek Falls Trailhead at the end of Forest Service Road (FR) 3062/FR 057, 17 miles north of Carson, WA

CONTACT: Mount Adams Ranger District, 509-395-3400, www.fs.usda.gov/giffordpinchot

Over the next 0.5 mile, you'll climb past a nice creekside picnic area on the right, cross a metal bridge over a lovely cascading creek (dry by late summer), and pass under a big rock formation on the left. By this time you should be hearing, and seeing through the trees, the main Lower Falls.

When you arrive at the falls, in an area of large boulders that provide plenty of seating, you'll see two levels of water plunging into a mossy bowl filled with maidenhair ferns. (In fact, a hidden, third level is even higher, making for a total drop of 200 feet.) The whole scene seems like something straight out of *The Lord of the Rings;* you expect to see archers on the hill, guarding their sacred pool. It's particularly impressive in early summer, when water flows are high.

Linger here awhile, and then head back the way you came, or consider taking the upper loop, recently maintained and signed by the Washington Trails Association. For the upper loop, follow the trail a steep 0.25 mile through a draw to a junction. Turn right and you'll climb another 0.5 mile—your last uphill for the day.

Right after the trail levels, look for a user trail leading right 50 yards or so to the top of some cliffs. Here, you'll get a view of the upper third of the big falls and down the canyon to some of the peaks of Trapper Creek Wilderness (Hike 22, page 114).

Walk another five minutes and you're back at the creek, where a trail leads right and to another view. From this point a path descends toward the top of the falls; it can be done, but be very careful, and keep dogs leashed and kids nearby. You'll notice that you can't see the lower viewpoint from here—you're seeing a whole new section of falls. A tiny bit of hiking remains, but it's just a few minutes to the Upper Falls. Though they are only about 6 feet high, they have a nice campsite.

When you do head back, stay with Trail #152 all the way down, just to see some new terrain. It's unspectacular but also uncrowded. Look for the trail on the left that will dump you out on the trail where you started, #152A, just above the trailhead.

Falls Creek Falls

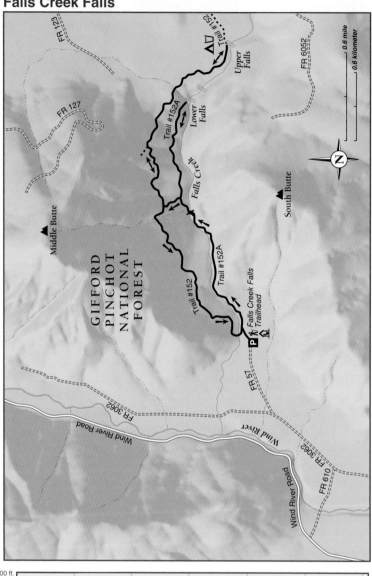

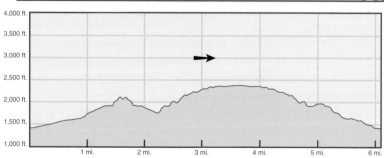

• •

GPS TRAILHEAD COORDINATES N45° 54.339' W121° 56.385'

DIRECTIONS Take I-84 from Portland to Exit 44. As soon as you enter the town, make your first right to get on Bridge of the Gods, following a sign for Stevenson. Pay the $2 toll (as of 2017), cross the river, and turn right (east) onto WA 14. Go 5.9 miles and turn left onto Wind River Road. Drive 14.5 miles, then turn right onto FR 30, and drive 0.8 mile. Turn right onto gravel FR 3062. Drive 2 miles and make a right onto FR 57, following a sign for Lower Falls Creek Falls Trail. The trailhead is at the end of the road.

Falls Creek Falls, which photos don't do proper justice

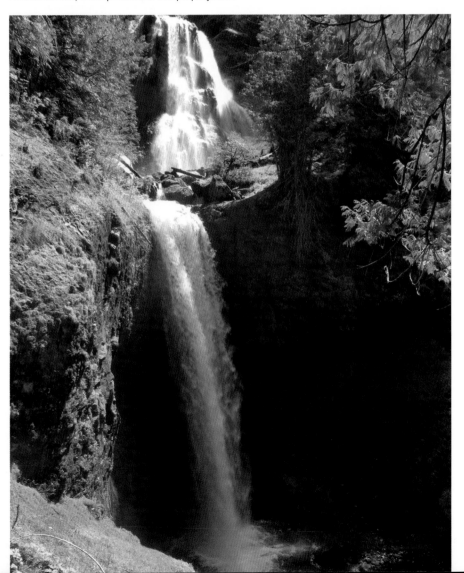

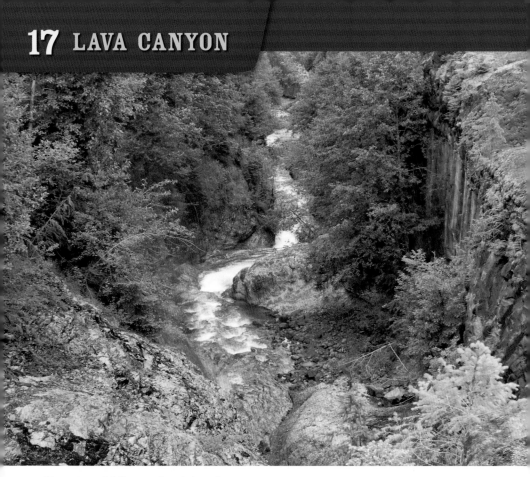

It's pretty much falls everywhere in Lava Canyon.

AN UNPARALLELED LOOK at geological forces at work, Lava Canyon is also a beautiful place to be, with numerous waterfalls, a dramatic bridge, some challenging hiking, and a short, barrier-free loop trail.

DESCRIPTION

First, a little history, so you'll know what you're looking at: In ancient times, a forest covered a deep valley. Then, 3,500 years ago, Mount St. Helens erupted, sending a massive mudflow down through the canyon, filling it with volcanic rock. Over the years, the river carved a path through the rock, forming a canyon with waterfalls, deep cuts, and towers of harder rock—Lava Canyon. Later mudflows covered all of that, and eventually forest grew back over the whole thing.

Then, on May 18, 1980, Mount St. Helens erupted again, melting 70% of its glaciers in an instant and sending millions of cubic feet of mud and rock blasting down the side of the mountain at about 45 miles an hour. That eruption cleaned out the forest and rock, exposing Lava Canyon for the first time in thousands of

DISTANCE & CONFIGURATION: Out-and-back or loop of 1.3–6 miles

DIFFICULTY: Easy for upper section, strenuous for whole thing

SCENERY: Waterfalls, canyon, geological wonders, suspension bridge

EXPOSURE: Mostly open, with several sections that are quite exposed. People have fallen to their death here, so if it has rained or snowed recently or you don't like heights, stick to the upper section. There's also a couple of ladders if you do the whole thing.

TRAFFIC: Very heavy on summer weekends, heavy during the week, moderate the rest of the season

TRAIL SURFACE: Paved, boardwalk, gravel, and ladders

HIKING TIME: 30 minutes for upper loop, 3 hours for whole thing

ELEVATION CHANGE: 500'–1,500'

SEASON: June–October; check ahead in June to make sure the road is snow-free.

BEST TIME: June for water flow, October or fall colors

BACKPACKING OPTIONS: None

DRIVING DISTANCE: 75 miles (1 hour, 45 minutes) from Pioneer Courthouse Square

ACCESS: Northwest Forest Pass required (see page 14)

MAPS: USFS *Mount St. Helens National Monument*

WHEELCHAIR ACCESS: Barrier-free trail in the upper section

FACILITIES: Restrooms at trailhead; no water

CONTACT: Mount St. Helens National Volcanic Monument, 360-449-7800, www.fs.usda.gov/mountsthelens

LOCATION: Lava Canyon trailhead at end of Forest Service Road (FR) 83, 18 miles east of Cougar, WA

years. As you drove in, you got a glimpse of this 1980 mudflow (also known as a lahar); now go see what it gave us.

From the trailhead, take the paved path leading left, which, though officially barrier-free, would require some work to push a wheelchair through. You can see here that the trees around you survived the 1980 eruption, but everything below was wiped out. Also, look around for trees that have rocks embedded in them—that's how strong the mudflow was, and this point is some 5 miles from its origin. The pavement will soon give way to boardwalk; two viewing platforms offer both information and dramatic views of the upper canyon.

Hike 0.4 mile to a junction with the loop trail. By now you have seen perhaps 15 warning signs telling you about various dangers and imploring you to stay on the trail. My favorite such sign is at this junction: DANGER is written in seven languages—and you have to get off the trail to read it. Anyway, be careful and stay on the trail.

Whichever loop you're doing, continue straight for now; in 100 yards you'll have a view of a waterfall and the swirling pools above it. In 0.2 mile you'll come to the suspension bridge, which is only 3 feet wide and 125 feet long. Kids, dogs, and people afraid of heights should not go beyond the suspension bridge, and everyone should be careful if it has rained recently. If you'd like to do only a 1.3-mile loop, cross the bridge and follow the trail back up to reach the first intersection after crossing another small bridge.

Lava Canyon

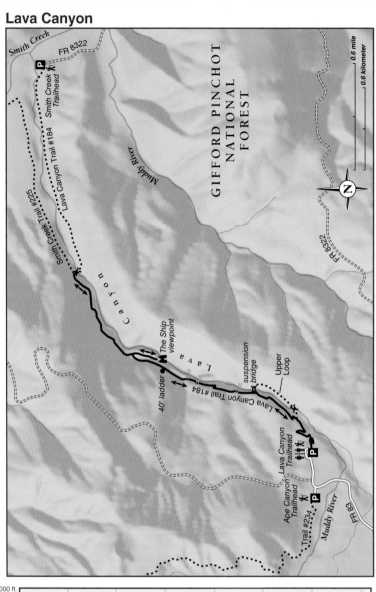

GIFFORD PINCHOT NATIONAL FOREST

Smith Creek

FR 8322

Smith Creek Trailhead

Smith Creek Trail #225

Lava Canyon Trail #184

Muddy River

FR 8322

0.6 mile

0.6 kilometer

Canyon

The Ship viewpoint

40' ladder

Lava

suspension bridge

Upper Loop

Lava Canyon Trail #184

Lava Canyon Trailhead

Ape Canyon Trailhead

Trail #234

Muddy River

FR 83

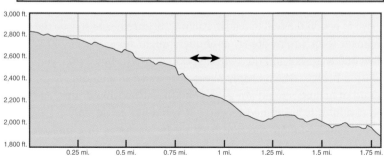

Otherwise, follow the trail down—and I do mean down—from the suspension bridge. In the next section of trail, you'll descend steep slopes, walk along unguarded ledges, cross a couple of creeks with no bridges (though one has a cable to hang onto), and climb down a 30-foot metal ladder. So if it's been raining, you have small kids, or you're tired or nervous about heights, think twice before you go past the bridge.

After a steep 0.5-mile descent that passes several beautiful waterfalls and an area where the river flows through a chute just a few feet wide, the trail mellows somewhat. After you've hiked a total of 1.1 miles, you'll climb down the ladder (be careful if your shoes are wet), and then cross a mossy stream. The rock formation on your right is known as The Ship; it was one of the formations left standing thousands of years ago when the river cut a new course through the ancient canyon. The top of The Ship was the floor of the valley before 1980. There's a little perspective, eh?

It's worth the effort to get to the top of The Ship. A couple hundred yards past the ladder, a trail on the right leads 0.2 mile up it; it's pretty steep and includes rock steps and yet another (smaller) ladder, but there are late-summer huckleberries up there, and it's a heck of a place for a picnic, with an excellent view back up the canyon.

At this point, you've seen the best of the hike, so it's a good spot to turn around. But if you'd like to keep going, Lava Canyon Trail #184 continues another 1.3 miles to the Smith Creek trailhead, losing 350 feet in elevation on the way. A bridge over the creek just 0.4 mile below the Ship trail is worth visiting.

When you head back up the trail, cross the suspension bridge and take the loop hike back onto a pre-1980 lava flow. When you cross a small metal bridge, turn left and you're 0.4 mile from your car.

• •

GPS TRAILHEAD COORDINATES N46° 9.945' W122° 5.275'

DIRECTIONS Take I-5 from Portland, driving 21 miles north of the Columbia River to Exit 21 (Woodland), then make a right onto WA 503 (Lewis River Road). Drive 31 miles, passing through the town of Cougar, until WA 503 turns into FR 90. Drive 3 miles on FR 90, then turn left onto FR 83, following a sign for Ape Cave and Lava Canyon. The Lava Canyon trailhead is 11.5 miles ahead, at the end of FR 83.

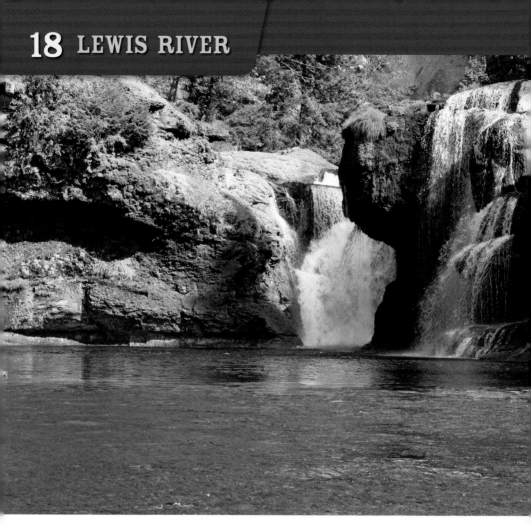

Lower Lewis River Falls is right by the campground at the trailhead.

HERE'S A PLEASANT, mostly flat stroll along a beautiful river with three dramatic waterfalls. Chances are they're unlike most falls you've ever seen. The long drive to the trailhead is worth it, especially if you get a campsite at the Lower Lewis River Falls Recreation Area and make a night of it.

DESCRIPTION

From the trailhead in the picnic area, follow a trail that starts just left of the restrooms. In 100 yards, turn right to reach several viewpoints above Lower Falls, one of the most dramatic falls around. The water looks like it's spilling off a shelf, and in fact it is—this is the edge of an ancient lava flow. Over the next stretch of trail, you're walking around the campground, so there are a lot of trails. Turning left will send you into the campground, but turning right will offer several opportunities to get down to the river. Once you're safely above the falls, you'll find some nice swimming spots.

DISTANCE & CONFIGURATION: Out-and-back of up to 5.2 miles

DIFFICULTY: Easy

SCENERY: Several waterfalls, wild stream flowing through a wooded canyon, old-growth forest

EXPOSURE: Shady

TRAFFIC: Heavy all summer long, especially on weekends

TRAIL SURFACE: Gravel at first, then packed dirt with some roots

HIKING TIME: 3.5 hours

ELEVATION CHANGE: 320'

SEASON: April–November; check ahead to see if the road is snow-free.

BEST TIME: Early summer or fall

BACKPACKING OPTIONS: A few decent sites along the river

DRIVING DISTANCE: 92 miles (2 hours, 10 minutes) from Pioneer Courthouse Square

ACCESS: Northwest Forest Pass required (see page 14)

MAPS: Green Trails *Map 365 (Lone Butte)*

WHEELCHAIR ACCESS: Campground loop only

FACILITIES: Restrooms at trailhead; drinking water at campground May–October

LOCATION: Lower Falls Day Use Area on Forest Service Road (FR 90), 32 miles east of Cougar, WA

CONTACT: Mount St. Helens National Volcanic Monument, 360-449-7800, www.fs.usda.gov /mountsthelens

About 0.5 mile after you leave the campground area, look for the remains of Sheep Bridge over the Lewis. According to the 1965 U.S. Geological Survey map of the area, Lewis River Campground used to be on the far side of the river, so that bridge offered access from the campground to this trail, as well as for driving sheep to pasture. You may also spot a rusted-out "steam donkey," a piece of equipment that was once part of a logging operation.

Around 0.8 mile from the campground, you'll pass the top of a small waterfall, and then at 1.2 miles you'll pass a trail heading up the hill to Wright Meadow; this is a 0.5-mile scenic loop that you can do on the way back, if you like. After passing the Middle Falls Trailhead, stay right to follow the main trail. Just past that trail, cross a bridge above Copper Creek Falls, which looks like a waterslide into the Lewis River—don't try it. A minute later you will arrive at Middle Falls, another shelflike falls. A side trail leads down to the creek here, but be careful on the slippery rocks.

Back on the main trail, you'll soon pass under some enormous cliffs then descend into an area with some seriously large trees. Western red cedars here reach close to 6 feet in diameter, and one Douglas-fir on the left must be 10 feet in diameter— definitely one of the biggest trees you'll see on any hike in this book.

Just past this area you'll come to a campsite on the right, then cross Alec Creek and enter the amphitheater of Upper Falls, which makes an 80-foot plunge. Logs and rocks in the sun here make for good picnicking or lounging; the best views of the falls are down by the river. A trail to the left leads 0.2 mile up the hill to a platform at the top of Upper Falls, a worthwhile side trip. Another 0.2 mile up, there's a view of Taidnapam Falls in the rocky gorge above Upper Falls.

Lewis River

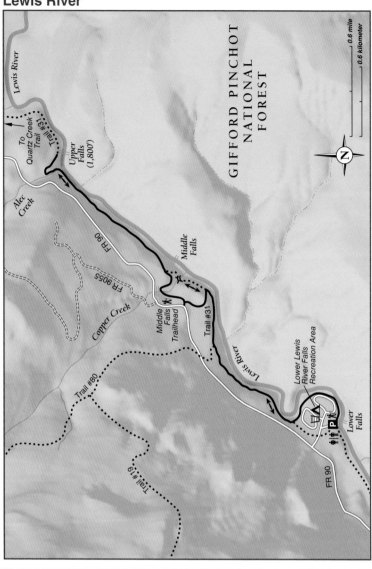

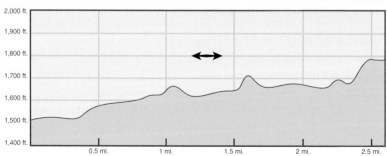

Extending up Quartz Creek

If you go another 0.7 mile past Taidnapam Falls—that would be 4 miles from the trailhead—you'll reach the end of Lewis River Trail at FR 90. Beyond that, the Quartz Creek Trail begins, entering some of the grandest old-growth forest around. The Washington Trails Association has been working for years to make this trail more accessible to hikers, but it still retains something of an adventure aspect, with creek crossings, steep inclines, and the occasional pile of logs to climb over.

The first 0.5 mile is along Quartz Creek and passes several nice picnic or camping spots. The trail then spends a mile climbing, then descending, to a ford of Straight Creek. This crossing will be sketchy during the early season, but there's a nice campsite on the east side of the creek. After Straight Creek, the trail climbs through younger forest before entering, after a mile, some awesome old growth.

Even longer backpacking loops are possible via this and the Quartz Butte Trail or the Boundary Trail into Mount St. Helens National Volcanic Monument; for more information, check with the U.S. Forest Service office.

• •

GPS TRAILHEAD COORDINATES N46° 9.293' W121° 52.782'

DIRECTIONS Take I-5 from Portland, driving 21 miles north of the Columbia River to Exit 21 (Woodland). Make a right onto WA 503 (Lewis River Road), which after 31 miles (2 miles past the town of Cougar) turns into FR 90. Continue 30 more miles on FR 90—you'll have to turn right just past the Pine Creek Information Center to stay on this road—to reach the Lower Lewis River Falls Recreation Area. Take the first right off the entrance road to reach the trailhead. You may notice that a mile before the campground on FR 90 there's a Lewis River trailhead, just past a bridge. You could start here if you like, but it adds 3 miles to the round-trip hike without the benefit of waterfalls.

19 SILVER STAR MOUNTAIN: Ed's Trail

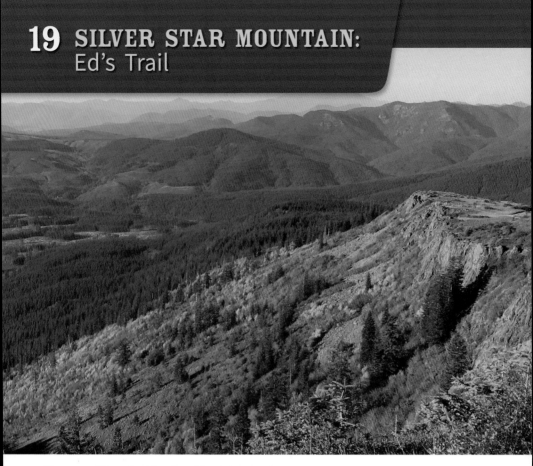

View toward Mount St. Helens from Silver Star in October

YOU MAY READ the directions to this one and think, "What a drive!" And the road *is* rough. But when you're on Ed's Trail approaching Silver Star Mountain, you'll be thinking, "This is too beautiful and mountainous to be so close to town!" This flower-soaked traverse through rocky alpine country is worth the hassle of getting here.

DESCRIPTION

Even the trailhead is scenic, and other than a few short stretches here and there, every foot of the trail is, too. From the trailhead, look for the path heading right, past a brown hiker sign. Follow this pathway through several brushy switchbacks to an old jeep road, then take that 150 yards to a wide gravel area with a view of Mount Hood through a notch in a ridge. Stop here, at the 0.5-mile point, and catch your breath.

Where the road swings back to the right and heads uphill, look for Ed's Trail #180A heading left, along the ridge. If you have little kids, consider taking this road out and back, as it would avoid some scrambling up ahead. We'll come back on the road, but it's better to follow Ed for now. Ed was Edward Robertson, a cofounder

DISTANCE & CONFIGURATION: 4.8-mile balloon loop

DIFFICULTY: Moderate

SCENERY: Wildflowers, open ridgetops, rocky crags, natural arch, several volcanoes

EXPOSURE: In the sun the whole time

TRAFFIC: Moderate on weekends, light otherwise

TRAIL SURFACE: Dirt, rocks, occasional stretches along rocky cliff edges, a brief section of scrambling

HIKING TIME: 3 hours

ELEVATION CHANGE: 1,460'

SEASON: June–October

BEST TIME: July for flowers, October for cool temperatures

BACKPACKING OPTIONS: Poor

DRIVING DISTANCE: 53 miles (1 hour, 50 minutes) from Pioneer Courthouse Square

ACCESS: No fees or permits required

MAPS: Green Trails *Map 396 (Lookout Mountain)* and *Map 428 (Bridal Veil),* though Ed's Trail isn't on either one

WHEELCHAIR ACCESS: No

FACILITIES: None at trailhead; restrooms at a campground along the way

CONTACT: Mount Adams Ranger District, 509-395-3400, www.fs.usda.gov/giffordpinchot

LOCATION: Silver Star trailhead at the end of Forest Service Road (FR) 4109, 16 miles southeast of Yacolt, WA

COMMENTS: The road to this one gets a little worse each year, and I really wish somebody would fix it. There are deep ruts, massive potholes, and times where you just have to pick your way through. I got my 1998 Subaru up there, but it took a while.

of the Chinook Trail Association, which built and maintains this trail; keep an eye out for a memorial plaque. Ed must have been a lover of flowers and open country, because his trail is an amazing piece of work: an ambling, gentle climb along a ridge that looks as if it's thousands of feet higher than it really is. That's because in 1902 fires razed the forest, and few trees have grown back—though more than 100 varieties of wildflowers and flowering shrubs have. So it's like you're getting a look at the decorated skeletons of the mountains, complete with bony spurs, cliffs, and rock formations normally covered by forest.

Climb toward some of these exposed formations, ascending 0.7 mile before the trail flattens and starts a tour of the rocky ridgetop. At 1.5 miles, pass through a rock arch and beside a small, overhanging cave that offers just about the only shade around on a hot day. Soon the trail takes off up the ridge face, and at a couple of points you go beyond hiking and more into something like scrambling. The first is a couple of switchbacks that can get slippery in bad weather; the second is an actual bit of low-grade rock climbing. But just after the top of the latter, you get your first view of the two-humped Silver Star ahead. Dramatic, huh?

Now the trail descends through meadows and into the trees, then climbs again to a junction with the road you left behind. (This whole Ed's Trail was just a scenic, adventurous diversion.) Follow the road to the left, staying left at a junction a couple hundred yards up. After 0.25 mile the road approaches a saddle between the two peaks. Head left for the big (shadeless) view at the official summit, and enjoy views

Silver Star Mountain: Ed's Trail

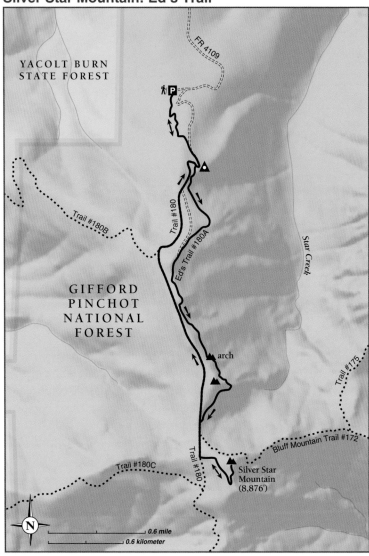

YACOLT BURN
STATE FOREST

FR 4109

Trail #180B

Trail #180

Ed's Trail #180A

Star Creek

GIFFORD
PINCHOT
NATIONAL
FOREST

arch

Trail #175

Bluff Mountain Trail #172

Trail #180C

Trail #180

Silver Star
Mountain
(8,876')

N

0.6 mile
0.6 kilometer

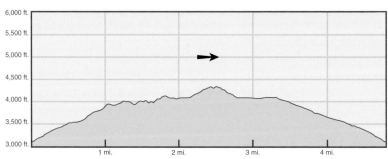

6,000 ft.
5,500 ft.
5,000 ft.
4,500 ft.
4,000 ft.
3,500 ft.
3,000 ft.

1 mi.   2 mi.   3 mi.   4 mi.

of the Columbia River Gorge, Mount Defiance (with radio towers), the back of Dog Mountain, Larch Mountain, the Portland area, and everything from Mount Jefferson to Mount Rainier. Look also for Bluff Mountain Trail (Hike 15, page 86) along the narrow ridges to the east. The view from the other peak isn't much different, but since you're up here go ahead and check it out.

By the way, Silver Star Mountain got its name because, when seen from above, the ridges running out from the summit form a five-pointed star.

The next rock to the south is Pyramid Rock. It's not impressive in and of itself, but in recent years there have been reports of at least one mountain goat hanging around there. So keep an eye out.

On your way back to the car, enjoy some different scenery while avoiding a treacherous descent on Ed's Trail. Simply skip the forested junction where you came out, and stay on the jeep road as it winds along the opposite side of the ridge. This will take you back to the far end of Ed's Trail, where you picked it up, and then you'll retrace your steps to your car.

• •

GPS TRAILHEAD COORDINATES N45° 46.344' W122° 14.678'

DIRECTIONS Take I-5 from Portland, driving 11 miles north of the Columbia River to Exit 11 (WA 502 E). Following signs for Battle Ground, go 6 miles and turn left onto WA 503/NW 10th Avenue. After 5.6 miles, make a right onto NE Rock Creek Road, which turns into Lucia Falls Road. Drive 8.8 miles on this road, then turn right onto NE Sunset Falls Road, follow it 2 miles, and make another right onto NE Dole Valley Road. Drive 2.4 miles on Dole Valley, then turn left onto Department of Natural Resources Road L-1100. Continue straight on L-1100 for 2.2 miles, bear left (downhill) at 4.3 miles, and then, at 6.7 miles, turn right (uphill) onto FR 4109. The trailhead is 2.6 miles up, at the end of this narrow, bumpy road.

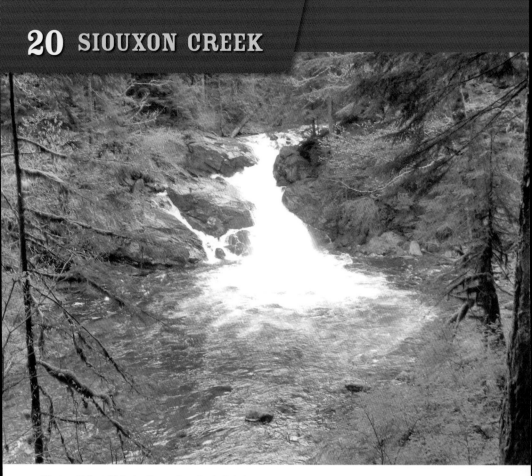

Siouxon Falls, with its inviting swimming hole below

AN EASY, PLEASANT stroll along a mountain stream, with old-growth forest and waterfalls all around, plus options that include a stream crossing and rugged climbing—what more could you want? Even the kids will like it; with supervision, they could go for a swim.

DESCRIPTION

The only spectacular thing about this hike is how easy and scenic it is. There are no panoramic viewpoints (unless you want to climb way up to one), no exotic geological features, and no serious hiking challenges—again, unless you want them. It's just a beautiful river in a peaceful, lush, tree-filled canyon, with waterfalls and campsites all over the place.

In fact, two mysteries have long intrigued me about this hike: one is why more people don't seem to know about it (though that seems to be changing), and the other is why most people stop at Chinook Falls when numerous beautiful spots lie farther up the creek and the most amazing falls of all (Wildcat) is just across it.

DISTANCE & CONFIGURATION: Out-and-back of up to 10.8 miles along the creek, with optional 7-mile loop

DIFFICULTY: Easy–moderate along the creek, strenuous to Siouxon Peak

SCENERY: Old-growth forest, waterfalls, pools in the river, mountaintop viewpoint

EXPOSURE: Shady all the way, optional creek wading, one set of slippery rocks

TRAFFIC: Moderate on summer weekends, light otherwise

TRAIL SURFACE: Packed dirt with some rocks and roots

HIKING TIME: 3–5 hours; more for the peak

ELEVATION CHANGE: 1,650'

SEASON: March–November; muddy in winter and spring, with occasional snow

BEST TIME: Early summer or fall

BACKPACKING OPTIONS: Several good sites along the creek

DRIVING DISTANCE: 55 miles (1 hour, 45 minutes) from Pioneer Courthouse Square

ACCESS: No fees or permits required

MAPS: Green Trails *Map 396 (Lookout Mountain)*

WHEELCHAIR ACCESS: No

FACILITIES: None at trailhead; water on trail must be treated.

LOCATION: Siouxon Creek Trailhead at the end of Forest Service Road (FR) 5701, 18 miles east of Amboy, WA

CONTACT: Mount St. Helens National Volcanic Monument, 360-449-7800, www.fs.usda.gov /mountsthelens

From the trailhead, you can choose from several paths into the woods. Take any one and turn right when you reach the main trail, Siouxon Creek Trail #130. You'll walk downhill briefly, cross West Creek on a log bridge, and then stroll over a small ridge to Siouxon Creek—and the first of many good campsites. At 0.9 mile you'll see, on the right, Horseshoe Ridge Trail #140, which makes a 7-mile, rugged, solitary loop . . . back to this trail. After 1.4 miles, your trail crosses Horseshoe Creek, so named because it drains a horseshoe-shaped ridge, the open mouth of which you're crossing. There will be a waterfall above and below you here; to get a view of the lower one and visit a fine campsite, take a side trail to the left just after the bridge.

Over the next 0.3 mile you'll climb slightly to a viewpoint (and very old bench) of Siouxon Falls, which could almost be called a really big rapids as opposed to a classic falls. Then the trail traverses flat ground for 0.5 mile, some 200 feet above the creek, before dropping to its side for another 0.5 mile. This is where some swimming might happen—just know that any dip will be brief, unless you're part polar bear.

At the 3-mile mark, you'll see two side trails in quick succession. The first, marked Wildcat Trail and on the left, leads down to the creek. This is one way to reach Wildcat Falls, but it involves a tricky crossing of Siouxon Creek that will be difficult for most people until late summer, at least. There's an easier (though longer) way a little farther up. The second trail you'll see, heading up and to the right, is the second appearance of Horseshoe Ridge Trail.

Go another 0.7 mile and you'll come to an unnamed creek on the right. Careful here, as the rocks tend to be slick. There's also a bridge over Siouxon Creek,

107

Siouxon Creek

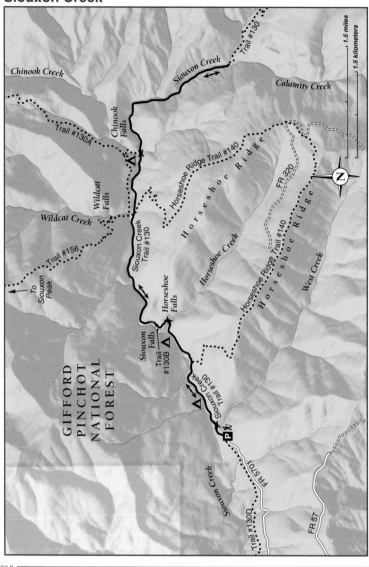

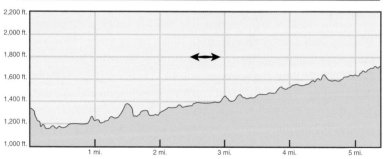

which at this point flows through a narrow gorge. Cross the bridge and go 0.3 mile to the beautiful, 50-foot Chinook Falls on Chinook Creek. There's another good campsite along this trail.

Here you could head back the way you came and, at just under 8 miles, call it a day. Or you could go visit Wildcat Falls by wading across Chinook Creek here and following an up-and-down trail to the left for 0.5 mile to Wildcat Creek. Go up that creek from a junction, and after 0.2 mile you'll arrive at the base of the 100-foot beauty. The views are even more dramatic farther up the trail. From there, you could try to ford Siouxon Creek and save some distance, but it never seemed like the right day for it to me. And if you're really looking for some exercise, go another 3.5 miles (and about 3,000 feet) up this trail to Siouxon Peak, following a route that's well marked on the Green Trails map.

At the very least, from the bridge near Chinook Falls, go a little farther up Siouxon Creek. I have no idea why no other guidebook recommends this, because it's just as beautiful up there, requires no more effort, and passes several more waterfalls. Another 1.7 miles of creekside trail end at a bridgeless crossing of Calamity Creek and gain only another 250 feet. Beyond Calamity Creek the trail climbs away from Siouxon, ending some 2 dull miles later on a road near Sister Rocks and Observation Peak.

• •

GPS TRAILHEAD COORDINATES N45° 56.797′ W122° 10.649′

DIRECTIONS Take I-5 from Portland, driving 11 miles north of the Columbia River to Exit 11 (WA 502 E). Follow WA 502 for 5.8 miles to Battle Ground, then turn left onto WA 503/NW 10th Avenue. Continue 16.7 miles on WA 503, passing through the town of Amboy. Just past the Mount St. Helens National Volcanic Monument headquarters, make a right on NE Healy Road. Healy Road turns into FR 54 at 2.4 miles; stay right at a fork at 5 miles, and then, 4 miles past that, turn left (uphill) on FR 57. After 1.2 miles on FR 57, turn left on FR 5701. The trailhead is 3.6 miles ahead, at the end of the road.

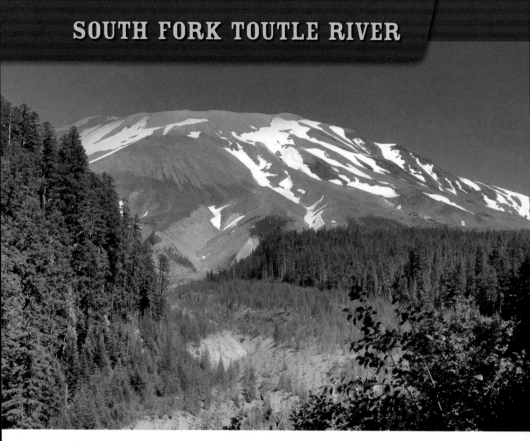

Upper Sheep Canyon and Mount St. Helens

WHENEVER PEOPLE ASK me what my favorite hike is—and everybody asks— I tell them that it depends on the season, but basically that this hike in late summer is in the top five, easily. Without driving all the way to the other side of Mount St. Helens, this is the most dramatic view you can get of the results of the mountain's 1980 eruption. You'll see where the mudflow was half a mile wide, as well as tour the majesty that survived the eruption.

DESCRIPTION

Back in 2003, this hike got a bit longer when the road beyond the Blue Lake Trail-head was washed out, cutting off a trailhead that was only 0.5 mile from Sheep Canyon and turning a 7-mile loop into a 10-mile loop. Then, in 2006, the Blue Lake Trailhead itself was destroyed, making this an 11-mile hike. Another in 2014 buried this trailhead, but we still get to use it. Assuming you can still get there when you read this, let's go do this wonderful, varied walk.

From the trailhead, follow a trail that parallels the old road until you reach the Toutle Trail #238. Go left here, up toward the mountain and Blue Lake, and after 0.6 mile, look for a crossing of a tiny creek up against a ridge to your left. There are

DISTANCE & CONFIGURATION: 11.2-mile balloon loop

DIFFICULTY: Strenuous

SCENERY: Old-growth forest, waterfalls in canyons, flower-filled meadows, close-up view of Mount St. Helens and the aftermath of its eruption

EXPOSURE: Alternately shady and sunny; one optional clifftop viewpoint

TRAFFIC: Light

TRAIL SURFACE: Rocky in places, packed dirt with roots, occasionally brushy with a poor tread, bridgeless (small) stream crossing

HIKING TIME: 7–8 hours

ELEVATION CHANGE: 2,535'

SEASON: June–October; in June, check ahead to make sure the road is snow-free.

BEST TIME: August and September

DRIVING DISTANCE: 80 miles (2 hours) from Pioneer Courthouse Square

BACKPACKING OPTIONS: One nice site on the loop, others nearby on Loowit Trail

ACCESS: No fees or permits required

MAPS: USFS *Mount St. Helens National Monument;* Green Trails *Map 364 (Mount St. Helens)* or *Map 364S (Mount St. Helens NW)*

WHEELCHAIR ACCESS: No

FACILITIES: None at trailhead; water on trail must be treated.

LOCATION: Blue Lake Trailhead at the end of Forest Service Road (FR) 8123, 14 miles north of Cougar, WA

CONTACT: Mount St. Helens National Volcanic Monument, 360-449-7800, www.fs.usda.gov /mountsthelens

usually ribbons marking a seasonal log crossing. Scramble up the other side to find the original trail in the woods, then start climbing gradually toward Blue Lake.

In just minutes, you'll pass well above the lake, which is visible through the trees to the right, then go slowly up and over a low ridge through a beautiful old forest. After a total of 2.1 miles, you'll start down, pass through a meadow, and intersect Blue Lake Horse Trail #237 on the right. Continuing on #238, you drop 0.7 mile to arrive at Sheep Canyon Trail #240, which comes up from the original trailhead and crosses #238 here.

Here, you have a few options: For the easiest route to Sheep Canyon and the South Fork Toutle River, follow #238 straight ahead 1.6 miles. But for the recommended loop, which will come back that way, turn right onto #240 and immediately cross a lovely creek, along which is the route's only campsite. Past that, you climb gradually through a lovely forest and into spectacular alpine high country. You'll gain 850 feet in 1.3 miles to reach an intersection with Loowit Trail #216, which goes all the way around Mount St. Helens. Turn left here, descend about 0.5 mile to traverse an ash-filled ravine with a wetland below you, and then climb 0.5 mile through a wonderful subalpine area of firs and hemlocks. In July you'll find bear grass going wild; in August the place will be ablaze with flowers, especially blue lupine and red paintbrush; and in fall the mountain ash and other plants will roar with color. And the views up here, at the foot of the mountain, are splendid. This is a fantastic stretch of trail.

South Fork Toutle River

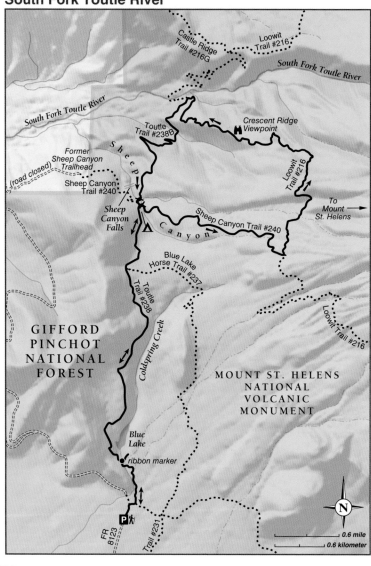

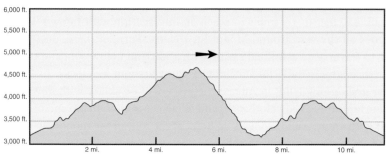

Just over the hump of a small ridge, you'll come to a big viewpoint on a boulder; this is Crescent Ridge Viewpoint. The South Fork Toutle, some 800 feet below you, is in the process of recarving its way through the 1980 mudflow. The drainage right at your feet was wiped out, too, when glaciers melted instantly. Coldwater Peak is visible across the way, as are the Johnston Ridge Observatory and a small portion of Coldwater Lake. The contrast between your side of the canyon and the other side, well within the blast zone, couldn't be more stark.

The trail now turns downhill, descending Crescent Ridge, 1.6 miles to a junction with Toutle Trail #238, just above the South Fork. It's in this stretch that the trail gets brushy and the tread is poor in places, mostly because the mountain wipes it out occasionally, so take your time to be sure of your footing. Explore to the right of the junction, checking out the minigorge the river has cut into the mudflow. Then go back to Toutle Trail #238, and follow its brushy and uneven path through old-growth forest. You'll climb over a small ridge in old-growth forest before arriving at the bridge over Sheep Canyon after 1.5 miles. Sheep Canyon was also gouged out by the 1980 eruption.

Cross that spectacular span, and for one final attraction, take a trail right for a couple hundred yards (toward the old trailhead) for a view of 100-foot-tall Sheep Canyon Falls. Come back up, turn right on Trail #238, and retrace your steps 3 miles back to your car.

NEARBY ACTIVITIES

If you'd like to learn more about the eruption and its fascinating aftermath, I can't recommend highly enough spending a day (at least) exploring the north side of the mountain, in particular the Johnston Ridge Observatory. It is typically open mid-May–October; see tinyurl.com/mshnvm for details.

• •

GPS TRAILHEAD COORDINATES N46° 10.028' W122° 15.709'

DIRECTIONS From Portland on I-5, drive 21 miles north of the Columbia River and take Exit 21 (Woodland). Turn right onto WA 503 (Lewis River Road) and drive 28 miles; then, between mileposts 35 and 36, turn left onto FR 8100, following a sign for Kalama Recreation Area. Drive 11.5 miles on FR 8100, make a sharp right turn at 8.6 miles onto FR 8123, and then continue straight 1.5 miles to the Blue Lake Trailhead, at the end of the road.

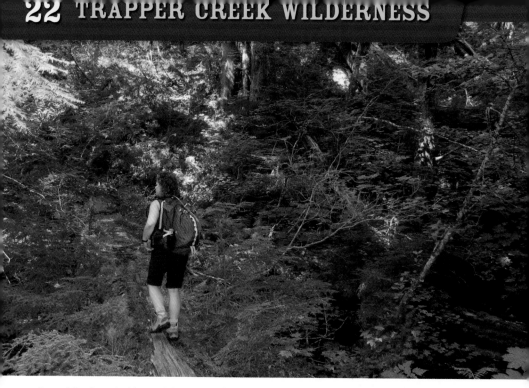

As you hike through old-growth forest, you'll be amazed such a lovely wilderness is so close to Portland.

MANY PEOPLE SEEM to have never heard of this hike, but everybody who goes there loves it. It's quiet and woodsy, with lots of creeks, two waterfalls, great campsites, and—if you want to gain some serious elevation—a great view from Observation Peak.

DESCRIPTION

Trapper Creek Wilderness covers a little more than 6,000 acres, and it's basically one U-shaped watershed, drained by Trapper Creek and its many tributaries. It's heavily forested with firs, hemlocks, maples, and cedars. Wildflowers abound in the spring and early summer, and the animals here include owls, black bears, cougars, and bobcats, very few of which you are likely to see.

To explore this area, you have numerous options: casually wander the old-growth forest, climb to a seldom-visited lake, slog up the hill to the big view, or take one of several semimaintained "adventure trails." Let this challenging 14.5-mile loop serve as an introduction, as it touches on all the other options, or plan for an overnight to break up the work a little.

From the trailhead, start into the woods on Trapper Creek Trail #192, which our loop follows 6 miles to its end. Right off the bat you'll intersect (but not take) Dry

DISTANCE & CONFIGURATION: 14.5-mile loop, but options abound

DIFFICULTY: Easy–strenuous

TRAFFIC: Moderate on summer weekends, light otherwise

SCENERY: Magnificent forest, two waterfalls, sweeping mountaintop view

EXPOSURE: A couple of lookouts; otherwise in the woods

TRAIL SURFACE: Packed dirt, rocks

HIKING TIME: 8 hours for big loop

ELEVATION CHANGE: Up to 3,575'

SEASON: July–October to climb the ridge, May–November for lower elevations

BEST TIME: September and October

BACKPACKING OPTIONS: Several nice sites

DRIVING DISTANCE: 66 miles (1 hour, 30 minutes) from Pioneer Courthouse Square

ACCESS: Northwest Forest Pass required (see page 14)

MAPS: USFS *Trapper Creek Wilderness,* Green Trails *Map 396 (Lookout Mountain).* The trailhead is actually on Green Trails *Map 396 (Wind River).*

WHEELCHAIR ACCESS: No

FACILITIES: None at trailhead

LOCATION: Trapper Creek Trailhead off Mineral Springs Road, 14 miles north of Carson, WA

CONTACT: Mount Adams Ranger District, 509-395-3400, www.fs.usda.gov/giffordpinchot

Creek Trail #194, which runs about 4 miles north along Dry Creek. After 0.9 mile on Trapper Creek Trail, you'll see Observation Trail #132 on the right; you'll be coming down this one if you do the big loop. For now, continue straight on Trapper Creek Trail—the forest gets even better as you get deeper into the canyon.

After another leg-friendly 0.7 mile, you'll cross Lush Creek and encounter Soda Peaks Trail #133, on the left. This leads to the one lake in the wilderness, Soda Peaks Lake; it's a climb of 2,500 feet in about 3 miles, and the trail doesn't loop back to this one. So unless you're looking for another hill to climb—or you want to do some lakeside backpack camping—stay on Trapper Creek Trail #192 to go up and around the end of a ridge, from which you'll get your first good views (or at least sounds) of Trapper Creek on the left.

About a mile later, barely climbing, you'll come to two trails: Big Slide Trail #195 and Deer Way Trail #209. Big Slide, like several other trails in the wilderness, was built and is maintained by the Mazamas, a Portland-based mountaineering club that has adopted this wilderness area. Some of these trails are steep scrambles, without such niceties as switchbacks, and they can be tough to follow. And when a log falls across them, rather than cut the log away (as the U.S. Forest Service does), the Mazamas might cut a little notch in the top of it to help you swing your leg over. So these trails are fun—and the Mazamas' signs are really cool—but they aren't what you'd call casual.

Deer Way Trail is basically an easy cutoff that avoids some elevation (plus scenery and campsites) for those in a hurry to get up the hill, so if that's your bag, take it. Otherwise, take Trapper Creek Trail, which dips down, for the first time, to almost touch Trapper Creek. Along the way, it passes Terrace Camp, a lovely spot with room for several tents. The trail continues steeply downhill, passing outrageous

115

Trapper Creek Wilderness

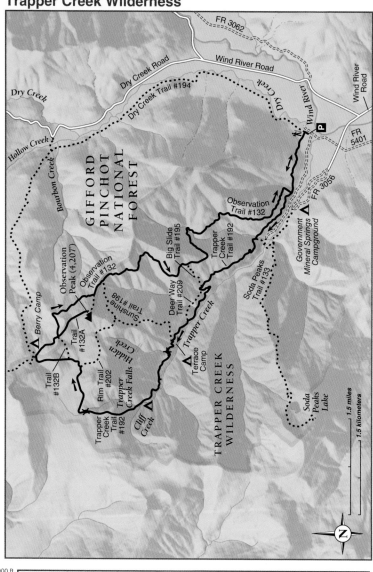

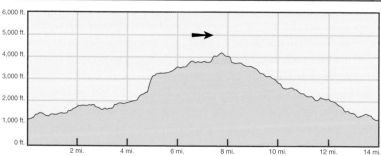

Douglas-firs—some of which are lying on the ground, causing the trail to wind through them—and another campsite, even closer to the creek.

After a total of about 3 miles, the trail seems to disappear at a small side creek. In fact, it continues over a well-worn log, but there's a fun little side trip here, if you're up for it. Pick—and climb and crawl—your way up this creek a couple hundred feet or so, and you'll be rewarded with a view of a tall, hidden waterfall.

Continue 0.4 mile, turning left at the far end of the Deer Way cutoff, and next you'll cross Sunshine Trail #198 with its cool handmade sign. This Mazamas masterpiece goes straight up about 2,000 feet in less than 2 miles. Staying on Trapper Creek Trail, you'll have it pretty easy for another 0.5 mile, crossing Hidden Creek (where the bridge has been shifting in recent years) and a steep side trail to view Hidden Creek Falls. Also in this area, look for nontraditional trail signs made by a Mazama named Basil Clark in the 1980s. One of his signs offers the mysterious ici! b&b. A trail on the left, at about 4 miles, leads to Rendezvous Flats, where you can enjoy some creekside loveliness; soon after, you'll pass a campsite at Cliff Creek. Then, if you like, you can start climbing.

You'll put in about 1,700 feet in 2.5 miles, much of it in viewless switchbacks that are better for walking meditation than for any form of entertainment. There's a mighty nice bridge over Trapper Creek, and about halfway up is a rocky ledge that makes a fine resting point with a view of Trapper Creek Falls off to the left. And this ought to cheer you up: see that ridge over there, the really big one? Observation Peak is 600 feet higher than that.

When this bit of climbing is done—you might notice a rare elevation sign (by Clark) indicating 3,200 feet—you'll cross Rim Trail #202 before Trail #132B, to the right, cuts off some distance to Observation Trail #132. Turn right here, take another right on Trail #132A in 0.5 mile, and, after just over 0.5 mile of additional climbing, you'll be at Observation Peak. Congratulations! You've hiked 8 miles and gained more than 3,000 feet. Look for Mount St. Helens and its blast zone to the north; from there, moving right, we have Mount Rainier, the Goat Rocks, and then Mount Adams. See if you can spot, well to the right of that, the meadow atop Dog Mountain, and across from that the radio towers atop Mount Defiance, the highest point in the Columbia River Gorge. Right of that are Mounts Hood and Jefferson, and closer in are the two Soda Peaks, host to the aforementioned lake. Nice, huh? Have yourself a cookie or something.

To get down, go back down Trail #132A and turn right on Observation Trail #132. You can simply follow this trail 5 uneventful miles to its end at Trapper Creek Trail #192, a mile up from the parking lot. Or you can test your knees going down a Mazamas trail. Just turn right on either Sunshine Trail #198 or the much shorter Big Slide Trail #195, and don't blame me if you have a hard time walking the next day. Seriously, if you want to tackle one of these, go *up* them instead.

Either way you go, you'll come to Trapper Creek Trail #192; your car will be to the left. Have another cookie.

NEARBY ACTIVITIES

It's all about springs in this area. When you drive back down Forest Service Road (FR) 5401 on your way out, take a right to go to Government Mineral Springs, and follow the signs to Iron Mike Well for mineral water from an iron pump. Or, when you get back to Carson, go to Carson Hot Springs Resort, with its hotel built in 1901 and its 1923 bathhouse and cabins. You can soak, get a massage, get wrapped in hot towels, and then enjoy the new hotel and golf course. Call 800-607-3678 or visit carsonhotspringresort.com for details.

• •

GPS TRAILHEAD COORDINATES N45° 52.891' W121° 58.828'

DIRECTIONS Take I-84 from Portland, driving 37 miles east of I-205 to Exit 44 (Cascade Locks). As soon as you enter town, take your first right to get on Bridge of the Gods, following a sign for Stevenson. Pay the $2 toll (as of 2017), cross the river, and turn right (east) onto WA 14. Drive 5.9 miles and turn left on Wind River Road, following a sign for Carson. Drive 14.5 miles, then continue straight, leaving Wind River Road and following a sign for Government Mineral Springs. Half a mile later, turn right on FR 5401; the trailhead is 0.4 mile ahead, at the end of the road.

Wildcat Falls is a bonus destination on the Siouxon Creek hike (Hike 20, page 106).

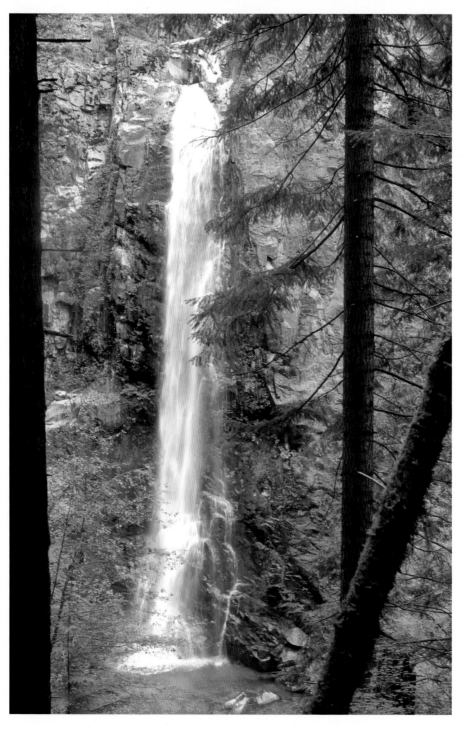

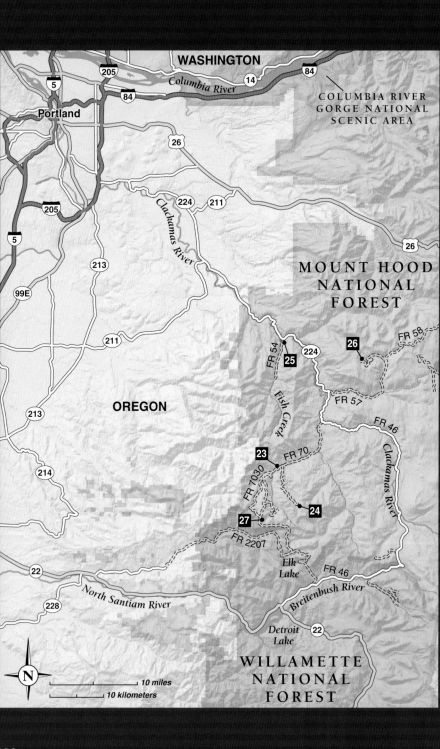

UP THE CLACKAMAS RIVER

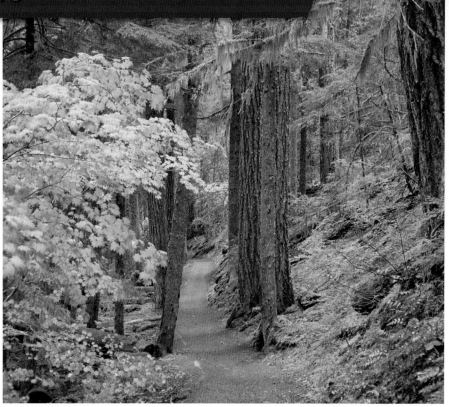

The wide, flat Bagby Trail winds through amazing old-growth forest.

UNLESS YOU'RE UNCOMFORTABLE being among naked people, this is one place you should absolutely visit, and even if you are, just avoid the bathhouses. The hike isn't much of a challenge, but it passes through sublime ancient-growth forest. And the springs feature cedar-log tubs, some of them private. It can get very busy on weekends (though alcohol is now banned at the springs), and an attendant at the trailhead lot should help reduce car break-ins.

DESCRIPTION

It seems that everybody in the area knows about Bagby, even those who have never been here. The name itself seems to stand for something about life in the Pacific Northwest: soothing, relaxing, a retreat from the hustle and bustle, a journey back to the days of the ancient forest and natural elements.

Well, it's not just that. It can get a little crazy on weekends, and the chances you'll be the only one there on any given day are slim. On weekends, you might have to wait to get your soak, unless you start early. If so, just wander around and enjoy the absolutely magnificent forest surroundings.

DISTANCE & CONFIGURATION: 3-mile out-and-back to springs, 3.6-mile out-and-back to Shower Creek

DIFFICULTY: Easy

SCENERY: Old-growth forest, mountain stream, wooden tubs of hot water

EXPOSURE: Shady

TRAFFIC: Heavy

TRAIL SURFACE: Packed dirt and crushed rock with some muddy spots in winter and spring

HIKING TIME: 2 hours (plus time for a soak)

ELEVATION CHANGE: 200'

SEASON: March–November; sometimes open in winter, but call ahead for conditions.

BEST TIME: Weekdays April–October

BACKPACKING OPTIONS: Several (crowded) sites just past the springs, with many more up in the wilderness

DRIVING DISTANCE: 67 miles (1 hour, 45 minutes) from Pioneer Courthouse Square

ACCESS: No charge just to park and hike; $5 soaking permit (cash only) can be bought at the trailhead or from the store at Ripplebrook on the way.

MAPS: USFS *Bull of the Woods Wilderness,* Green Trails *Map 524 (Battle Ax)*

WHEELCHAIR ACCESS: No

FACILITIES: Pit toilets but no water at trailhead

CONTACT: Clackamas River Ranger District, 503-630-6861, www.fs.usda.gov/mthood

LOCATION: Bagby Hot Springs Trailhead on Forest Service Road (FR) 70, 39 miles southeast of Estacada, OR

COMMENTS: Don't leave any valuables in your car at this trailhead.

From the trailhead parking lot, start up the wide trail and cross the bridge over Nohorn Creek, named for an early pioneer in the area. The hiking is pleasant, the river pools inviting, and the forest inspiring. You might notice some old metal loops tacked high in the trees; those once held telephone wires that connected fire lookouts back in the 1930s. Cross a bridge over Hot Springs Fork Collawash River, and you're almost to the springs.

When you come to the springs area, the first thing you'll notice is the 1913 ranger cabin, which is listed on the National Register of Historic Places but isn't open to the public. It was a central communications station for those fire lookouts and housed firefighters in season. I should mention that this cabin of 16-inch cedar logs was hand-built by one ranger, Phil Putz, who first visited the area after walking 39 miles in one day. Do you think he was happy to arrive at the springs? The path behind the cabin leads to a monumental downed tree; check out the inside, which rotted away long before the giant was felled to keep it from squashing the bathhouses.

The bathhouse on the right has one big tub, with room for five or six adults. The one on the left has an open area with several tubs and five private rooms, each with a two-person log tub. The water comes out of the springs at 136°F and runs through a system of log flumes. To fill a tub, you just open up the valve and let the hot water in, then grab a bucket, fill it with cold water from a nearby tub, and get the temperature where you want it. Typically, a full tub needs four or five buckets of cold water to make it tolerable. As it cools off, just open up the valve

Bagby Hot Springs

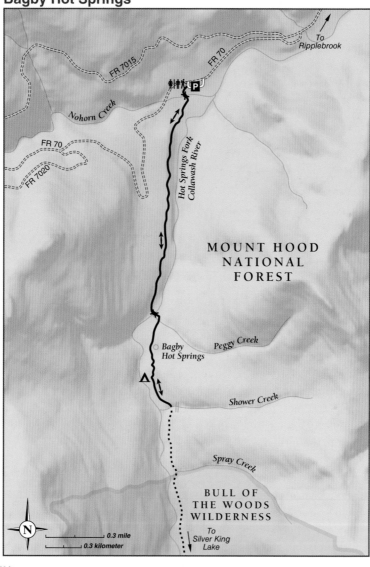

MOUNT HOOD NATIONAL FOREST

BULL OF THE WOODS WILDERNESS

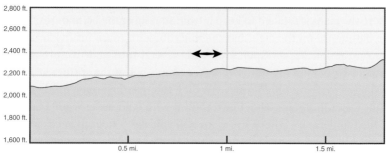

and let some more hot water in. It's fantastic. Many bathers don't wear swimsuits, but outside the private rooms you're supposed to. With a private concessionaire in charge, this seems to be running better recently. If people are waiting, you'll also be asked to limit your soak to 1 hour.

Even if there's nobody around when you get to the springs, consider taking some time to explore farther up the trail before you soak. It's old growth all the way, up Hot Springs Fork, past Shower Creek and Spray Creek, and eventually into Bull of the Woods Wilderness. You should go at least as far as Shower Creek (0.3 mile past the springs and just 0.1 mile past a camping area on the right) to enjoy the 50-foot falls and a little wooden platform somebody built underneath it so that folks could take a shower. Beyond that, the trail continues 6 miles and ascends 1,800 feet to reach Silver King Lake, in the heart of the wilderness. Trails fan out from that area to many other great locations.

• •

GPS TRAILHEAD COORDINATES N44° 57.440' W122° 9.594'

DIRECTIONS Take OR 224 from Portland, traveling 44 miles southeast of I-205, through the town of Estacada, to the ranger station at Ripplebrook. Turn right on FR 46, drive 3.6 miles, and make another right, onto FR 63. Drive 3.5 miles and turn right on FR 70. The trailhead is 6 miles ahead, on the left.

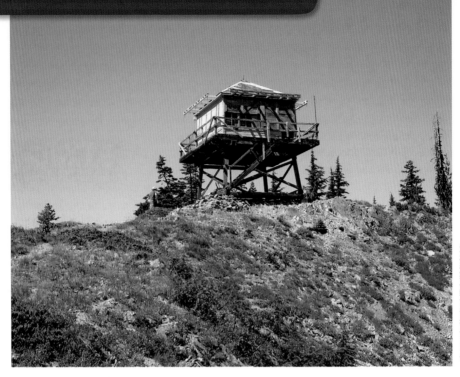

Old U.S. Forest Service fire lookout tower

photographed by Sistak/Flickr/CC BY-SA 2.0 (creativecommons.org/licenses/by-sa/2.0)

THIS IS LIKE two great hikes in one. Choose either an easy stroll through old-growth forest past rhododendrons to two beautiful lakes or a more challenging climb to a fire lookout tower with a panoramic view. Either way, it will introduce you to a magnificent wilderness area.

DESCRIPTION

This trail has it all. Come in late June, as soon as the snow has cleared, and enjoy a mind-boggling display of rhododendrons among the old-growth forest on the way to Pansy Lake. (Bring bug repellent.)

Come in late summer and pick huckleberries up on the ridge. Or come in fall, when the ridge is awash in color and the mountains might see their first snow. Just make sure you get here; the long drive is more than worth it.

Bull of the Woods Peak is the second-highest point in the 27,000-acre Bull of the Woods Wilderness, which boasts more than a dozen lakes bigger than an acre, 68 miles of hiking trails, and even the world-famous northern spotted owl, which you almost certainly won't see.

From the start, on Pansy Lake Trail #551, you're walking through a beautiful forest on a basically flat trail. In 0.8 mile, you'll cross some nice little creeks, traverse

DISTANCE & CONFIGURATION: 2.2-mile out-and-back to Pansy Lake; 7-mile loop to Bull of the Woods

DIFFICULTY: Easy to Pansy Lake, strenuous to Bull of the Woods

SCENERY: Old-growth forest, mountain lake, rhododendrons, huckleberries, mountaintop panorama

EXPOSURE: In the shade to top of ridge, then wide open

TRAFFIC: Moderate on summer weekends, light otherwise

TRAIL SURFACE: Packed dirt with some roots, then a few rocks up top

HIKING TIME: 1 hour to Pansy Lake, 4 hours for everything

ELEVATION CHANGE: 2,100'

SEASON: Late June–October

BEST TIME: August and September

BACKPACKING OPTIONS: Sites at Pansy Lake; better ones at other lakes in the wilderness (more info at end of profile)

DRIVING DISTANCE: 75 miles (2 hours, 10 minutes) from Pioneer Courthouse Square

ACCESS: No fees or permits required

MAPS: USFS *Bull of the Woods Wilderness,* Green Trails *Map 524 (Battle Ax)*

WHEELCHAIR ACCESS: No

FACILITIES: None

LOCATION: Pansy Creek Parking on Forest Service Road (FR) 6341, 46 miles south of Estacada, OR

CONTACT: Clackamas River Ranger District, 503-630-6861, www.fs.usda.gov/mthood

gauntlets of rhododendrons, and ignore an unsigned trail on the right before reaching a signed trail junction. Dickey Lake Trail #549, coming down the hill from your left, is the return portion of the loop; take a right, following a sign for Pansy Lake.

Just before the lake, you'll pass a sign that says TWIN LAKES, but ignore it (for now) and continue straight to visit Pansy Lake. A campsite on the right has excellent sitting rocks for picnicking or getting a quick rest and snack before you start up the hill.

Now return to the trail and take what's now a right turn, following the TWIN LAKES sign. You'll climb gradually for a while, passing a nice view back down to the lake, and then start a series of switchbacks. Just under a mile from the lake, you'll gain 500 feet before you intersect Mother Lode Trail #558, in a saddle between Pansy Mountain and Bull of the Woods. Turn left onto Mother Lode.

While the switchbacks you just did were obviously steep, this trail is what I call "sneaky steep," which means that it doesn't look like much, but you'll feel the elevation gain. You're gaining about 700 feet in 1.1 miles, and since you're now going above 5,000 feet, you may start to feel the relative lack of oxygen. The forest in here is beautiful, though, and should take your mind off the climb. If you're wondering why the moss doesn't grow on the bottom 10 feet of the trunks, it's because that's how high the snow usually gets.

When you gain the top of the ridge and intersect Welcome Creek Trail #554, turn left, and with one more push through some switchbacks, you'll pop out at the top of Bull of the Woods, with its old U.S. Forest Service fire lookout tower. Walk up onto the deck and have a look around.

Bull of the Woods

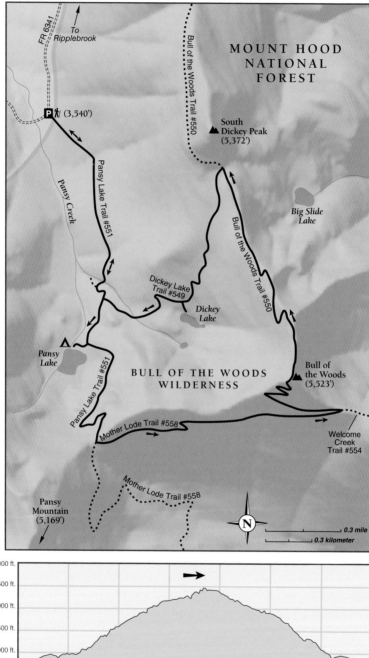

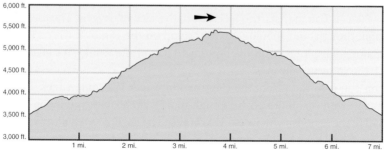

You'll see Big Slide Lake below you, but Mount Jefferson, 20 miles away, dominates the view. On a clear day, you can see all the way from the Three Sisters on your right to Mount Rainier on your left. As the crow flies, it's about 175 miles from the Sisters to Rainier. Rest here and feel proud.

To continue the loop, find a trail junction in the trees on the opposite side of the watchtower from Mount Jefferson—this is Bull of the Woods Trail #550. Follow it to your right, along the ridge. You'll see occasional great views and many, many flowers in the next 1.1 miles, at which point you'll intersect Dickey Lake Trail #549. Take Dickey Lake Trail down and to the left, and you'll quickly lose elevation. Just past 0.5 mile, peer through the trees on your left to see Dickey Lake—a lake spied through branches is always a magical sight. Also look for a trail that leads down to the lake itself; it's just past a meadow on Dickey Lake Trail.

After another 0.5 mile, most of it through a sea of rhododendrons, you'll get back to the trail where this whole thing started, Pansy Lake Trail #551. Turn right and you'll be back to your car in no time.

Backpacking in the Wilderness

Without getting into too much detail, I'll just say that Bull of the Woods is an awesome place to go backpacking. Get yourself a map and make a couple nights of it. Pansy Lake, on this hike, is just the beginning. Lake Lenore, about 2 miles east of the lookout, is particularly appealing. The Welcome Lakes area burned a few years back and isn't as nice. One great trip, with a reasonable car shuttle, would be to enter here, swing south by Twin Lakes and Silver King Lake, and come out for a soak at Bagby Hot Springs (see previous hike).

• •

GPS TRAILHEAD COORDINATES N44° 53.993' W122° 6.977'

DIRECTIONS Take OR 224 from Portland, traveling 44 miles southeast of I-205, through the town of Estacada, to the ranger station at Ripplebrook. Bear right to take FR 46 and, 3.6 miles later, head right again to access FR 63. After 5.7 miles, turn right on FR 6340, following a sign to Bull of the Woods and Pansy Basin. At a junction 3.5 miles on, continue straight, still on FR 6340. Then, 4.4 miles past that junction (7.9 miles after FR 63), turn right on FR 6341, ignoring a sign to the left for Bull of the Woods Trail. The parking area is 3.6 miles ahead, on the right; the trailhead is across the road, on the left.

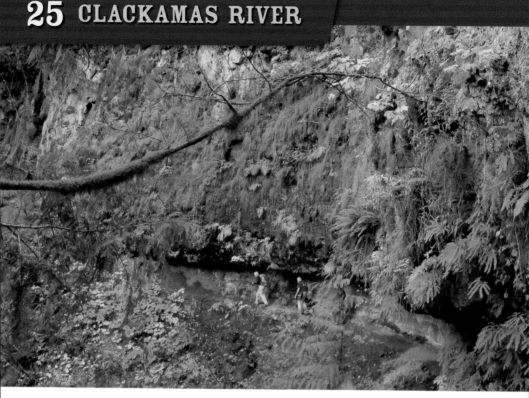

Along the upper stretches of Clackamas River Trail

CONVENIENT, NOT TOO tough, and not terribly long, Clackamas River Trail is a great way to stretch your legs and enjoy the scenery among old trees and along a beautiful river. With only one car, do an out-and-back from either trailhead to Pup Creek Falls; with two cars (or one and bikes), do the whole thing with a car shuttle.

DESCRIPTION

On that rare nice day in early spring—*nice* meaning it's not pouring—when you want to get out and do some hiking, here you'll find fairy slipper orchids and Clackamas lilies in bloom. And if it's blazing hot in summer and you want to visit a cool, shady place, or it's autumn and you want to see the fall colors—whatever the time—it's always a nice day to go out and hike the Clackamas River Trail. If you can bring a second car to stash at Indian Henry, it'll be that much better. A lot of folks put bikes there and ride them back afterward. Otherwise, you can do essentially the same distance and make a fine day of it. (You'll avoid a potentially wet-footed creek crossing if you come in from a single car at Fish Creek.)

From Fish Creek, you'll start out in a flat section with the river a short distance to your left. After 0.5 mile you'll come to a river-access point with moss-covered

DISTANCE & CONFIGURATION: 8.2-mile point-to-point, 8-mile out-and-back to Pup Creek Falls

DIFFICULTY: Moderate

SCENERY: Old-growth forest, whitewater river, fascinating rock formations, waterfalls

EXPOSURE: Shady all the way, with occasional stretches on narrow trail high above the river

TRAFFIC: Heavy on nice-weather weekends, light–moderate otherwise

TRAIL SURFACE: Packed dirt with roots and rocks; one creek ford if you do the whole thing

HIKING TIME: 5 hours for either option

ELEVATION CHANGE: 1,550'

SEASON: Year-round; muddy and possibly snowy in winter and spring

BEST TIME: May for flowers and big water, October for fall colors

BACKPACKING OPTIONS: A few good sites

DRIVING DISTANCE: 44 miles (1 hour, 20 minutes) from Pioneer Courthouse Square

ACCESS: $5 parking fee at Fish Creek May–November; Northwest Forest Pass is accepted, but Senior and Access Passes are not. No fee at Indian Henry.

MAPS: Green Trails *Map 492 (Fish Creek Mountain)*

WHEELCHAIR ACCESS: No

FACILITIES: Restrooms at Fish Creek Trailhead; campgrounds at Fish Creek and Indian Henry; water along the way must be treated.

CONTACT: Clackamas River Ranger District, 503-630-6861, www.fs.usda.gov/mthood

LOCATION: Fish Creek Trailhead on Forest Service Road (FR) 54, 15 miles southeast of Estacada, OR

COMMENTS: Because of a history of recent fires, this trail is particularly prone to landslides; call the ranger station to check conditions.

rocks and a sandy beach—perfect for chilling out or perhaps, if you've brought small kids, for turning around. Soon after, you'll come into the first exceptional old-growth forest, featuring 5-foot-thick Douglas-firs and even bigger western red cedars. In the next mile or so of trail, you'll do a little climbing and occasionally find yourself with some pretty serious drops to and views of the river to your left. Much of this early section burned in 2004, so you can check on how it's recovering.

If you're wondering about a good place to picnic or spend the night, you will find a campsite 1.5 miles in, but a better one is 2.5 miles up. There's a stupendous western red cedar right by the water here and plenty of places to sit and gaze at the river. OR 224 is right across the river, by the way, but you'll hardly notice it. Again, if you've brought kids, think about turning around here, because in the next mile you'll go up, down, then up again (a couple hundred feet each time); pass an area where trail crews rebuilt after a big slide; and occasionally find the river a potentially treacherous 200 feet below you.

After you've hiked a total of 3.8 up-and-down miles and descended a hill to find yourself under power lines, you'll come to a trail on the right, just before Pup Creek. This leads 0.2 mile up the creek to a view of beautiful Pup Creek Falls, with a total drop of some 230 feet. If you didn't stash a car at Indian Henry, turn around here and you'll have an 8-mile hike. If you are doing a shuttle, keep on trucking.

The ford of Pup Creek, even at low-water times, can be a bit tricky. In spring it would be hard to keep your feet dry, so consider bringing some sandals and hiking

Clackamas River

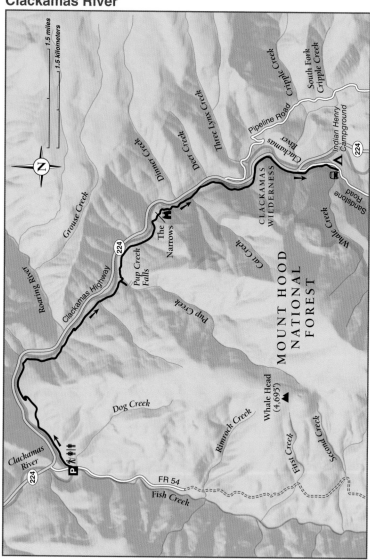

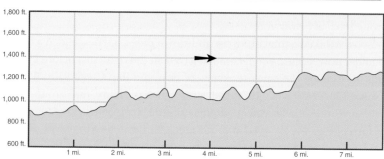

poles. Just beyond it, the trail goes under the power lines for a bit, meaning you can get some sunshine and find some flat land to enjoy lunch or a break.

In 0.9 mile a side trail will lead left to another beach, and right after that you'll climb to a view up the Clackamas that includes The Narrows, a spectacular gouge in ancient lava. Down the other side of this hill, a side trail to the left will lead 0.1 mile to The Narrows themselves. Also here, you'll find a nice campsite and enter the new Clackamas Wilderness, created by the Mount Hood Wilderness Act of 2009.

By the way, if you've seen some cables crossing the river in a few spots and wondered what that's about, they were put in by Portland General Electric for cable-car access across the river to maintain their power lines.

In the last 3 miles to Indian Henry Campground, you'll cross several side creeks (the biggest one named Cat Creek), see numerous giant trees, get sprayed by a waterfall, pass two more campsites and a mossy "weeping wall," and go under a cliff and several amazing rock formations—in other words, enjoy a chorus of forest pleasures. I would offer more details, but I've never managed to maintain a GPS connection in here, and besides, let's leave something of mystery in these woods. It's a beautiful and easy stretch of trail that I encourage you to explore.

NEARBY ACTIVITIES

If you haven't had enough riverside fun, stop by Promontory Park and its 350-acre North Fork Reservoir (40600 SE OR 224, Estacada, OR). The park, which is open mid-May–mid-September, has a marina; a campground with showers; and a store where you can get all your fishing supplies and licenses, rent boats, and enjoy ice cream when you're done fishing. (Small Fry Lake is for kiddie fishing only.) Campsites are $20 per night and can be reserved at 503-622-7229. For more info on the park and marina, call 503-630-5152. You can also visit tinyurl.com/clackcamp.

• •

GPS TRAILHEAD COORDINATES
Fish Creek Trailhead N45° 9.456' W122° 9.051'
Indian Henry Campground N45° 6.529' W122° 4.526'

DIRECTIONS Take OR 224 from Portland, traveling a total of 33 miles southeast of I-205. Fifteen miles past Estacada, just after crossing Armstrong Campground and a bridge over the Clackamas River, turn right onto Fish Creek Road. Pass Fish Creek Campground, cross another bridge, and park in the parking lot on the right, 0.5 mile up from OR 224 on FR 54. The trail starts across the road, on your left. To leave a car at the other end, drive another 6.5 miles on OR 224 and make a right onto Sandstone Road toward Indian Henry Campground. The trailhead is 0.7 mile up, on the right.

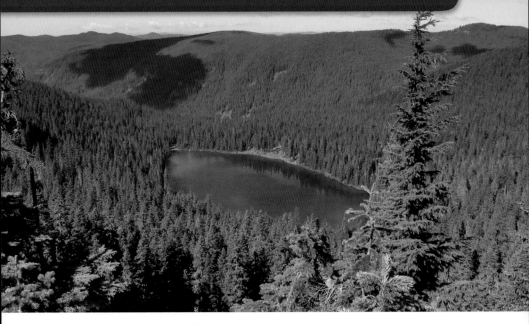

Serene Lake from the viewpoint on the way to Cache Meadow

THIS HIKE REQUIRES an extended drive to a long, up-and-down forested loop, but it comprises six lakes, a flower-filled meadow, late-summer huckleberries, views of five Cascades volcanoes, and a beautiful forest that you may have largely to yourself. Lovely shorter options exist, but if you want to do the whole thing, it's a long day, so consider backpacking or car-camping at Hideaway Lake, near the trailhead.

DESCRIPTION

It used to be that you could drive to Frazier Turnaround, knocking some 3.6 miles off this hike. And technically, you still can. But I can no longer, in good conscience, send people down this road—I've been cursed for doing so—and besides, hiking in this new way adds another lake and more lovely forest to the experience.

Consider camping at Hideaway Lake before you do this hike; start early in the morning to beat the crowds, and you can go for a swim when you get back in the heat of the afternoon. Although this loop never goes below 4,000 feet or above 5,000 feet, its cumulative elevation gain is more than 2,000 feet.

At the trailhead for Shellrock Lake Trail #700, you may at first wonder why you're here. Hiking 0.5 mile through a clear-cut doesn't exactly scream "wilderness," but there are plenty of flowers, and at least the trail is nearly flat. The reward for your patience is big, beautiful Shellrock Lake, with campsites galore and stocked trout—a fine, easy destination if you have kids or don't care to put in the miles.

DISTANCE & CONFIGURATION: 1.4-mile out-and-back to Shellrock Lake, 5-mile out-and-back to Rock Lakes, 12.6-mile balloon for the whole thing

DIFFICULTY: Easy to Shellrock, moderate to Rock Lakes, strenuous for the whole loop

SCENERY: Peaceful old-growth forest, several lakes, big meadow, nice viewpoint

EXPOSURE: Shady most of the way, with a few open spots

TRAFFIC: Moderate on summer weekends, light otherwise

TRAIL SURFACE: Packed dirt with roots and rocks

HIKING TIME: 1 hour to Shellrock Lake, 3 hours to Rock Lakes, 8 hours for the whole loop

ELEVATION CHANGE: 2,200'

SEASON: July–October

BEST TIME: August and September

BACKPACKING OPTIONS: Excellent sites on the shore of 3 lakes

DRIVING DISTANCE: 70 miles (2 hours, 20 minutes) from Pioneer Courthouse Square

ACCESS: No fees or permits required

MAPS: Green Trails *Map 492 (Fish Creek Mountain)* and *Map 493 (High Rock)*

WHEELCHAIR ACCESS: No

FACILITIES: Nearby at Hideaway Lake Campground; none at trailhead. Water on trail should be treated.

LOCATION: Shellrock Lake Trailhead on Forest Service Road (FR) 5830, 42 miles southeast of Estacada, OR

CONTACT: Clackamas River Ranger District, 503-630-6861, www.fs.usda.gov/mthood

To keep going, walk along the right side of the lake, and climb the hill, following a sign for Frazier Turnaround. It gets rocky in places, and mildly steep, until 1 mile past the lake, where you'll hit Grouse Point Trail #517. Turn right (downhill) here, and in a moment you'll arrive at Frazier Turnaround, the old trailhead.

Look for Serene Lake Trail #512 going downhill and to the left, and follow it 0.8 mile down to a junction. The loop keeps going here, but you should definitely go left a flat 0.25 mile to Middle Rock Lake, which has a few nice campsites. Turn right when you get to the lake, cross the outlet creek, and walk to the far end of the lake. Then follow a short trail up the hill to Upper Rock Lake, the smallest of the three and host to a dreamy private campsite. That trail gets a little brushy and can be tough to follow in early summer. The side trip to Middle and Upper Rock Lakes adds just over a mile to your day.

From the main trail, keep going the way you were headed, and in a couple hundred yards you'll come to a trail leading right, to Lower Rock Lake, which has one inferior campsite. Lower and Middle Rock Lakes are stocked with trout, by the way, so if you're into fishing, get a license and bring your rod. If you have small kids or you feel done for the day, you're now 3 miles from your car. But for an even nicer lake, and then some, keep going.

You'll put in another 0.8 mile going downhill then turn up (steeply at times) for most of a mile to gain the top of a ridge, thick with bear grass. Just over the top of the hill (now 4.3 miles from the trailhead), you'll come to Serene Lake and a signed trail leading left to a sunny campsite on the shore. Serene Lake is just what its name

Roaring River Wilderness

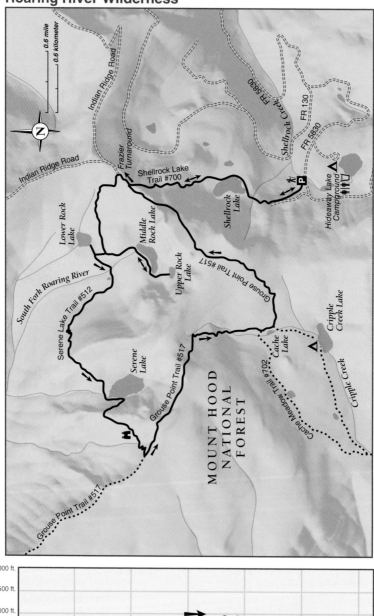

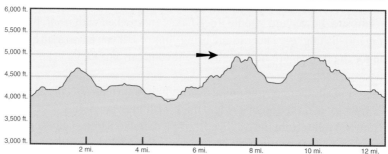

implies; anglers pull 15-inch trout from its deep, cold, clear water, and the same boulders, grassy shallows, downed trees, and thickly vegetated shoreline that hide the fish also make for outstanding scenery. This is the finest lake of the loop. Follow the right-hand shoreline to continue our hike.

If you're camping, you can choose from several excellent spots, one that in 2013 had an Adirondack chair and table at the trail junction (who put them there?); one at the far end on a point that sticks out into the lake; and another on the left side. There's also a huge boulder about 100 yards along the shoreline past the junction—an awesome spot to jump into the (very cold) lake. A decent trail circles the lake, but you'll have to cross a couple of rockslides to make the full circuit.

Beyond Serene Lake, the trail climbs about 600 feet in less than a mile to the top of a ridge and a junction with Grouse Point Trail #517. Turn left here, climb 200 more feet, and in 0.7 mile you'll reach a clear-cut that was put in for helicopters to drop off firefighters—thankfully it hasn't been needed for a while. A cliff affords a sublime view back down to Serene Lake and out to Mounts St. Helens, Rainier, Adams, and Hood. The two bare peaks to the right are the Signal Buttes. Also, as you look north toward Mount Hood, you're seeing an area of about 8 miles, as the crow flies, with only one road and two trails to break it up.

The trail now drops 700 feet in a mile, and when you get to the flower-filled Cache Meadow, you'll find an intersection. The right-hand trail leads out to another road; another heads into the meadow, where you can see the lily-filled Cache Lake to the left. To continue the loop, stay on the main trail, keeping the meadow on your right, and go 200 yards to the site of an old shelter. From here, you can cross the seasonal creek on your right and go 0.2 mile to Cripple Creek Lake, yet another mountain beauty with a couple of campsites.

A minute past the shelter site, turn left to stay on Grouse Point Trail #517, and take it uphill 1 mile (you'll get all of that 700 feet back) until you come to an abandoned road. Keep heading up, and in just under a mile you'll be back at the trail leading down to Shellrock Lake and your car. Just keep an eye out, in the clear areas along the road, for a view back to Mount Jefferson. That makes this a six-lake, five-volcano hike.

• •

GPS TRAILHEAD COORDINATES N45° 7.627' W121° 58.238'

DIRECTIONS Take OR 224 from Portland, traveling 44 miles southeast of I-205, through the town of Estacada, to the ranger station at Ripplebrook. Half a mile past the ranger station, turn left onto FR 57. After 6.8 miles, turn left onto FR 58. Drive 3 miles, then turn left onto FR 5830 and follow it 5.7 miles, staying left at one unsigned junction, to the Shellrock Lake Trailhead, on the right just past Hideaway Lake Campground.

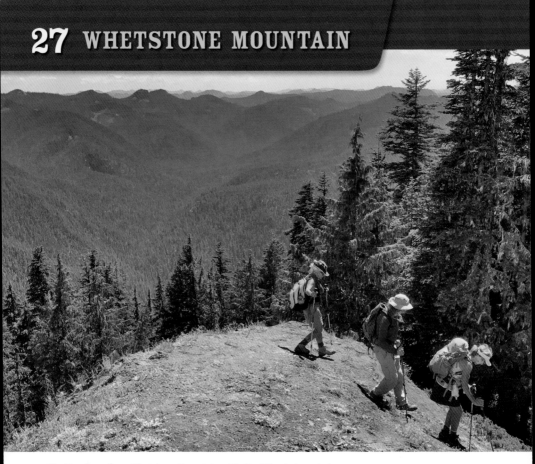

Starting down from Whetstone Mountain, with Opal Creek down below

IT'S A LONG, tedious drive. And it isn't much of a hike if you're looking for a ton of exercise. But what a view you get from Whetstone Mountain! And for what it's worth, you can do an up-close comparison of a clear-cut and old-growth forest. This hike is also a gateway into both Opal Creek Wilderness and Bull of the Woods Wilderness.

DESCRIPTION

Whetstone Mountain got its name in pioneer days because of a prevalence in the area of a rock that was useful for sharpening knives. The peak hosted a fire lookout tower for many years, but both it and the useful rock appear to be long gone. What's left, though, is an easy-to-reach viewpoint that rivals anything in the area.

You can actually see your destination from the extensive trailhead, which sits in the middle of a lovely clear-cut. Whetstone is the forested ridge right in front of you, and a little to the left in the distance you can see flat-topped Battle Ax Mountain (see next hike). Your route to Whetstone is to head toward it, swing left, gain that ridge you see, and then ascend the other side to the tiny, rocky summit.

DISTANCE & CONFIGURATION: 4.8-mile out-and-back

DIFFICULTY: Moderate

SCENERY: Old-growth forest on the way up, sweeping mountain view up top

EXPOSURE: Shady all the way; some mildly sketchy side-hill sections

TRAFFIC: Moderate on summer weekends, light otherwise

TRAIL SURFACE: Some rock at the very top

HIKING TIME: 3 hours

ELEVATION CHANGE: 1,360'

SEASON: June–October

BEST TIME: June for rhododendrons, October for fall colors

BACKPACKING OPTIONS: None on this trail but plentiful in Bull of the Woods Wilderness (Hike 24, page 126)

DRIVING DISTANCE: 74 miles (2 hours, 20 minutes) from Pioneer Courthouse Square

ACCESS: No fees or permits required

MAPS: Green Trails *Map 524 (Battle Ax)*, USFS *Bull of the Woods Wilderness*

WHEELCHAIR ACCESS: No

FACILITIES: None at trailhead; the last restroom you will see is at Bagby Trailhead.

CONTACT: Clackamas River Ranger District, 503-630-6861, www.fs.usda.gov/mthood

LOCATION: Off Forest Service Road (FR) 7020, 47 miles southeast of Estacada, OR

COMMENTS: Consider doing this hike as part of an overnight trip to the area—it takes almost as long to get here as it does to hike the trail.

When you start out hiking downhill, don't be concerned—you're on the right trail. You'll descend about 0.25 mile, passing rhododendrons (which bloom in late June) and huckleberries (ripe mid-August). This area was cut around 1980 and then replanted, so you have a chance to see how it's recovering. About 0.2 mile in, when you enter Bull of the Woods Wilderness, you'll see the amazing difference between cut and uncut forest, and you'll get a bigger-picture view of it later.

Around the time you start uphill, about 0.3 mile in, look for a meadow on the right with a spring, then cross a couple of its outlets. Just past 0.5 mile, you'll reach the base of a rockslide with a pond on your left, then go through a few switchbacks—one with a view of Mount Hood on the left—as you get up onto the ridge.

At the ridgeline, just over a mile into the hike, you'll intersect Whetstone Mountain Trail #3369. You've been on Whetstone Trail #546, and if you're wondering, you've gone from three digits to four because you've just hiked from Mount Hood National Forest to Willamette National Forest. Turn right on Trail #3369, and start a slow ascent along the north side of the ridge, with occasional views down and to the left into Opal Creek Wilderness. In a couple of places, you'll be walking on a side-hill section of trail with a fairly steep drop to the left, but the good news is you'll also be, in August, walking through huckleberry heaven.

When you've gone about a mile since the turn, you'll reach another right turn, this time up the short, steep trail to the rocky summit; going left here would drop you 3.5 miles to an intersection early in the Opal Creek Wilderness hike (Hike 30, page 152). Gaining Whetstone's summit requires a few steps on rocky terrain but

Whetstone Mountain

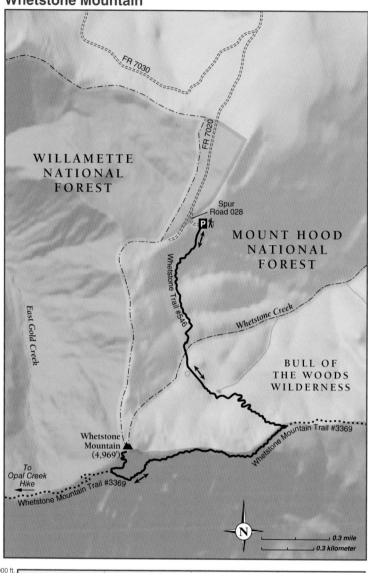

FR 7030

WILLAMETTE
NATIONAL
FOREST

FR 7020

Spur
Road 028

MOUNT HOOD
NATIONAL
FOREST

Whetstone Trail #546

East Gold Creek

Whetstone Creek

BULL OF
THE WOODS
WILDERNESS

Whetstone
Mountain
(4,969')

Whetstone Mountain Trail #3369

To
Opal Creek
Hike

Whetstone Mountain Trail #3369

N

0.3 mile
0.3 kilometer

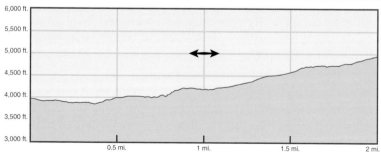

nothing challenging. Besides, when you get there, the summit is so small and so high relative to its surroundings, you may feel like you're airborne.

Catch your breath; then let's do the visual tour. The easy way to start is to find Mount Hood to the northeast. Left of that is Mount Adams, and left of that is Mount Rainier. To the right of Hood, and seemingly at your feet, a ridge heads east toward unseen Silver King Lake, in the heart of Bull of the Woods (Hike 24) and at the top of the Bagby Hot Springs hike (Hike 23). The right side of that ridge is the drainage for Battle Ax Creek, which joins Opal Creek at Jawbone Flats, almost directly beneath you.

In the distance to the east is knob-topped Olallie Butte, and right of that is Mount Jefferson, 25 miles away but seemingly right behind Battle Ax, which is 5 miles away. Still moving right, look for crumbly Three-Fingered Jack; the next pointy one to the right is Mount Washington, followed by tiny-looking Coffin Mountain and then the Three Sisters and Broken Top. Way out there is Diamond Peak, just north of Crater Lake. Near as I can figure, the straight-line distance from Diamond to Rainier is about 225 miles.

Quite a view, eh? Worth the drive? Thought so. If you're looking for some backpacking options, you won't find anything good on this trail, but Bull of the Woods is filled with lakes, trails, and campsites—just turn left at the intersection on the ridge, instead of right as you did to get here. But if you're thinking of a car shuttle to Opal Creek, consider this: you could hike from this trailhead to that one in about 6 miles, but the drive on FR 46 is more than 60 miles.

• •

GPS TRAILHEAD COORDINATES N44° 52.522' W122° 12.157'

DIRECTIONS From Portland on OR 224, drive 44 miles southeast of I-205, through Estacada, to the ranger station at Ripplebrook. Turn right onto FR 46 and then, 3.6 miles later, right again onto FR 63. After 3.5 miles turn right onto FR 70 and drive 7.6 miles; turn left onto FR 7020. Drive 6.7 miles and turn left onto Spur Road 028, which is 0.6 mile past where Road 7030 comes in from the right. The trailhead is at the end of Spur Road 028, 0.1 mile ahead.

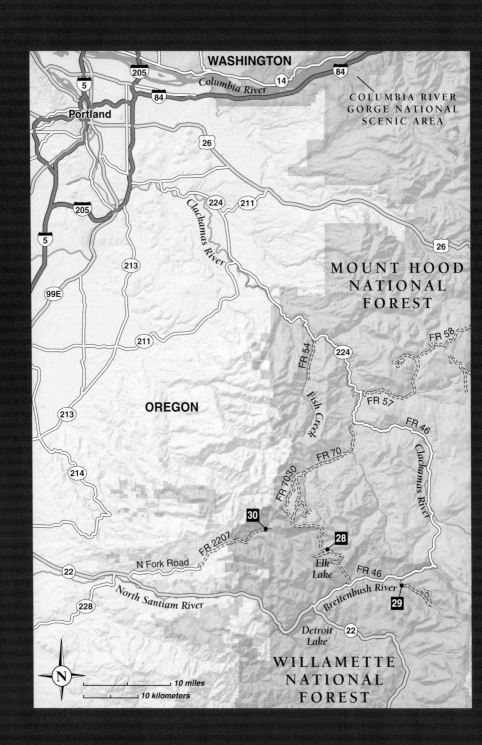

UP THE SANTIAM RIVER

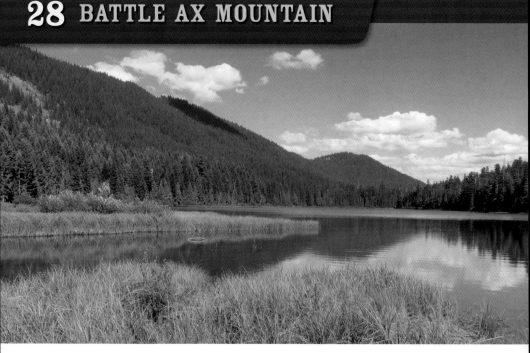

Elk Lake, near the Battle Ax trailhead, has campsites.

WHY HIKE BATTLE AX? Four reasons: one of the greatest views among all the hikes in this book, few fellow hikers, tent-only camping by a lake, and easy access to fantastic, lake-filled wilderness.

DESCRIPTION

Let's start with the road, because there's a chance that when you mentioned Battle Ax Mountain or Elk Lake to friends, they told you they had their teeth rattled out of their heads while driving up there. First, the road has been worked on quite a bit in the last few years, and second, I got my 1992 Nissan Sentra up there with no problem. Sure, I was going 5 miles an hour at times, but I made it just fine. While you're up there, consider spending the night at the campground, which costs only $10 but has a reputation for a little weekend rowdiness. It's a great base for exploring the whole area.

Now, the hike. If you drive to the trailhead, you'll knock 1.4 miles off your walk, and I'll describe it as if you did that. (If you're parked at the campground, just walk back up to the fork and go left to reach the trailhead.) It isn't too exciting at first, winding up Bagby Trail #544 through thick forest. The initial 0.6 mile gains 500 feet to reach a pair of small ponds, and 0.2 mile past them it flattens out to start a 1-mile traverse along the northeast side of Battle Ax. So, at this point, you're actually walking away from the peak, which will be visible over your left shoulder.

Halfway across this traverse, you'll enter an impressive rockslide where, if you give a shout, you'll notice that the sound really bounces around. The far end of this

DISTANCE & CONFIGURATION: 5.1-mile loop from trailhead, 6.5-mile loop from campground

DIFFICULTY: Strenuous

SCENERY: Forest, rock formations, mountain vistas

EXPOSURE: Lots of time in the open; some rocky slopes and side hills

TRAFFIC: Light

TRAIL SURFACE: Rocky in places

HIKING TIME: 4 hours

ELEVATION CHANGE: 1,765'

SEASON: June–October

BEST TIME: August and September

BACKPACKING OPTIONS: Plenty in the vicinity, though limited on this trail; see end of profile for details.

DRIVING DISTANCE: 108 miles (2 hours, 20 minutes) from Pioneer Courthouse Square

ACCESS: No fees or permits required

MAPS: USGS *Bull of the Woods Wilderness*

WHEELCHAIR ACCESS: No

FACILITIES: Restrooms (but no drinkable water) at nearby Elk Lake Campground

CONTACT: Detroit Ranger District, 503-854-3366, www.fs.usda.gov/willamette

LOCATION: Elk Lake at the end of Forest Service Road (FR) 4697, 12 miles northeast of Detroit, OR

COMMENTS: The road to this trailhead is pretty bumpy; check ahead for current conditions.

slide offers a great view back to Battle Ax; don't worry, you're not going up that side of it. You'll next cross a series of brushy, spring-fed forks of Battle Creek, with views north into the heart of Bull of the Woods Wilderness.

When you're 1.8 miles from the trailhead, the trail intersects Battle Ax Mountain Trail #3340, heading up and to the left. You'll also see, on the right, one of the more pitiful campsites of your life. It's a nice place for a rest or snack before you start climbing, but if you're looking to camp overnight, check the backpacking options on the next page.

While you're resting and snacking, perhaps you'd like to know where Battle Ax got its name. One theory is that it's shaped like an ax. Another is that an old woodsman named it for a brand of chewing tobacco that was popular in the 1890s.

To get up Battle Ax, take the trail left from this junction, and soon you'll be climbing and in the sun, as the forest thins out and you approach 5,000 feet in elevation. Another rockslide offers a view southeast to Mount Jefferson, as does a rocky bowl 0.3 mile up. After 0.5 mile of climbing, you'll cross over the ridge, and then your view will be west, down Battle Ax Creek—not to be confused with Battle Creek (on the other side)—and into the Opal Creek Wilderness.

Now you'll switchback up 0.6 mile, gaining a final 600 feet to put you at the north end of the broad, flat summit. Look for remnants of the old fire lookout, and a 1947 benchmark from the U.S. Coast and Geodetic Survey.

A big rock at the southern end of the peak offers a great view back down to Elk Lake, 1,800 feet below. Otherwise, you can see from Mount Hood to the Three Sisters. Try to spot the distinctive Coffin Mountain and Whetstone Mountain (see previous hike), both of which are on the far side of Opal Creek Wilderness (Hike 30, page 152).

Battle Ax Mountain

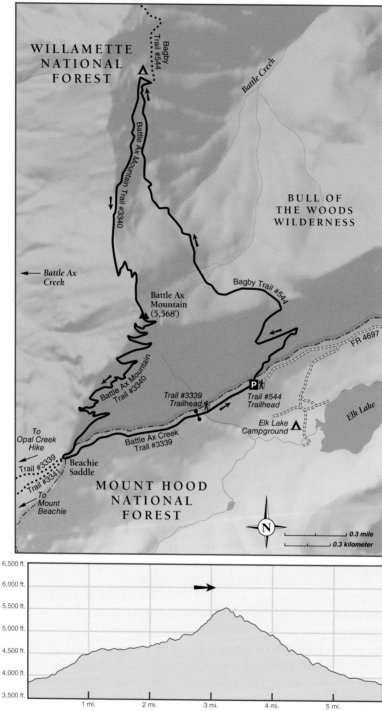

To go down, we'll aim for Beachie Saddle, between Elk Lake and Battle Ax Creek. Take the trail that heads right (when looking at the lake) from near the southern end of the summit, and descend a series of rocky, dusty, sun-drenched switchbacks. Some of this trail is also mildly exposed on steep, rocky side hills—nothing life-threatening, but a fall would ruin your day.

A little less than a mile downhill, you'll pass some neat rock formations. Check out Mount Beachie, across the way. It looks like somebody took a saw to the summit, cut out a rectangular chunk, and planted a tree in it. You can go up there later, if you want.

A mile and a half below the summit, you'll come to Beachie Saddle and an old road that is now Battle Ax Creek Trail #3339, to your right; this leads 4 miles down to Jawbone Flats in the middle of Opal Creek Wilderness, passing lots of old railroad and mining relics along the way. So the walk from Elk Lake to Jawbone Flats on the trail is about 5.5 miles; the drive is 46 miles. Above you is Mount Beachie, with a well-shot-up sign marking the start of that 1.5-mile, 800-foot climb.

To get to your car, head left and down the gravel road, which is at times a trail and at times something less than that. You'll pass the trailhead for Battle Ax Creek Trail #3339—imagine driving there—0.2 mile before our original trailhead, which is 0.7 mile from the campground and the lake you now deserve to jump into.

Backpacking Options

You're at the corner of two wilderness areas, so why not use this hike as a way into the backcountry? Options abound in Bull of the Woods, as do lakes—there are a dozen at least an acre in size. From the pitiful campsite at the first junction you came to, it's about 3 miles to Twin Lakes, which are in the middle of the wilderness. Get a map and go for it; with a car shuttle, you could even end the hike at Bagby Hot Springs. Or go down Trail #3339 into Opal Creek Wilderness.

· ·

GPS TRAILHEAD COORDINATES N44° 49.513' W122° 7.500'

DIRECTIONS Take I-5 south from Portland to Exit 253. Drive east 49 miles on OR 22 to Detroit, then turn left onto FR 46. After 4.4 miles, turn left on FR 4696—note that from here on, many intersections have no signs. Drive 0.6 mile and turn left on FR 4697, following it 2.2 miles to a T intersection; turn right. Drive 1.8 miles and make a left. This is where the road gets rough(er). Follow it 2.1 miles to another left, then 0.3 mile to a fork just above the campground: Here, you can bear right and drive 0.4 mile to reach the trailhead, on the right, or you can turn left and drive 0.3 mile to park in the campground.

The author relaxes on the log bridge over the South Fork of the Breitenbush.

WITH ITS COMBINATION of old-growth majesty and New Age spirituality, this area is one of the most serene and inspiring places in Oregon.

DESCRIPTION

Like a refuge of tranquility amid a sea of logging operations, the area along the South Fork Breitenbush River is often described with words like *peaceful* and *magical.* The hot-springs resort (see Nearby Activities) is itself a draw, but pleasant walks through the forest and along the river beckon.

Starting at the Resort Lot

One option is to register for a day pass at the resort and start your hike at the Spotted Owl Trailhead, off the parking lot. After 1.1 miles, during which you cross meandering Devils Creek, you come to Cliff Trail. Turn right and climb a fairly steep 0.5 mile, including some semiexposed sections along a cliff, to Devils Ridge Trail, which climbs steeply to Devils Lookout and Devils Peak (details below). If you'd rather stay on Spotted Owl Trail instead of turning on Cliff Trail, you'll come to Emerald Forest Trail in 0.5 mile at a junction described below.

DISTANCE & CONFIGURATION: Out-and-back or point-to-point options of 1–8 miles

DIFFICULTY: Easy–strenuous

SCENERY: Ancient forest, river, narrow gorge, mountain viewpoint, tubs filled with hot water

EXPOSURE: Shady all the way, except some rocky areas on the hilltops

TRAFFIC: Light–moderate

TRAIL SURFACE: Packed dirt, a few roots

HIKING TIME: 30 minutes–5 hours

ELEVATION CHANGE: Up to 2,500' if you do Devils Rest

SEASON: April–November

BEST TIME: September and October for fall colors and fewer crowds

BACKPACKING OPTIONS: A few options along the South Fork Breitenbush

DRIVING DISTANCE: 107 miles (2 hours) from Pioneer Courthouse Square

ACCESS: Northwest Forest Pass (see page 14) required to park on Forest Service Road (FR) 4685, day-use fee to park at hot springs (see Nearby Activities, page 151)

MAPS: Green Trails *Map 525 (Breitenbush);* free maps at resort office

WHEELCHAIR ACCESS: No

FACILITIES: None at trailhead; full services at hot springs with a fee

CONTACT: Breitenbush Hot Springs Resort, 503-854-3320, breitenbush.com; Detroit Ranger District, 503-854-3366, www.fs.usda.gov/willamette

LOCATION: 53000 Breitenbush Road SE, Detroit, OR

COMMENTS: Even if all you plan to do is hike, you need to check in at the resort if you are parking there; there's now a welcome house at the parking lot.

Breitenbush Gorge

For the shortest hike, walk about a mile round-trip to see Breitenbush Gorge, a 40-foot-deep chasm the river rips through. From the upper trailhead on FR 4685, start downhill and turn right at a sign for the gorge. Cross Roaring Creek on a log bridge and look for a river viewpoint on the left. After 0.3 mile, pass through an open area where a 1999 storm blew down lots of trees.

To find the gorge from this area (the junction is unsigned), walk a couple more minutes and look for two parallel logs pointing downhill between a big cedar and a root ball with ferns and hemlock saplings. The "trail" drops 100 feet or so to a viewpoint. Here the gorge has several big logs lying across it. A little trail heading left and under some logs leads to a view of the upper part of the gorge.

Emerald Forest and Devils Ridge

The most recommended hike starts at the lower parking area on FR 4685. Walk 0.1 mile downhill, and turn left onto South Breitenbush Gorge National Recreation Trail. You will only hear the river at this point; for views you'll have to "settle" for towering Douglas-firs, hemlocks, and western red cedars; cloverlike oxalis; and early-summer wildflowers. Rhododendrons bloom in June.

After 0.7 mile, you'll come to a trail on the right, signed EMERALD FOREST. (If you continue straight and bypass this trail, it's a 1-mile flat hike to the gorge.) Take the Emerald Forest Trail 0.1 mile downhill to the South Fork Breitenbush River,

Breitenbush Hot Springs Area

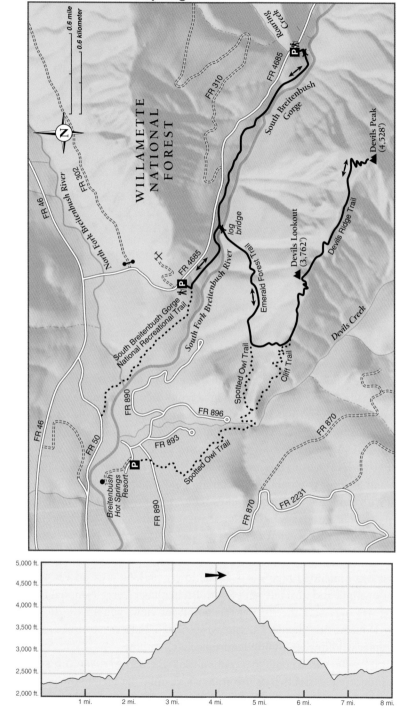

which hikers could once cross on a one-log bridge. The 1999 storm rolled the bridge over on its side, closing it. But subsequent storms blew several more trees down over the river, and someone added a handrail. On the other side, climb 0.5 mile on the Emerald Forest Trail through as pretty a forest as you'll ever see.

Your path intersects Devils Ridge Trail 0.8 mile past the bridge. Along the way, you may notice a sign for the Neotropical Migratory Bird Conservation Program, which was a program of small grants that improved habitats for birds in Central and South America, many of which come here for the summer. Making a right, toward Spotted Owl Trail, would lead you 1.6 miles to the hot springs. But if you're looking for some serious exercise and a spectacular view, turn left onto Devils Ridge Trail, which becomes quite steep in its 0.3-mile climb to a junction with Cliff Trail.

From this intersection, you can turn right and loop back, again toward Spotted Owl Trail and the resort, passing a viewpoint atop steep cliffs about 0.2 mile from here. Or you can turn left and keep doing the horribly steep thing. You'll pass a decent viewpoint after climbing 200 feet in 0.2 mile and then Devils Lookout after climbing 700 feet in 0.6 mile. Beyond Devils Lookout, Devils Peak is 1 mile away and 800 feet up, but you actually *lose* elevation on the way, and it gets crazy steep, but you get a view of Mount Jefferson.

NEARBY ACTIVITIES

Breitenbush Hot Springs Resort (503-854-3320, breitenbush.com) is open to day-use visitors daily (except for occasional closures of up to a week), 9 a.m.–6 p.m. Reservations are required and give you access to the pools, steam room, and well-being programs for a sliding-scale fee of $13–$26. Overnight rates include meals and range from $69 to $165. You can also camp here in the summer.

• •

GPS TRAILHEAD COORDINATES
Breitenbush Hot Springs Resort N44° 46.896' W121° 58.527'
Lower Trailhead (FR 4685) N44° 46.508' W121° 57.214'
Upper Trailhead (Gorge) N44° 45.972' W121° 55.666'

DIRECTIONS Take I-5 from Portland, driving 35 miles south of I-205 to Exit 253 (Detroit Lake). Turn left (east) on OR 22 and follow it 49 miles to Detroit. Turn left onto FR 46. For the hot springs, drive 9 miles on FR 46 and turn right onto a bridge just past Cleator Bend Campground. Over the next 1.2 miles, keep left at three junctions to reach the resort parking lot. For the trailheads on FR 4685, drive 2.5 miles from FR 46 (so 11.5 miles from Detroit), turn right onto FR 4685, and drive 0.6 mile to the trailhead, on the right. The trailhead nearest the gorge is another 1.3 miles up the road, on the right.

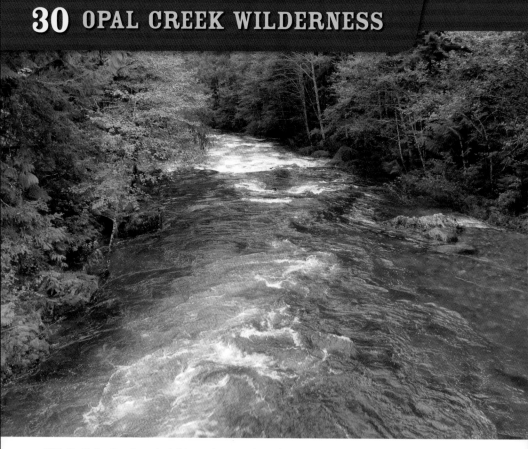

Little North Santiam from the bridge to the Kopetski Trail

OPAL CREEK'S HISTORY stretches from ancient times to a modern-day legislative showdown, but its value can hardly be measured. It's an almost completely preserved sample of what the Northwest used to be, a place that hasn't been logged and where the water runs clear. The largest such low-elevation area in the state, it doesn't even require that you work hard to see most of it.

DESCRIPTION

For thousands of years, the Santiam Indians maintained their summer camp at the confluence of what we now call Opal and Battle Ax Creeks. In the 1850s, pioneers started mining for silver and gold. Not much of either was found, but there were enough other minerals to keep mining alive here until the early 1980s. A mining town was built at the confluence in the 1920s, and it came to be known as Jawbone Flats; the story has it that while the men were out mining, the women were back there "jawboning." In 1992, the mining company donated 4,000 acres of land to a nonprofit group now known as the Opal Creek Ancient Forest Center, asking that it be preserved. A big fight ensued, and in 1998 the 35,000-acre Opal Creek Wilderness

DISTANCE & CONFIGURATION: 7-mile out-and-back to Opal Pool, 10-mile out-and-back to Cedar Flats, 13-mile out-and-back to see it all

DIFFICULTY: Easy–moderate

SCENERY: Uncut forest, clear-water pools, historic mining structures

EXPOSURE: Shady

TRAFFIC: Heavy on summer weekends, moderate otherwise

TRAIL SURFACE: Packed road for 3.1 miles; otherwise dirt, roots, rocks

HIKING TIME: 4 hours to Opal Pool, 5.5 hours to Cedar Flats, 6 hours to see it all

ELEVATION CHANGE: Up to 1,240'

SEASON: April–November

BEST TIME: July–September for weather, October for fall colors

BACKPACKING OPTIONS: Plentiful

DRIVING DISTANCE: 92 miles (2 hours) from Pioneer Courthouse Square

ACCESS: Northwest Forest Pass required (see page 14); can be purchased at trailhead

MAPS: USFS *Opal Creek Wilderness*

WHEELCHAIR ACCESS: No

FACILITIES: Outhouses at trailhead; composting toilet in meadow at Jawbone Flats

CONTACT: Opal Creek Ancient Forest Center, 503-892-2782, opalcreek.org

LOCATION: Opal Creek Trailhead at the end of Forest Service Road (FR) 2209, 22 miles northeast of Mehama, OR

COMMENTS: The U.S. Forest Service has initiated parking restrictions for this trailhead. Basically, you're allowed to line up only a quarter mile back from the trailhead on the south side of the road and park for 15 minutes at the booth to buy your pass, if needed. So please carpool or come during the week.

and Scenic Recreation Area was established. Today the center operates educational programs at Jawbone Flats, and a sprawling system of mostly easy trails brings visitors into the magical land of what used to be.

From the gate, start by walking slightly downhill on an old road. Most of the big trees are still ahead, but a Douglas-fir on the right is thought to be between 700 and 1,000 years old; a side trail leads to it at about 0.2 mile. But take care—walking too close to the base will actually contribute to its demise. Soon after, another old road leads down to the right, to two mine shafts on either side of the Little North Santiam River. At 0.3 mile, a high bridge crosses Gold Creek; 0.1 mile past that, you'll see Whetstone Mountain Trail #3369 on the left. This 3.5-mile trail climbs 3,000 feet to a superb view from atop Whetstone Mountain, but if you want to see that, it's much easier to do the Whetstone Mountain hike instead (Hike 27, page 138). About 0.2 mile past that trailhead, you'll cross a series of "half bridges" and another old mining shaft on the left just past them.

The most impressive forest along the road occurs between 1 and 1.5 miles out, where you'll find 6-foot-thick Douglas-firs. At a wide spot in the road 1.5 miles out, look for a trail to the right that leads 100 yards to a rocky viewpoint. At 2 miles, you come to a trail on the right leading into an area filled with old mining equipment and the burned-out remains of a sawmill's steel and masonry boiler; there is a steam engine here said to be reclaimed from the USS *Oregon* battleship. Behind the one

Opal Creek Wilderness

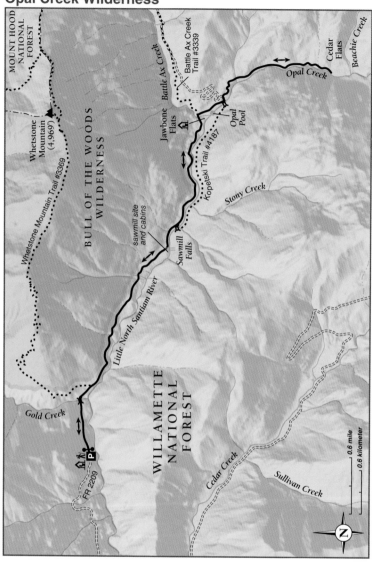

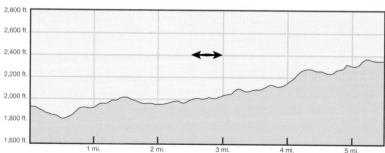

building still standing, a trail leads 100 feet to a falls, known as both Sawmill Falls and Cascadia de los Niños ("Waterfall of the Children").

Just past the sawmill site, you'll come to a junction. You can head straight ahead on the road to reach a river-access point, on the right 0.2 mile farther on; Jawbone Flats is 1.2 miles past that. There you'll find several cabins from the 1920s and 1930s (some can be rented overnight from opalcreek.org) and two cabins built since a fire in 1999. To reach the local highlight, Opal Pool, take the road straight through the camp, following signs to make a right turn and pass a collection of old vehicles that includes, oddly, a U.S. Navy fire truck. The pool is 0.1 mile past the cars.

Back at the first fork in the road, I recommend taking the right turn, across a bridge and then left, onto Kopetski Trail #4187. (Then-congressman Mike Kopetski sponsored the Opal Creek Forest Preserve Act of 1994.) Along this trail, several side trails lead left to the Little North Santiam; you'll also pass several campsites on both sides of the trail; the best of them are on the left, down by the river. The trail will also be muddy and swamped if it has rained recently.

Continue 1.4 miles to a sign directing you to the sublime Opal Pool, on the left. In summer you may see people jumping off the rocks into the amazingly clear, cold water. You're now looking at Opal Creek itself, probably the clearest water you'll ever see. Just past the pool, the trail swings left to cross a bridge then climb briefly to a junction with the trail coming up from Jawbone Flats. Go left to head back toward your car, or go right, sticking with the Kopetski Trail to head for Cedar Flats. This is a new trail section, built in 2013 because a bridge just up Opal Creek was wiped out by a flood. It passes one place with mild exposure then crosses Flume Creek between two waterfalls; this latter bit is sketchy if the water is high.

A mile up from the junction—a total of 5 miles from the gate—the trail more or less ends at Cedar Flats, where Beachie Creek flows into Opal Creek from the left and three 1,000-year-old cedars frame the trail. You'll also find good camping in this area.

I say "more or less ends" because the trail beyond there is not maintained, but it is possible to go off exploring. Look for a log over Beachie Creek (or wade it if that is gone), and then just go with it. Sometimes there's a trail; sometimes there are logs to walk on; sometimes there are logs to climb over. If a trail dead-ends near a log, hop up on it, walk a ways, and look around; you just might find some more trail. There is at least one more waterfall and one more pool like Opal Pool up there. Some folks just wander up the creek itself, which can be OK at low-water times; you might even find Poster Falls, made famous by a poster during the save-the-forest campaign. A mile up is Franklin Grove, another collection of cedars and as far as this "trail" goes.

Opal Creek has still more to offer. Battle Ax Creek Trail #3339 goes 4 miles and 1,800 feet up from Jawbone Flats to a junction near Elk Lake and the Battle Ax Mountain hike (Hike 28, page 144), passing old mining equipment and railroad sections along the way. From the start of Kopetski Trail, near the first bridge, another trail leads up Stony Creek to a hidden waterfall. There's even a trail that branches off Whetstone Mountain Trail, heading up Gold Creek; beyond Whetstone Mountain, you can hike 14 miles through Bull of the Woods Wilderness to Bagby Hot Springs (Hike 23, page 122).

NEARBY ACTIVITIES

A mile back on OR 22, you may have noticed The Gingerbread House (503-859-2247). It's on your left as you head home, at the junction of OR 22 and OR 226 in Mehama. Stop in for some fresh, warm gingerbread with ice cream after your hike, and your day will be complete.

* *

GPS TRAILHEAD COORDINATES N44° 51.591' W122° 15.864'

DIRECTIONS Take I-5 from Portland, driving 35 miles south of I-205 to Exit 253 (Detroit Lake). Turn left (east) onto OR 22 and follow it 22 miles, then turn left onto North Fork Road, following a sign for Little North Santiam Recreation Area. In just over 15 miles, the pavement ends and the road becomes FR 2207. Veer left onto FR 2209 at a junction; the trailhead is at the end of the road, 5.6 miles after you leave the pavement.

Some of the finest forest around, on the road to Jawbone Flats

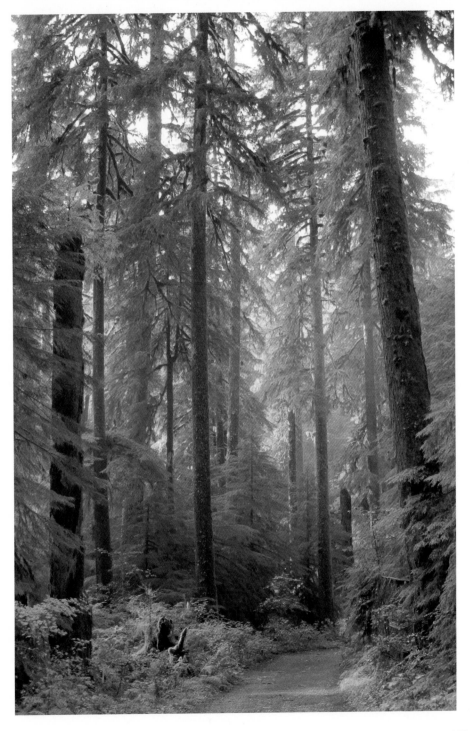

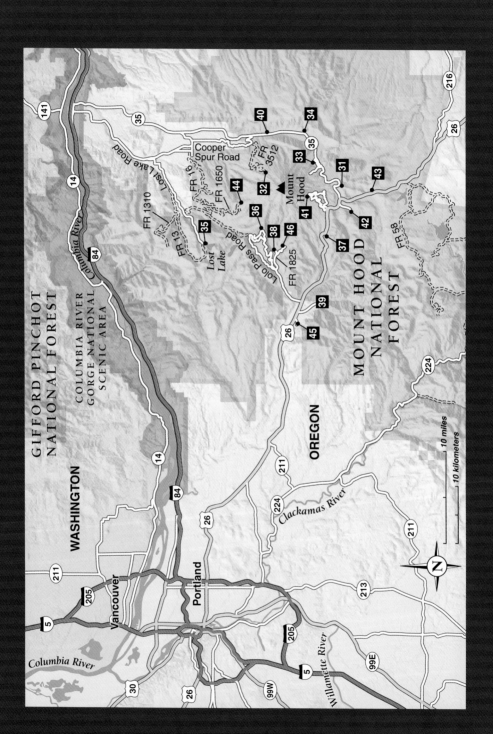

AROUND MOUNT HOOD

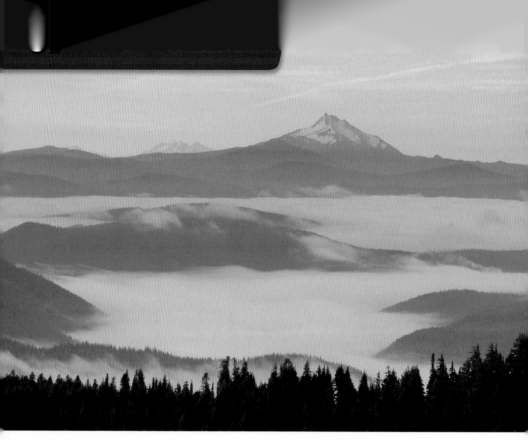

Early morning view of Mount Jefferson with Three Sisters beyond

THIS CONVENIENT HIKE is all about the forest, traversing some of the finest high-elevation old growth around and ending at an Oregon landmark.

DESCRIPTION

There are more-spectacular hikes in the Mount Hood area, but none offers the same combination of solitude and old-growth beauty. It's also perfect for a picnic or just a dose of sunshine, in a high-altitude meadow with Mount Hood towering above.

From the trailhead, walk across FR 3531 and into the woods on Pacific Crest Trail (PCT) #2000. Stop to admire the relief map of the PCT in Oregon and contemplate some of the distances. People who hike the whole PCT in five or six months average about 20 miles a day—and when they get to Oregon, it's often more like 30. You'll get in 4–5 miles today—a distance most PCT long-haul hikers fly through.

At the sign, take the leftmost fork of the trails before you, walking north on the PCT toward Mount Hood. You'll take a few steps across historic Barlow Road and, after 0.1 mile, carefully cross OR 35. The trail continues in a small draw on the far side.

The first part of the trail isn't too exciting, but in 0.5 mile you enter a glorious stand of mostly noble fir, with its long, branchless trunks. In early summer the

DISTANCE & CONFIGURATION: 10-mile out-and-back, 5-mile point-to-point with shuttle

DIFFICULTY: Moderate

SCENERY: Forest, meadows, views of Mount Hood, two river canyons

EXPOSURE: Forest on the way up, open on top

TRAFFIC: Light

TRAIL SURFACE: Packed dirt with some roots

HIKING TIME: 3.5 hours one-way

ELEVATION CHANGE: 1,640'

SEASON: July–October

BEST TIME: August and September

BACKPACKING OPTIONS: One good creekside site along the way

DRIVING DISTANCE: 62 miles (1 hour, 20 minutes) from Pioneer Courthouse Square

ACCESS: Northwest Forest Pass required May 1– October 30; Oregon Sno-Park Pass required November 1–April 30 (see page 14)

MAPS: Green Trails *Map 462 (Mount Hood),* USFS *Mount Hood Wilderness*

WHEELCHAIR ACCESS: No

FACILITIES: None; water along trail must be treated.

CONTACT: Hood River Ranger District, 541-352-6002, www.fs.usda.gov/mthood; Pacific Crest Trail Association, pcta.org

LOCATION: Barlow Pass at the intersection of Forest Service Road (FR) 3530 and OR 35, 5 miles east of Government Camp, OR

COMMENTS: You can combine this hike with the Twin Lakes trip (Hike 43, page 213). This is also a great hub for snowshoeing and cross-country skiing.

ground is blanketed with wildflowers. In late summer you'll see several species of huckleberries, and in fall, red-and-orange vine maple. If you're quiet, especially early in the day, you'll hear birds and possibly see deer or elk. It's just a pleasant place to be, and the altitude gain—less than 400 feet per mile—is entirely manageable.

The blue diamonds on the trees early in the hike mark winter trails for cross-country skiers and snowshoers. Their height gives you a sense of how much snow falls in these parts. The white diamonds mark the PCT from Mexico to Canada.

At the 2-mile mark, you'll enter a more diverse forest that includes firs and hemlocks, then cross a creek beside a small campsite at 2.7 miles. A little more than 3 miles into the hike, you'll reach an overlook of Salmon River Canyon and the headwaters of the Salmon River. The Salmon is the only river in the lower 48 states classified as a Wild and Scenic River from its headwaters to its mouth. The river flows from a glacier above Timberline Ski Area, snaking its way down to the Sandy River along US 26. Two hikes along the lower Salmon—Salmon River Trail and Wildwood Recreation Site—are described elsewhere in this book (Hikes 39 and 45, pages 196 and 223, respectively).

Just past here, the forest will start to open up; in July and August, you'll see meadows filled with wildflowers, especially purple lupine and the spectacular beargrass, which looks like a giant cotton swab. In a few minutes, your trail intersects Timberline Trail #600 in just such a meadow, with Mount Hood rising above you. Relax here if you like, then turn around. Or continue 0.3 mile left on Timberline Trail to reach a spectacular lookout with views of the White River Canyon, hundreds of feet deep. If you turn around here, it will be a 10.2-mile day.

Barlow Pass

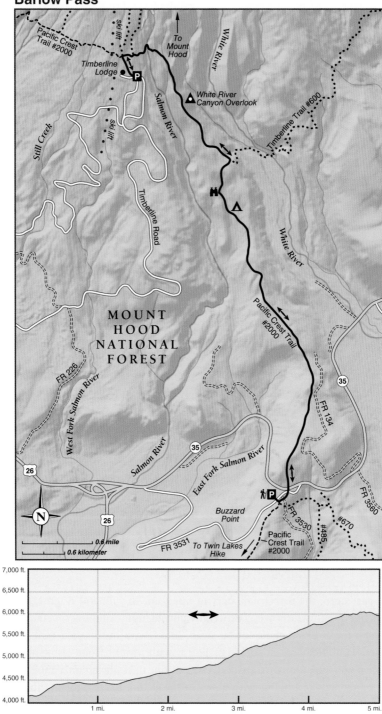

If you've opted to park a car up at Timberline, keep going up Timberline Trail (which, at this point, is also the PCT) toward the mountain. It's 1.25 miles to the lodge—700 feet up—so it's not *too* much more work. However, most of the climbing is along the first part of the trail, which is also, at points, as sandy as a beach. So it can get arduous. And if cold weather is in the forecast, it's a sure thing up here, so bring a coat. There's nothing to stop the wind this high on the mountain.

You first go along the edge of the White River Canyon and then through meadows and across the tiny Salmon River; this crossing has no bridge but is manageable. Look for views south to Mount Jefferson, some 45 miles away, and a sign on the PCT with mileages to Canada and Mexico. You'll also encounter Mountaineer Trail, which loops up to Silcox Hut then back down to Timberline Trail west of the lodge, in a section that's part of Hike 41, Timberline Lodge (see page 204). When you get close to the lodge, trails will go every which way, so just aim for the hot chocolate, and finish the hike with style.

You can hike just the upper part of this walk from Timberline Lodge—an especially good idea if you have kids with you. This is an easy, scenic alternative with little elevation gain; it's about 1 mile round-trip to the White River Canyon overlook.

If you're wondering about those PCT thru-hikers, the main "herd" typically passes through here in late August or early September—look for (usually) young, thin, filthy people with small backpacks. It's fun to do something nice for them and practice some "trail magic" by offering them chips or candy bars or taking out their garbage.

NEARBY ACTIVITIES

If your vehicle has some clearance, you can drive Barlow Road for miles, eventually making your way to The Dalles—though the road improves dramatically long before that. The drive is fun for the historical value and a few campsites along the way.

Though it's crowded, spend some time exploring Timberline Lodge (503-272-3311, timberlinelodge.com). Watch the film *The Builders of Timberline* to hear the story of how artists and artisans came together during the Depression to create this masterwork. Then learn the details of their accomplishment, especially those of the Head House and its massive central stone tower.

• •

GPS TRAILHEAD COORDINATES
Barlow Pass Trailhead N45° 16.957' W121° 41.116'
Timberline Lodge N45° 19.841' W121° 42.551'

DIRECTIONS Take US 26 from Portland to OR 35, following signs for Hood River. Drive 2.5 miles north on OR 35 and turn right onto FR 3531. The trailhead is 0.2 mile ahead.

163

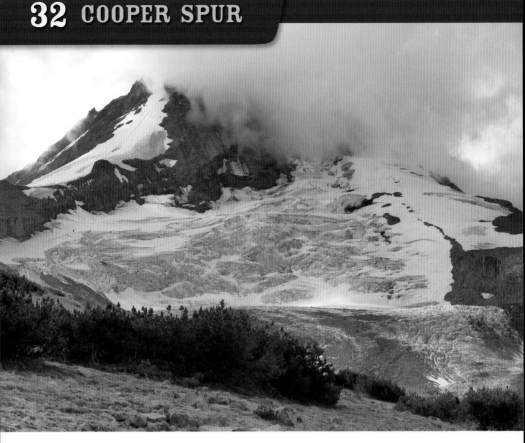

Eliot Glacier looms large from beyond Cooper Spur Shelter.

THOUGH IT'S NOT the toughest trail in this book, it is the highest—right up into the realm of the mountain climber. But while you'll be in the world of rock and snow, you won't wear yourself out getting here—well, not completely. You'll also get to see the oldest buildings on Mount Hood and the results of a massive landslide and a recent forest fire.

DESCRIPTION

If you want to get way, way up there, this is your hike. In the days before Timberline Lodge and the road to it were built, Cooper Spur was the standard climbing route to Mount Hood's 11,239-foot summit, and people still climb it that way today.

The whole area, in fact, is historically significant. Just up a hill from the trailhead, at the end of the road, is Cloud Cap Inn. Built in 1889 by two prominent Portland families as a recreation destination, it's the oldest building on Mount Hood. The hotel venture never took off, however, and by World War II the property was given to the U.S. Forest Service. In 1956 the Crag Rats, a Hood River–based climbing and rescue organization, took it over, and they maintain it to this day. Although

DISTANCE & CONFIGURATION: 6.8-mile balloon loop

DIFFICULTY: Strenuous

SCENERY: Old-growth forest, glaciers, wide panoramas, the upper reaches of Mount Hood

EXPOSURE: Mostly out in the open, with plenty of wind

TRAFFIC: Heavy on summer weekends, moderate otherwise

TRAIL SURFACE: Packed dirt, sand, rocks

HIKING TIME: 4.5 hours

ELEVATION CHANGE: 2,800'

SEASON: July–October

BEST TIME: August and September

BACKPACKING OPTIONS: One site at Cooper Spur Shelter, but access to water is tough from here. Other options along the Timberline Trail, but why not just camp at the trailhead? It's $15 a night.

DRIVING DISTANCE: 98 miles (2 hours, 15 minutes) from Pioneer Courthouse Square

ACCESS: Northwest Forest Pass required (see page 14)

MAPS: Green Trails *Map 462 (Mount Hood)*, USFS *Mount Hood Wilderness*, USGS *Mount Hood North*

WHEELCHAIR ACCESS: No

FACILITIES: Outhouse and water at trailhead

CONTACT: Hood River Ranger District, 541-352-6002, www.fs.usda.gov/mthood

LOCATION: Cloud Cap Saddle Campground at the end of Cloud Cap Road, 19 miles south of Parkdale, OR

COMMENTS: No matter the forecast, bring warm clothing—weather at this altitude can change quickly. Also, Cloud Cap Road (Forest Service Road [FR] 3512) can get a little rough and tedious, but virtually all cars can handle it.

officially the public isn't allowed in, if you're nice to the folks there, they might let you pop in for a bit. The Forest Service also offers public tours on occasion.

In 2008 a forest fire swept through this area, and dramatic measures were taken to save the buildings, including wrapping them in a protective material. As you start the hike, you'll get to see how the forest is recovering and appreciate the folks who saved the area's historic legacy.

More history later—now for the hike. The trail starts at the far end of the campground. Take Timberline Trail #600 up and to the left, and enter a rare snow-zone, old-growth forest, where mountain hemlock and Pacific silver firs get bigger than you'd think possible in an area that usually has 10 feet of snow by the end of December. Walk 1.2 miles to reach a junction after winding through the rocks and sand; following a sign for Cooper Spur Trail #600B, turn right and uphill—and get used to the climbing.

Just a hundred yards up, back among the twisted whitebark pines on your right, sits the Cooper Spur Shelter, at the end of a small side trail. This thing has been standing for some 70 years; imagine what weather it's been through. You can pitch a tent here or even sleep in the shelter, but you should follow a trail a minute or two beyond it to an amazing view of the Eliot Glacier. Then have a snack and keep climbing. The trail will switchback through the sand and rocks, and the glacier will gradually come into view to the right. You'll hear it pop and rumble as it carves the

Cooper Spur

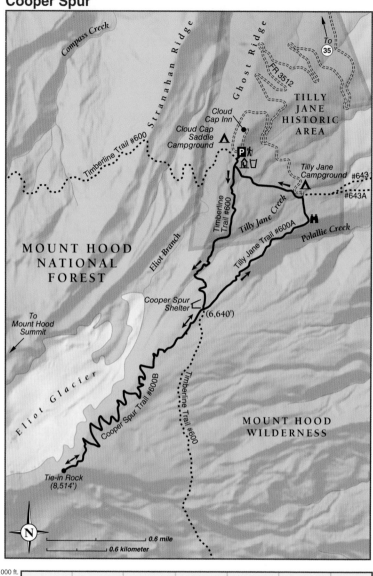

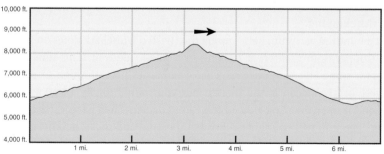

side of the mountain, and if you're lucky, especially on late-summer afternoons, you'll see big boulders tumbling down its face.

After 2 miles of tough climbing, gaining 1,900 feet, you'll come to the top of the ridge, where you should look for a rock with some impressive carvings. JULY 17, 1910 is engraved in the stone here, commemorating a Japanese climbing party's ascent. Since you've climbed all the altitude at this point, you might as well go another 0.2 mile along the ridgetop—just be aware that this ridge is thin, rocky, and usually windswept. If it's also snow-covered, stop here.

Just before the (permanent) snow line, you'll come to a plaque attached to the side of what's known as Tie-in Rock, so named because it's here that climbers tie themselves to one another to venture out onto the glacier. Heed my warning, though: Do *not,* under any circumstances—short of having ropes, crampons, and relevant experience—go out onto the glacier. Be satisfied with having reached the top of your local hiking world, and relax among the sheltering rocks to take in the view.

From left to right, with Mount Hood behind you, you can see Eliot Glacier on your left; Newton Clark Glacier on your right; Gnarl Ridge at your feet; and, way off in the distance, the bare face of Table Mountain in the Columbia River Gorge, Mount St. Helens, Mount Rainier, and Mount Adams. Lookout Mountain is on a ridge to the east. There's a building below you and to your right, which is the top of a ski lift at Mount Hood Meadows Ski Area.

Now look up at Mount Hood. The Cooper Spur climbing route begins on the snowfield right in front of you and proceeds up through the rocks, tending slightly to your left. (As climbers like to say, it's not as steep as it looks.) Look for a prominent rock called The Chimney, just below the summit, and Pulpit Rock more to your right. The Crag Rats say that whenever somebody falls on the Cooper Spur climbing route, they generally wind up within about 200 feet of the same falling spot at the top of Eliot Glacier.

When you've descended to the junction where you originally turned right, continue straight, leaving Timberline Trail #600 for Tilly Jane Trail #600A. Hike 0.6 mile and you'll come to an overlook of a large, bare bowl on your right. That's what was left behind by the Polallie Slide, a massive debris flow and flood in December 1980 that wiped out parts of OR 35.

A short distance on, you'll find yourself at some old buildings. This is part of the 1,400-acre Tilly Jane Historic Area, which is immensely popular with cross-country skiers and snowshoers, who come up a 2.7-mile trail from near Cooper Spur Ski Area and spend the night here. (In fact, during winter you can rent the Tilly Jane A-Frame, which is managed by the Oregon Nordic Club, at reserveamerica.com.) And if you're wondering about that name, Tilly Jane was the nickname of the matriarch of the Ladd family, one of the builders of Cloud Cap Inn and the former owners of what's now the Ladd's Addition neighborhood in Portland.

In this area you'll also find a campground, an amphitheater that's been there since at least the 1950s, and a 1938 guard station, managed by the Oregon Nordic Club and available for rent in the winter. A sign at the parking lot tells more about the local history.

To get back to your car, just put Mount Hood on your left and follow Tilly Jane Trail #600A for 0.5 mile back to the trailhead. You'll find the trail over by the amphitheater, heading across the creek.

NEARBY ACTIVITIES

When you get back to OR 35, go north (left) and indulge yourself at some of the berry and fruit stands in the Hood River Valley. Some let you pick your own. See hoodriverfruitloop.com for details.

• •

GPS TRAILHEAD COORDINATES N45° 24.141' W121° 39.297'

DIRECTIONS Take US 26 from Portland, driving 51 miles east of I-205; turn left (north) on OR 35, following signs for Hood River. Continue 17 miles on OR 35, then turn left at a sign for Cooper Spur Ski Area. (You can also take I-84 east and OR 35 south via Hood River to this spot; it's about the same amount of time.) Drive 2.4 miles; at Cooper Spur Mountain Resort, turn left onto Cloud Cap Road, and follow another sign for Cooper Spur Ski Area. In 1.4 miles, continue straight, leaving the pavement. Go 8.3 winding miles on Cloud Cap Road (FR 3512) to a T junction, and turn right. The trailhead is 0.5 mile ahead on the right, in Cloud Cap Saddle Campground.

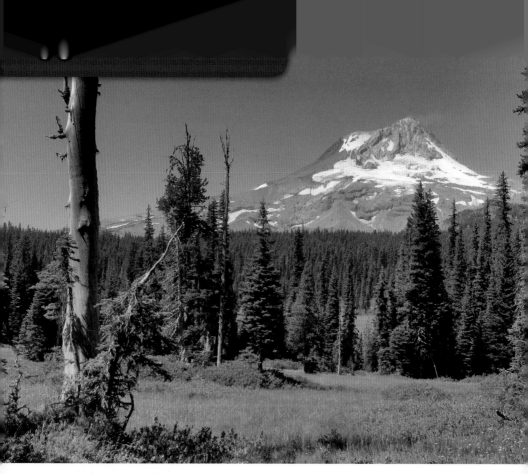

Mount Hood from Elk Meadows

ONE OF THE most spectacular sights in the Mount Hood area, sprawling and flower-filled Elk Meadows is relatively easy to reach. Beyond it lies Gnarl Ridge, with its awesome close-up view of the mountain.

DESCRIPTION

If I were to tell you there's a place where you can skip through meadows and over creeks, picking berries all the way, and wind up in a flower-filled wonderland with a snow-covered peak above it, and that if you wanted, you could climb up through more meadows to a rocky point with a huge view of everything around, right up where the water blasts out from under the glaciers, you'd be interested in that, right?

That's this hike. And if all you're doing is going to Elk Meadows, there's only one moderate hill between you and your destination. In fact, you and the kids could walk a flat mile, see two mountain streams, and have a ball. And you could do the whole thing in an easy day or spend the night on an easy introductory backpack.

From the trailhead, follow Sahalie Falls Trail #667C through moss-draped forest, pocket meadows with wildflowers, and huckleberries that ripen in late August. You

DISTANCE & CONFIGURATION: 2-mile out-and-back Newton Creek, 5.5-mile out-and-back to Elk Meadows, 12-mile loop to see it all

DIFFICULTY: Moderate to Elk Meadows, strenuous to Gnarl Ridge

SCENERY: Meadows, mountain streams, extreme close-ups of Mount Hood, fire-recovery area

EXPOSURE: In and out of the trees, with two bridgeless creek crossings

TRAFFIC: Moderate on summer weekends, light otherwise

TRAIL SURFACE: Dirt, some roots and rocky areas

HIKING TIME: 3.5 hours to Elk Meadows, 8 hours for the whole loop

ELEVATION CHANGE: 1,200' to Elk Meadows, 2,460' to Gnarl Ridge

SEASON: July–October

BEST TIME: August and September

BACKPACKING OPTIONS: Several good ones

DRIVING DISTANCE: 69 miles (1 hour, 30 minutes) from Pioneer Courthouse Square

ACCESS: No fees or permits required

MAPS: Green Trails *Map 462 (Mount Hood),* USFS *Mount Hood Wilderness*

WHEELCHAIR ACCESS: No

FACILITIES: Outhouse at trailhead; water on trail must be treated.

LOCATION: Elk Meadows and Sahalie Falls Trailhead on Elk Meadows Trailhead Road, 10 miles east of Government Camp, OR

CONTACT: Hood River Ranger District, 541-352-6002, www.fs.usda.gov/mthood

COMMENTS: This makes an excellent snowshoe or ski trip; start at the Clark Creek Sno-Park on OR 35. The Green Trails map shows winter trails.

---

may notice that some of the meadows aren't entirely natural (they're filled with stumps); these are Nordic ski runs, part of Mt. Hood Meadows ski resort.

Pass Umbrella Falls Trail #667 on the left, and now you are officially on Elk Meadows Trail #645. After hiking 0.5 mile, you'll cross Clark Creek on a bridge, which skiers and snowshoers can attest is a lot more interesting with about 2 feet of snow on it. There's also a campsite at this crossing, but better ones await.

Keep going straight—ignore the trails leading left—and after another 0.6 mile you'll cross Newton Creek—on logs, one hopes. If you're here early in the season and the logs aren't in place yet, this crossing (and a later one) might be tricky. Check portlandhikers.org for the latest conditions.

While we're here, a few words about the names of these creeks: they both flow from Newton Clark Glacier. What many people don't realize is that Newton Clark was just one guy, a teacher and surveyor who moved from South Dakota to Hood River Valley in 1877 and lived until 1918. He also has a county in South Dakota named for him.

Safely across Newton Creek, you're at the hill. Hike 1 mile to gain almost 700 feet in a series of long switchbacks; consider this the price of admission to Elk Meadows. Just over the top, you'll come to a four-way intersection: for Elk Meadows, go straight 0.4 mile, sticking with Trail #645 until the second intersection with #645A on the left; for a side trip to Elk Mountain, turn right, into an area that burned in 2006.

The trail to Elk Mountain isn't spectacular in and of itself, but it's quiet and woodsy, and it leads to a view east across OR 35 and south to Mount Jefferson. To

Elk Meadows

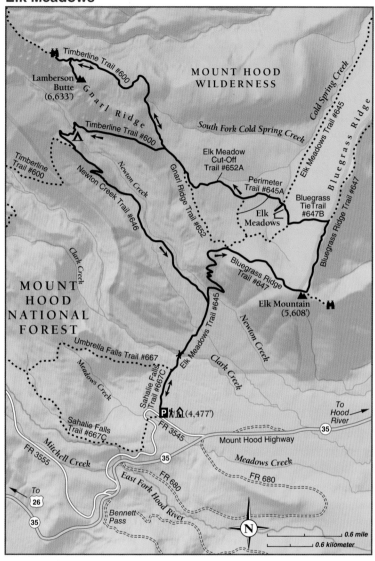

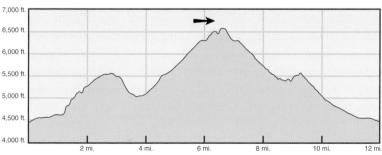

get to the lookout, climb 0.6 mile on Bluegrass Ridge Trail #647, then stay straight at a junction with Elk Mountain Vista Trail #647C; the lookout is 0.3 mile ahead. When you come back, take Bluegrass Ridge Trail, now to the right, and follow it 0.5 mile along the ridgetop—through the heart of the burned area—before turning left at a large stone cairn and plunging 0.4 mile down Bluegrass Tie Trail #647B, back to Trail #645. Turn right, and in 0.2 mile you'll be at Perimeter Trail #645A on the edge of the meadows.

Elk Meadows is almost unbelievable. It's basically a circular area of meadows about 0.5 mile in diameter, with islands of trees throughout and streams crisscrossing it. For the good of the flowers and grass, resist the temptation to go meadow-stomping, but by all means find a log or rock on the perimeter and take a load off. To complete a loop around the meadows, or to head for Gnarl Ridge, follow Trail #645A, with the meadows to your left.

After about 50 yards on Perimeter Trail #645A, you'll come to a trail leading left. Follow it out into the middle of the meadows, where a stone shelter hosts backpackers most summer nights (additional tent sites are behind the shelter in the woods). It's a lovely place for a picnic, with a great view of Mount Hood across the way.

After returning from the shelter, take a left on Perimeter Trail #645A, and start climbing along the side of the meadow, passing a couple more campsites along the way. In about 0.5 mile, you'll come to a junction with Gnarl Ridge Cut-Off Trail #652A. To return to your car, turn left, finish the loop around the meadows, and then turn right at the junction with Elk Meadows Trail #645. But to climb toward Mount Hood, stay straight on Gnarl Ridge Trail.

During a little more than a mile of gradual climbing, you'll join Gnarl Ridge Trail #652 and then reach Timberline Trail #600. Here you have another choice to make: turn left to start back toward the car, or turn right to climb another 900 feet in 1.5 miles to the top of Gnarl Ridge. That trail leads through more meadows and an ever-thinner forest, with views of Mount Adams to your right and Lookout Mountain (see next hike) behind you. You can also clearly see the whole of Bluegrass Ridge, the scene of that 2006 fire.

The gravelly viewpoint of Gnarl Ridge offers one of the finer vistas around. The glaciers of Mount Hood loom above you, with the headwaters of Newton Creek bursting out from under them, and across the way you can make out a ski-lift building on the resort. Mount Jefferson and the Three Sisters are out beyond that. A short trail leads up to Lamberson Butte (6,633 feet), the official summit of the ridge.

Keep wandering up Timberline Trail—it's out in the open for quite a while now and leads just a couple of miles over to Cooper Spur (see previous hike). Or head back down to the junction, and turn right onto Timberline Trail #600. A gradual descent will bring you back to another crossing of Newton Creek, where again (one hopes) logs will help you across. On the far side, pass a fine campsite next to a spring creek, climb about 0.3 mile, and then turn left at the ridgetop onto Newton Creek Trail #646. Two miles down that heavily huckleberried trail, your path intersects the trail you started all this wandering on: Elk Meadows Trail #645. Turn right to hike less than a mile back to the trailhead.

I know this is a lot of numbers, letters, and junctions—just bring this book and the Green Trails map with you, make up your own loop if you want, and enjoy the ride.

NEARBY ACTIVITIES

For a little piece of Oregon history, pay your respects at the Pioneer Woman's Grave, off OR 35 on Forest Service Road (FR) 3531, just east of its intersection with US 26 (GPS: N45° 16.928′ W121° 42.004′). Workers building the old Mount Hood Loop Highway found the woman buried beneath a crude marker; her remains have since been moved twice, and to this day people lay crosses or flowers on the pile of rocks marking her grave.

. . . .

GPS TRAILHEAD COORDINATES N45° 19.399′ W121° 38.125′

DIRECTIONS Take US 26 from Portland, driving 51 miles east of I-205. Turn left (north) on OR 35, following signs for Hood River. Drive 7.5 miles and turn left onto FR 3545, at the second entrance for Mt. Hood Meadows ski resort (the one for the Nordic Center). The trailhead is 0.5 mile ahead, on the right. If you prefer to take I-84 to Hood River, then OR 35 south for 31 miles to the same intersection, that is some 30 miles farther but only about 15 minutes more time.

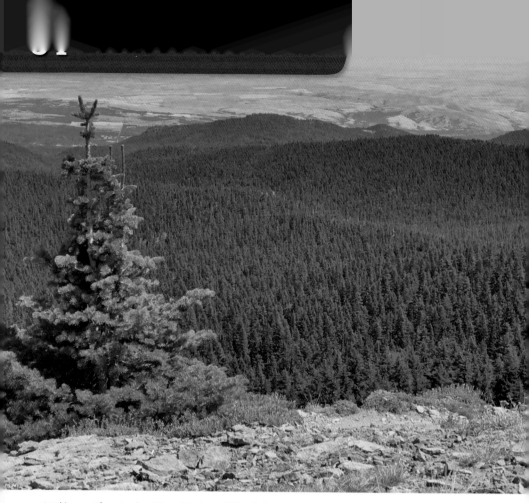

Looking east from Lookout Mountain toward Flag Point

ONE OF THE easternmost points in this book, Lookout Mountain is also one of the widest and most wonderful viewpoints, stretching from south of the Three Sisters all the way to Mount Rainier and including desert, lakes, and the Columbia River.

DESCRIPTION

First, for the out-and-back route, which is a lot more work but comes with a lot of benefits: From the trailhead on OR 35, the first couple of miles are relentlessly uphill. On Gumjuwac Trail #480, you'll gain 1,400 feet in 1.8 miles to reach a view of Mount Hood and then catch a little break over the last 0.5 mile to Gumjuwac Saddle. All this is in the forest: slow, steady, soft, and shady.

If you're thinking of driving Forest Service Road (FR) 3550 to this point, you'd better have some clearance. But if you insist, turn right at the BADGER LAKE sign mentioned in the directions to High Prairie, then bounce about 3 miles to

DISTANCE & CONFIGURATION: 3-mile loop (starting from High Prairie), 9.6-mile out-and-back (starting at OR 35)

DIFFICULTY: Easy for loop, strenuous for out-and-back

SCENERY: Meadows, forest, one of the great vistas around here

EXPOSURE: Shady; exposed rock at the top

TRAFFIC: Moderate on weekends, light otherwise

TRAIL SURFACE: Packed dirt, rock

HIKING TIME: 1 hour for loop, 5 hours for out-and-back

ELEVATION CHANGE: 2,900' if you start at OR 35

SEASON: July–October

BEST TIME: August and September

BACKPACKING OPTIONS: Not great; some sites around Senecal Spring

DRIVING DISTANCE: 70 miles (1 hour, 40 minutes) from Pioneer Courthouse Square; add another 20 minutes for the shorter loop.

ACCESS: Northwest Forest Pass (see page 14) required at High Prairie Trailhead

MAPS: Green Trails *Map 462 (Mount Hood)*, USGS *Badger Lake*

WHEELCHAIR ACCESS: No

FACILITIES: Outhouse at High Prairie Trailhead; nothing at OR 35

LOCATION: OR 35, 13 miles east of Government Camp, OR

CONTACT: Barlow Ranger District, 541-467-2291, www.fs.usda.gov/mthood

the saddle. The name *Gumjuwac* comes from a sheepherder named Jack. Apparently, Jack liked gum shoes; hence "Gum Shoe Jack," which somehow morphed into "Gumjuwac" over the years.

At Gumjuwac Saddle, on FR 3550, Gumjuwac Trail crosses the road and drops to the other side of the ridge, into Badger Creek Wilderness. But to keep going to Lookout Mountain, cross the road and take Divide Trail #458 to the left. You'll encounter a lovely spring 0.9 mile up; on this stretch you'll also have a view of Lookout Mountain straight ahead (the summit is actually to the right and appears lower than the one on the left). And you'll see why this trail is called Divide Trail. Technically, it splits two watersheds—Hood River from The Dalles—but it also exhibits the amazing contrast between east and west. Coming up Gumjuwac Trail, it's all shady, with a view of glacier-covered Mount Hood, but on this side you'll encounter meadows, flowers, and views of the desert. As you climb with Mount Hood on your left, look for views over your right shoulder to Badger Lake. Watch for wildlife, too: I once saw two falcons chasing each other around here, and another time I scared up an owl in the woods.

After the spring, the trail gets a little steeper; also note that a recent fire led to a slight reroute of this section, meaning most maps are not completely up-to-date. Keep climbing, and just below a summit of sorts, continue straight and uphill where High Prairie Loop #493 cuts left. This will put you on a rocky outcrop with an amazing view; many people stop here, but it's not the top of Lookout Mountain. To get there, put Mount Hood behind you and keep going, staying on Divide Trail. You'll walk along a rocky ridge and keep right where an old road goes left and then climb

Lookout Mountain

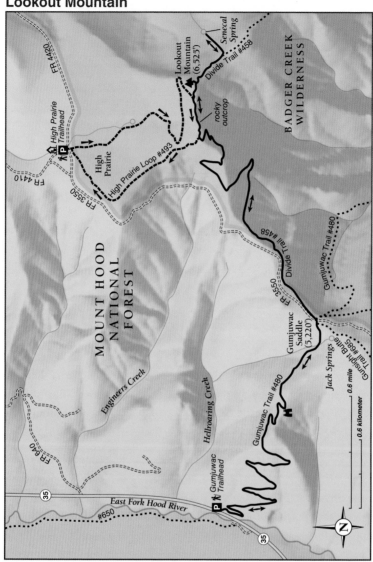

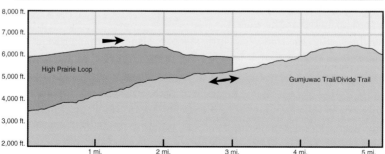

a short way to a trail leading left, to the wide-open summit and the foundation of an old fire lookout. For a description of the view, see below.

There's one more spring up here that's worth visiting. To reach Senecal Spring—named for a U.S. Forest Service ranger from the turn of the 20th century—take Divide Trail 0.2 mile past the summit, and turn left on a trail that's barely visible and whose sign is often lying on the ground. The (very cold) spring is 0.25 mile below Divide Trail.

The Shorter Loop

If you're more into driving up long hills than walking up them, choose High Prairie Loop. Lookout Mountain has many trails, some of which aren't marked on maps. So take our map with you and remember that just about all these trails go to the same two places: Lookout Mountain and the trailhead.

From the parking area on FR 4410, walk straight across the road and up the wide path—so well worn it's practically paved—into the meadows filled with daisies and lupines. Stay on the trail to preserve the flowers. The trail you see immediately on your right, labeled for horses, is High Prairie Loop #493; ignore it for now.

Follow the wide trail ahead 0.7 mile until, in an area of reddish rock, it splits into three. Take the far-left option, the widest trail, and you'll loop around to a point with a view east of the Cascades, out into the Oregon High Desert. The road then swings back around to the right and intersects Divide Trail #458. Turn left on Divide Trail, climb a bit, and follow a narrow trail to the left to reach the summit. Like Gumjuwac Trail, this approach is listed on our elevation profile.

To finish this loop after the summit, take Divide Trail along the ridge past the old road another 0.1 mile, then drop left briefly to turn right onto High Prairie Trail #493. In just under a mile you'll be back at the trailhead.

The Summit

The view from Lookout Mountain's 6,525-foot summit is one that you just can't get from the western side of the Cascades, or for that matter from most points in the Cascades. From left to right, on a clear day, you can see Diamond Peak; the Three Sisters; and Mounts Jefferson, Hood (absolutely huge, just 7 miles across the way), St. Helens, Rainier, and Adams. From Diamond Peak to Mount Rainier, as the crow flies, it's about 225 miles. You can also see, if you look closely, a stretch of the Columbia River to the northeast and the Flag Point Lookout to the east.

If you came up from Gumjuwac, you might as well see some new country on the way back by checking out High Prairie: From the summit, walk toward Mount Hood on Divide Trail, retracing your steps from the trip up. At 0.1 mile, turn right on the signed Trail #493 (here an old road), and follow it down into the meadows. Then just come back and head for the car. If you want to make a loop up here, keep going down that road 0.7 mile, and take a trail to the left, just before the trailhead. Following that for a mile will put you back on Divide Trail.

GPS TRAILHEAD COORDINATES
Gumjuwac Trailhead N45° 20.396' W121° 34.197'
High Prairie Trailhead N45° 21.124' W121° 31.866'

DIRECTIONS Take US 26 from Portland, driving 51 miles east of I-205. Turn left (north) on OR 35, following signs for Hood River. For the longer hike, on Gumjuwac Trail, drive 11 miles on OR 35 and park along the shoulder on the right, just after the road crosses the East Fork Hood River. There's not much space here, but you can find more 100 yards north on the other side of the highway.

For the shorter loop, at High Prairie, drive 2.5 miles farther on OR 35 and turn right onto FR 44. Drive 3.7 miles and turn right, following a sign for High Prairie, onto gravel FR 4410. Over the next 4.6 miles—during which the road occasionally rides like a washboard—take the larger, more uphill road at all the junctions. At a sign for Badger Lake, on the right, follow FR 4410 around to the left; the parking area is 100 yards ahead.

Note that you can also take I-84 and OR 35 via Hood River to these trailheads; that way is some 20 miles longer but about the same time. Heck, make it a loop and get a beer in town.

Badger Lake and the Badger Creek Wilderness from Lookout Mountain

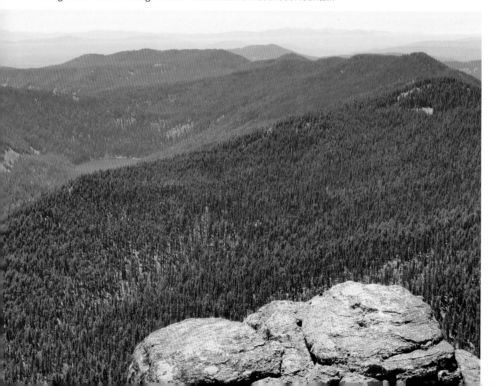

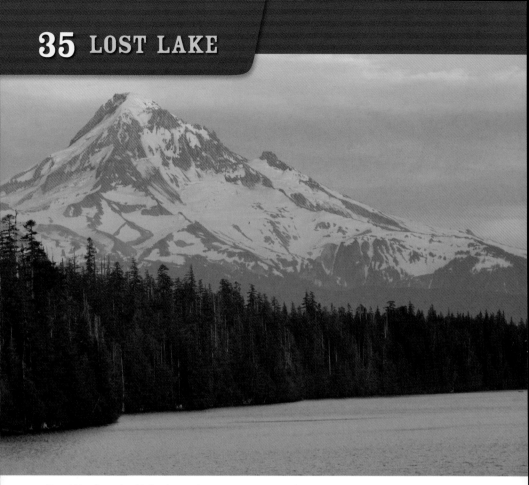

Mount Hood over Lost Lake at sunset

THE SOMEWHAT RUSTIC resort at Lost Lake is a great place to spend a night or two, with boats for rent, picnic tables with grills, a campground, and a beautiful lake stocked with trout. It's also a lovely walk around the natural 240-acre lake, including an interpretive, barrier-free, old-growth trail and one of the most photographed views of Mount Hood—all this, plus two optional longer hikes, one of them to a fine lookout point.

DESCRIPTION

Whether you're looking for a pleasant family campout or a good day of hiking, Lost Lake has what you need; that's why there are often so many people there. But as is always the case, their numbers decrease in direct proportion to how far you walk and your ability to avoid weekends.

Around the Lake

For the 3.3-mile trail around the lake, start in front of the general store. Walk to the boat dock and turn right. The first 0.25 mile of Lost Lake Trail #620, which parallels

DISTANCE & CONFIGURATION: 3.3-mile loop around the lake, 4.6-mile out-and-back to Lost Lake Butte, 16-mile out-and-back to Buck Peak

DIFFICULTY: Easy around the lake, moderate to Lost Lake Butte, strenuous to Buck Peak

SCENERY: Lake, beaches, views of Mount Hood, huge trees

EXPOSURE: Shady except at lake and atop butte

TRAFFIC: Heavy on summer days, nuts on weekends

TRAIL SURFACE: Packed dirt and boardwalk

HIKING TIME: 1.5 hours around lake, 2.5 hours to Lost Lake Butte, 9 hours to Buck Peak

ELEVATION CHANGE: Virtually none around the lake, 1,270' to the butte, 2,500' to Buck Peak

SEASON: June–October; call the resort to make sure the road is snow-free before June.

BEST TIME: August and September

BACKPACKING OPTIONS: Sites along the Pacific Crest Trail on the way to Buck Peak

DRIVING DISTANCE: 88 miles (1 hour, 45 minutes) from Pioneer Courthouse Square

ACCESS: $8/vehicle day-use fee

MAPS: Green Trails *Map 461 (Government Camp)*; resort maps available free at Lost Lake General Store

WHEELCHAIR ACCESS: 2 miles of lakeside trails, including old-growth boardwalk

FACILITIES: Full-service camping resort

LOCATION: 9000 Lost Lake Road, Hood River, OR

CONTACT: Lost Lake Resort, 541-386-6366, lostlakeresort.org

the road, is dotted with lakeside picnic tables. Soon you'll come to a platform with a view of Mount Hood that may look quite familiar from calendars or postcards. Come back here at the end of the day for the best photographic light.

Beyond the platform, the trail leaves the road and you're actually out in the woods. In late summer, your progress may be slowed by plump, ripe huckleberries. Keep an eye out for signs identifying tree species.

After just less than a mile, you'll come to a marshy area where the trail becomes a boardwalk. At 1.6 miles there's a rockslide with excellent swimming. After another mile, you'll see Huckleberry Mountain Trail #617 leading right 2.5 miles to an intersection with the Pacific Crest Trail (PCT). More on that in a bit.

Just past Huckleberry Mountain Trail, after rounding the southern end of the lake, you reach a junction and have a choice. You can keep going on this trail and stick with the lakeshore, passing fishing platforms and campsites. But I suggest you veer right and away from Lakeshore Trail #660, then stay left as you approach a group of buildings. This will put you on a road; Old Growth Trail #657 begins 100 yards ahead on a boardwalk and immediately passes between two of the largest cedars you're likely to ever see—both in the neighborhood of 12 feet in diameter.

This 1-mile trail is great for kids because it's not too long and includes educational signs explaining the roles that nurse logs, the forest canopy, weather, and animals play in a forest's life. Some of these trees are hundreds of years old and more than 200 feet tall. When the boardwalk runs out, continue another 0.3 mile, and follow Lakeshore Express Trail to the left. It goes through the campground and down to the lake; turn right to get back to the store.

Lost Lake

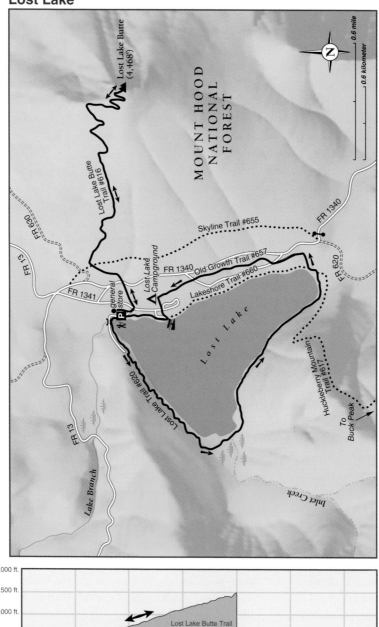

Lost Lake Butte (4,468')

MOUNT HOOD NATIONAL FOREST

FR 630
FR 13
FR 1341
FR 13
Lake Branch

Lost Lake Butte Trail #616

Skyline Trail #655
FR 1340
FR 620
Old-Growth Trail #657
FR 1340
Lakeshore Trail #660

Lost Lake Campground
general store
P

Lost Lake Trail #620

Lost Lake

Huckleberry Mountain Trail #617

To Buck Peak

Inlet Creek

0.6 mile
0.6 kilometer

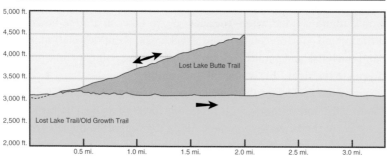

Lost Lake Butte Trail

Lost Lake Trail/Old Growth Trail

5,000 ft.
4,500 ft.
4,000 ft.
3,500 ft.
3,000 ft.
2,500 ft.
2,000 ft.

0.5 mi.　1.0 mi.　1.5 mi.　2.0 mi.　2.5 mi.　3.0 mi.

Lost Lake Butte

To climb Lost Lake Butte for the best view in the area, start in the general store's parking area. Walk back up the road and, at the turnoff for the main exit, look for a sign and a trail heading into the woods. You'll come to an unsigned trail intersection; turn right and uphill here. A hundred yards later, you'll cross another road—aim for a sign that reads LOST LAKE BUTTE TRAILHEAD. It can get confusing here, but when in doubt, keep going uphill. It's a steady climb of 1,300 feet in 2 miles to the former site of a fire lookout. You will know you're on the right path when you cross Skyline Trail #655, 0.2 mile beyond all the roads.

Mount Hood, of course, is the dominant view to the south, but you can also see as far north as Mount Rainier. Then come back down the way you went up, and get yourself a cool drink or some ice cream at the store as a reward for all your effort. (Constant access to refreshments is one of the great things about Lost Lake.)

Note: A one-day fishing license, required for visitors age 14 and up, costs $16.

To Buck Peak

This one's a bit of a slog, but it offers some amazing forest, a little introduction to the PCT, and a lookout at the end. Across Lost Lake from the general store, start up Huckleberry Mountain Trail #617, which, at least according to all the maps, goes nowhere near anything called Huckleberry Mountain. I can't explain it.

The trail is steep for the first mile, gaining 700 feet, and passes some undesirable campsites along the way. A flatter mile leads to the PCT junction; turn right. Soon you'll pass a much better campsite at Salvation Spring, which for years had a handwritten (and misspelled) sign reading SALVATOIN SPRING. I hope it's still there.

Now the trail climbs gently for a mile through towering forest to a saddle between Preachers Peak and Devils Pulpit. A U.S. Forest Service ranger named the former for his father, a local minister; the latter got its name because somebody remarked that if a preacher is here, the devil can't be far away!

Passing between those peaks, the PCT offers views of Lost Lake and Mount Adams to the east as it loses elevation 0.5 mile to a rock pile on the left. Here you can scramble up for a rare view west into Bull Run watershed, the uncut, off-limits drainage that supplies Portland's water. You can just make out Bull Run Lake to the left.

At a total of 6.8 miles since the trailhead (about 2.5 miles since you got on the PCT), you'll round a ridge where the view north takes in a large bowl with two peaks at the far end—the one on the right, Buck Peak, is our destination. Work your way around the bowl, and 1 mile north from the viewing point, an unsigned, brushy trail heads up to the right; this is your 0.5-mile summit trail.

The view from 4,751-foot Buck Peak takes in Mounts Hood, Adams, Jefferson, and Defiance (the forested one with the radio towers), as well as Lost Lake and the upper parts of the Hood River Valley. Along the summit to the left are the rusty remains of an old lookout tower, in a small meadow that makes a fine picnic site.

To return, retrace your steps, finish the loop around the lake, perhaps go for a swim, and go get ice cream at the store.

NEARBY ACTIVITIES

The Apple Valley Country Store (2363 Tucker Road, Hood River, OR; 541-386-1971; applevalleystore.com) is one of my favorite places in the world. They use local fruits to create a wide variety of treats, and annual events include barbecues and fall weekends when pear dumplings are served. (Trust me—you want a pear dumpling.)

• •

GPS TRAILHEAD COORDINATES N45° 29.789' W121° 49.141'

DIRECTIONS Take I-84 from Portland to Exit 62 (West Hood River). Make a right at the end of the off-ramp, then immediately turn right again, onto Country Club Road, following signs for several wineries. At the end of the road, 3 miles later, turn left at a stop sign onto Barrett Drive. Continue 1.3 miles and turn right on Tucker Road. Go 2 miles up Tucker and turn right on Dee Highway, where a sign reads PARKDALE. Drive 6.5 miles, then turn right onto Forest Service Road (FR) 13, following signs for Lost Lake. The resort is 14 miles ahead, at the end of FR 1341—just keep following the signs for Lost Lake.

The magical forests along the Pacific Crest Trail above Lost Lake

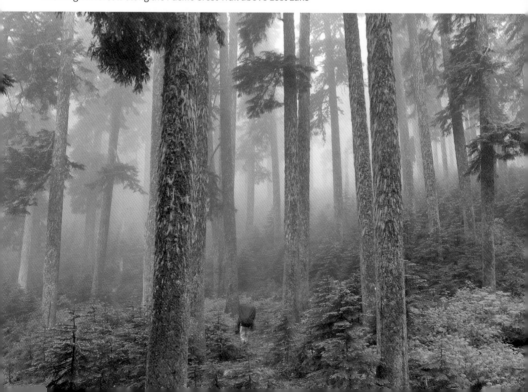

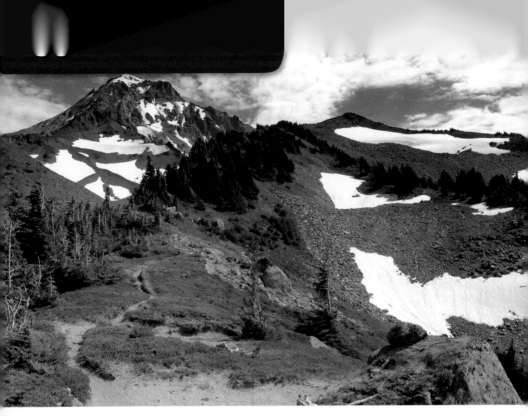

McNeil Point leaving Timberline Trail for Mount Hood's high country

THIS TRAIL OPENS with a great view, passes through a cathedral forest to wildflower meadows and alpine ponds, then gets up close and personal with Mount Hood. If you go all the way up, you can hear glaciers pop and rumble.

DESCRIPTION

This is a honey of a hike. Start out on Top Spur Trail #785, which climbs gradually 0.5 mile to a veritable highway interchange of trails. First you'll reach the Pacific Crest Trail (PCT); turn right. At a four-way junction with Timberline Trail #600, the PCT, on the right, leads down 2.2 miles to the Ramona Falls trail (Hike 38, page 192). To head for McNeil Point, follow Timberline Trail #600 uphill and to the left. But it's well worth it to see the magnificent view from the open side (not actually the top) of Bald Mountain, a mere 0.4 mile the other way (the middle path) on Timberline Trail. Head out there to take in the sweeping view of Mount Hood and the Muddy Fork Sandy River. Then keep going, toward Mount Hood, and look for a signed cutoff trail that goes over the ridge to your left, just before the trail heads back into the woods (if you come to a gate, you just missed it). The cutoff extends about 100 yards over the ridge and back to Timberline Trail; turn right for McNeil Point.

This stretch of Timberline Trail lies in a true cathedral forest—the tall, straight trees, mostly hemlocks, have no branches on their lower portions, creating a forest

DISTANCE & CONFIGURATION: 12-mile out-and-back

DIFFICULTY: Easy to Bald Mountain viewpoint, strenuous to McNeil Point

SCENERY: Old-growth forest, meadows, rugged mountainside

EXPOSURE: Shady, with a few stretches on rock and snow

TRAFFIC: Heavy on summer weekends, light otherwise

TRAIL SURFACE: Packed dirt with roots, a few small stream crossings, some rocks and snow

HIKING TIME: 5.5 hours

ELEVATION CHANGE: 2,220'

SEASON: July–October

BEST TIME: August and September

BACKPACKING OPTIONS: Excellent

DRIVING DISTANCE: 57 miles (1 hour, 30 minutes) from Pioneer Courthouse Square

ACCESS: Northwest Forest Pass required (see page 14)

MAPS: USFS *Mount Hood Wilderness*; trailhead and early part of hike are on Green Trails *Map 461 (Government Camp)*, and the rest is on Green Trails *Map 462 (Mount Hood)*.

WHEELCHAIR ACCESS: No

FACILITIES: None at trailhead; water on trail must be treated.

CONTACT: Zigzag Ranger District, 503-622-3191, www.fs.usda.gov/mthood

LOCATION: Top Spur (McNeil Point) Trailhead off Forest Service Road (FR) 1828, 12 miles northeast of Zigzag, OR

COMMENTS: Bring warm clothing if you're going to McNeil Point. It's above the treeline, and weather changes quickly up here.

scene that's both open and lofty. Adding to the pleasure are the many huckleberry bushes that make up the ground cover; their juicy morsels are typically ripe in late August. You'll hardly notice that you've started climbing in earnest.

On Timberline Trail, pass McGee Creek Trail #627 on the left (more on it later), and at the first big view of Mount Hood you come to (you'll have gone 2.3 miles), look for the large, unnamed waterfall across the valley on Hood's flank. At 3.5 miles, you'll cross a fork of McGee Creek and, if it's around August, arrive in the land of wildflowers. Lupines, daisies, pasqueflowers, lilies, and butterflies will welcome you to the high country. Just a bit farther are a couple of ponds, which make ideal places to stop for lunch and also host some fine campsites. You can skip and frolic in this area and call it a day, or you can keep going to even higher country.

At 3.9 miles, soon after Mazama Trail #625 has come in from the left, you'll see the old McNeil Point Trail, now closed for revegetation. Timberline Trail next passes through one more patch of forest—look for the Mount Adams view on the far side—and then intersects the new trail to the point, heading up and to the right.

If you just want more meadows without more climbing, stay on the main trail as it swings left, negotiate a stream crossing that can be mildly dangerous in high water, and connect with the outer reaches of the Vista Ridge trip (Hike 44, page 218) for Cairn Basin and Eden Park. If you're set on McNeil Point, turn right and climb the braided trail that seems to wander a bit. It all goes to the same place, so just stick to the ridge.

About 0.5 mile up, the trail crosses a rockslide and, in most years, a snowfield. Be careful on both these terrains: they aren't steep, but remember that even big

McNeil Point

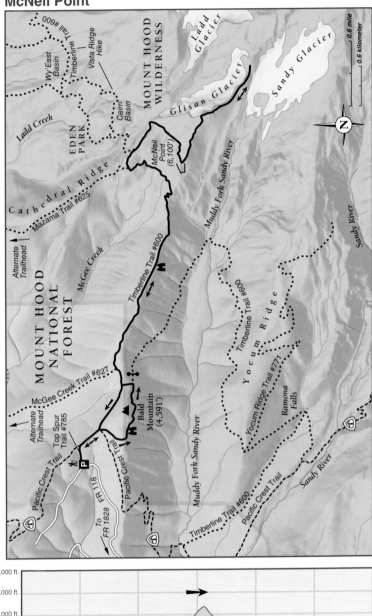

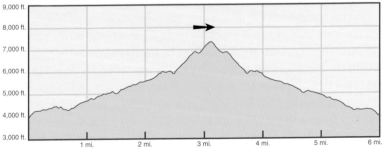

rocks move and that even packed snow is slippery. The trail keeps ascending the ridge face, crossing occasional small patches of snow. At a Y junction, head right for the official McNeil Point, or go left to stay higher. Note some side trails leading down and to the right, to campsites in the trees below.

One mile from the turnoff at the creek, you'll reach the 1930s-era stone shelter at McNeil Point. From here the view is stupendous: Mount Hood soaring above you, the valley of the Muddy Fork Sandy River stretching out below you, and the other Cascade volcanoes beyond. As you look at Mount Hood, the sprawling glacier on your right is Sandy Glacier, and the trickle coming out the bottom of it is the beginning of the Muddy Fork Sandy, which flows into the Columbia River down at Troutdale. See if you can also spot Lost Lake to the north and Bald Peak, which you just visited, looking like a green gash on the side of a hill. Evidence of the 2011 Dollar Fire on Mount Hood is clearly visible to your right.

Also, as you look at Mount Hood, you'll notice more trail above you, heading into the Really High Country. It's not on any maps, but if you follow it you'll (1) soon run out of breath as you approach 7,000 feet in elevation with virtually no switchbacks and (2) find yourself on a narrow, rocky ridge between Glisan (on your left) and Sandy (on your right) Glaciers. Somebody formed quite the bivouac among the rocks up there.

You may hear or see reports of another, more direct trail between McNeil Point and Timberline Trail, connecting with the latter at a point west of the ponds. Avoid that trail. It's steep, rocky, difficult, and unnecessary. The one described here is easier and more scenic, and it doesn't tear up sensitive habitat

Alternative Trailheads

The Top Spur Trailhead just wasn't made to handle the number of people using it. So go during the week, carpool, or even consider some of the other trailheads that access the same area. The best option, for me, is McGee Creek Trail #627; it's 0.2 mile longer with 400 more feet of elevation. To get there, stick with Lolo Pass Road all the way to the pass, take the second right onto FR 18, and the trailhead is a mile ahead on the right. Just 1.5 mile farther along that road is the Mazama Trail, which climbs 2,100 feet over 3.1 miles to the Timberline Trail.

• •

GPS TRAILHEAD COORDINATES N45° 24.467' W121° 47.149'

DIRECTIONS Take US 26 from Portland to Zigzag; turn left onto Lolo Pass Road. Go 4.2 miles; turn right onto Muddy Fork Road, signed for campgrounds and trailheads. The trailhead is 7.1 miles ahead, on the right.

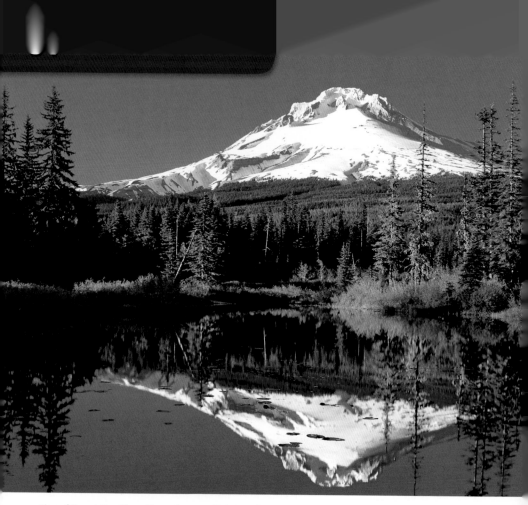

View of Mount Hood from the aptly named Mirror Lake

YOU CAN GO a short way on this hike and join the weekend throngs at a lovely little lake with a great view of Mount Hood. Or you can put in a little more effort and leave most of the crowds behind to claim an even better view at the top of—believe it or not—Tom, Dick, and Harry Mountain.

DESCRIPTION

When you come around the corner on US 26 and see 75 cars parked on the side of the road, know that it's not a fair; it's the Mirror Lake Trailhead. The interest in this trail is well justified, so think about starting early or going on a weekday to have a decent chance for some quiet time (and keep an eye out for that new trailhead; see Comments, above right).

The lower portions of Mirror Lake Trail #664 have rhododendrons that bloom pink in late June, and the upper portions are cool and shady, keeping you from warming up too much as you head up the hill. But it isn't even much of a hill, gaining

DISTANCE & CONFIGURATION: 2.8-mile out-and-back to lake, 6-mile out-and-back to ridge

DIFFICULTY: Easy to lake, strenuous to ridge

SCENERY: Rhododendrons; deep forest; small, placid lake; big view

EXPOSURE: Shady on the way up, open at lake, wide-open atop ridge

TRAFFIC: Heavy all summer, insane on weekends

TRAIL SURFACE: Packed dirt, rocks

HIKING TIME: 2 hours to lake, 4 hours to ridge

ELEVATION CHANGE: 780' to lake, 1,520 to ridge

SEASON: Late June–October

BEST TIME: August and September

BACKPACKING OPTIONS: A few sites at lake

DRIVING DISTANCE: 54 miles (1 hour, 15 minutes) from Pioneer Courthouse Square

ACCESS: Northwest Forest Pass required May 15–October 1 (see page 14)

MAPS: Green Trails *Map 461 (Government Camp)*, USFS *Mount Hood Wilderness*, USGS *Government Camp*

WHEELCHAIR ACCESS: No

FACILITIES: Portable restroom at trailhead

CONTACT: Zigzag Ranger District, 503-622-3191, www.fs.usda.gov/mthood

LOCATION: Mirror Lake Trailhead on US 26, 2 miles west of Government Camp, OR

COMMENTS: Though this trail is popular as a snowshoe destination, parking at the trailhead November 1–April 30 is prohibited; your car will be towed. Even in summer, parking outside the signs marking the lot will get you towed. When this book was written, a project was under way to create an entirely new trailhead for this hike, off US 26 in a new parking area near Skibowl. Projected completion was October of 2018; see tinyurl.com/mirrorth for the latest.

less than 800 feet in 1.4 well-graded miles. Just below the lake, you'll come to the outlet creek and a trail junction. You can go either way to loop 0.4 mile around the lake, but if you're headed up the ridge, bear right.

The lake itself is a beauty. The beaches are on the right side, the (unimpressive) campsites are on the left, and the view of Mount Hood you're looking for is at the far end, on the boardwalk in a marshy area.

To get to the top of Tom, Dick, and Harry Mountain, walk to the far right side of the lake (as you face it when you arrive), and follow a trail that goes right and steadily climbs the face of the ridge. Your destination is actually right above you, but you have to walk almost 2 miles to get there. As for the mountain's name, it indicates the three peaks on the ridge—not, as some would suggest, the fact that every Tom, Dick, and Harry hikes this trail.

The trail is really just two lengthy switchbacks, each almost a mile long. It's time to turn left when you get to some serious rock cairns. The forest opens a little more here, and as you approach the summit the trail gets a smidgen steeper. When you reach a rocky area (neither steep nor dangerous), you're almost there.

The view from atop this ridge is really something, considering how close you still are to your car. For starters, look at how pitifully small—and how far down—Mirror Lake is. It never ceases to amaze me how quickly you gain elevation when hiking. Right across the highway is Mount Hood, in all its glory. It's actually blocking

Mirror Lake

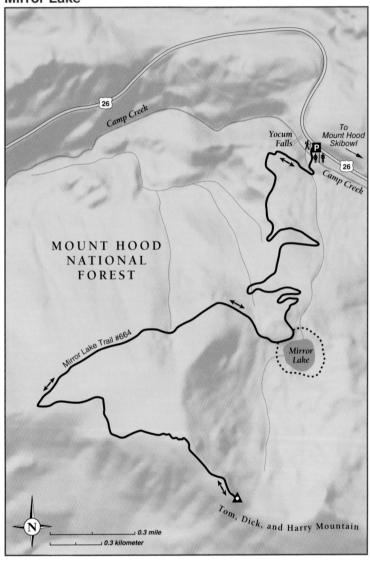

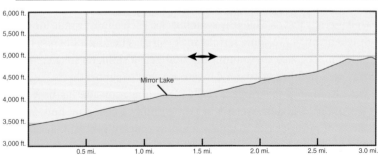

Mount Adams. To the left is Mount St. Helens. What looks like a shoulder on St. Helens is in fact Mount Rainier, some 100 miles north of you.

If you're still feeling energetic, resist the temptation to explore the other two peaks on this ridge—Tom and Dick, as it were. They're off-limits because they're home to protected peregrine falcons. A random historical note: In the opening scene of the film *Wild*, Reese Witherspoon (as Cheryl Strayed) tossed a boot off a cliff. Though it was set on the PCT, that scene was filmed up here somewhere (they used the chairlift at Skibowl, the cheaters). Some two years later, a hiker found (and kept) the boot way down in the rocks below.

NEARBY ACTIVITIES

The easternmost peak of Tom, Dick, and Harry Mountain is the summit of Mt. Hood Skibowl, which, in the summer, is like a constant carnival. You can bungee-jump, ride the alpine slide, play minigolf, drive go-carts, take a trip in a helicopter, or ride the chairlift to the top of the hill and hike or mountain-bike down. The entrance is 1 mile east of the Mirror Lake Trailhead on US 26. Call 503-222-BOWL (2695) or visit skibowl.com for details.

. . . .

GPS TRAILHEAD COORDINATES N45° 18.410' W121° 47.534'

DIRECTIONS Take US 26 from Portland, driving 45 miles east of I-205. Park at the trailhead, on the right. It's 0.5 mile past the historical marker for the Laurel Hill Chute, also on the right. And take note of the new trailhead coming, at least in theory, in the fall of 2018. See Comments, page 189.

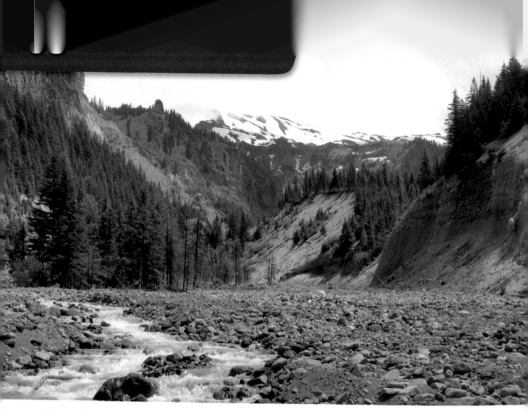

The Sandy River winds through a recent lahar (mudflow).

THIS IMMENSELY POPULAR trail is a fairly easy hike to a beautiful waterfall, with campsites and room for a picnic when you get there.

DESCRIPTION

This hike starts on a trail that looks like a highway; that's because it's basically flat and thousands of people make the trek to the falls every year. Walk 0.2 mile and cross Sandy River Trail #770; continue on Ramona Falls Trail #797, admiring a large, cracked boulder near the junction. A short walk rewards you with a view of Mount Hood up the main stem of the Sandy River. You'll also see the results of a massive 2007 flood. The deep cut you see here didn't exist before that, and at one point about a mile up you can see the former trail reappearing on the far edge of a big bend in the gorge.

At 1.2 miles, you reach the Sandy River crossing. In the fall, you can cross without the logs if there hasn't been much rain. Otherwise, be super careful, and look for other spots to cross. Check for recent trip reports in the forums at oregonhikers .org. After crossing, follow the ribbons across the debris flow, putting in 0.25 mile to reach a junction with Trail #797 as well as the Pacific Crest Trail (PCT) as it makes its way around the west side of Mount Hood. The signage here is a little goofy, because both trails are #797 *and* the PCT. This is also where your loop starts, so for now turn right onto the PCT, and continue your gradual climb over moss-covered ground and

DISTANCE & CONFIGURATION: 7.1-mile balloon to falls, 16-mile balloon up Yocum Ridge

DIFFICULTY: Easy

SCENERY: Stream, historic cabin, waterfall, possible trip to high country

EXPOSURE: Woods with occasional open spots

TRAFFIC: Heavy, especially on summer weekends

TRAIL SURFACE: Packed dirt

HIKING TIME: 4 hours to falls, 9 hours to Yocum Ridge

ELEVATION CHANGE: 1,100' to falls, 3,600' to Yocum Ridge

SEASON: May–October

BEST TIME: July–September

BACKPACKING OPTIONS: Campsites near falls and on Yocum Ridge

DRIVING DISTANCE: 53 miles (1 hour, 20 minutes) from Pioneer Courthouse Square

ACCESS: Northwest Forest Pass required (see page 14)

MAPS: Green Trails *Map 461 (Government Camp),* USFS *Mount Hood Wilderness,* USGS *Bull Run Lake*

WHEELCHAIR ACCESS: No

FACILITIES: None at trailhead; campground with water and toilets less than a mile away

CONTACT: Zigzag Ranger District, 503-622-3191, www.fs.usda.gov/mthood

LOCATION: Ramona Falls Trailhead at end of Muddy Fork Road, 7 miles northeast of Zigzag, OR

COMMENTS: Until 2014, the U.S. Forest Service put in a seasonal bridge over the Sandy River every May; it has been replaced by logs thrown together mostly by hikers. Keep this in mind, especially early in the season, after a big rain, or if you are bringing kids. Also, many hikers have had their cars broken into at this trailhead—leave valuables at home, and consider leaving the door unlocked so they won't take out your window.

under large rhododendrons. A mile past the junction, you'll reach the top of a bluff from which the Sandy River is more audible. Look for eroded cliffs across the way, which offer a cross-section of Mount Hood's volcanic deposits.

When you're 1.5 miles past the junction (3 miles from your car), you hit the Timberline Trail and another bizarre intersection. To your left is the Timberline/Ramona Falls Trail. To your right is the PCT/Timberline Trail, heading toward the river; follow it for a short descent to a pretty sad campsite near the shore. The PCT crosses the Sandy here and starts a long climb toward Timberline Lodge; it's worth walking out to the crossing to stand on the debris flow and catch views up the canyon toward Hood and some big-time waterfalls. Follow pink ribbons if you get confused.

Back at the campsite, look for log steps leading up the hill to a 1935 ranger station, built to keep hikers out of the Bull Run watershed. The rangers are long gone, and the cabin has been boarded up for years, but there are some tent sites nearby, along with a view of Sandy River Canyon, about 100 yards uphill. Now head back to the junction.

Back on the Ramona Falls Trail, turn left, go 0.3 mile, and pass through a gate that keeps horses from the falls area. From here you can descend left to find campsites; camping is not allowed at the falls. Pass through the gate and enter the falls area.

Ramona Falls is a perfect example of how a tiny stream can make one heck of a waterfall. The falls are best compared to a pyramid of Champagne glasses: as the water cascades over broken columns of basalt, it spreads across a 120-foot-wide expanse, the force of the water sending a cool, misty spray into the air (see page 231

Ramona Falls

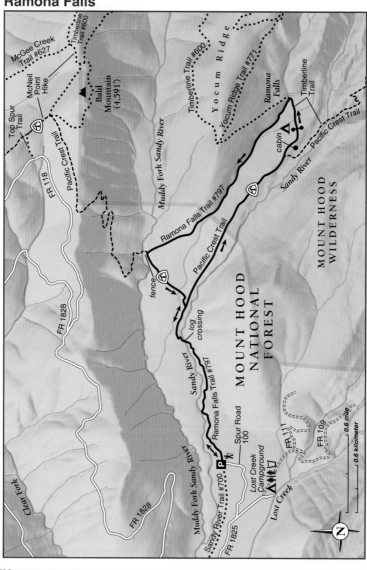

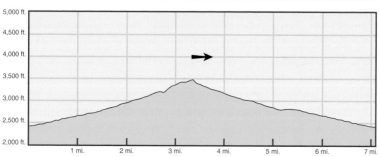

for a photo of the falls). No wonder so many people come here with kids, dogs, and picnic supplies. Just beware of the gray jays that haunt the area—they'll take food right out of your hands. Cloudy days are best for photographing the falls.

There's a nice story behind the name. In 1933, a U.S. Forest Service employee came across the falls while scouting the area for a trail. He was courting his future wife and named the falls after a popular romantic song of the time called "Ramona."

Continue over the bridge to reach a junction at the far end. Here, the Timberline Trail and Ramona Falls Trail part ways. To head back to your car, go straight. Or, if you're looking for an adventure, make a right onto Timberline Trail #600, the 42-mile wonder trail around Mount Hood. You can follow this trail 5 or so miles around the headwaters of the Sandy River's Muddy Fork to wind up on the flanks of Bald Mountain (also part of the McNeil Point hike, page 184). That trail, though, has suffered over the years from mudslides and washouts, and it can be sketchy, especially the river crossings and washouts. Call to check conditions.

What you can certainly do is put in just over 0.5 mile on Timberline Trail and then head right, up Yocum Ridge Trail #771, an occasionally steep affair that gains 2,100 feet in 4.1 miles. The reward for that effort is an amazing bit of alpine splendor, far enough from any trailhead that it receives relatively few visitors. You'll pass a pond in 2.5 miles, a campsite at 2.9, unbelievable Yocum Meadow at 4.1, and an incredible viewpoint at 4.7 miles—2,650 feet above Timberline Trail. That's the end of the official trail, but you can put in another 0.8 mile and 650 feet of elevation to another viewpoint.

To complete the simpler loop back to the parking lot from Ramona Falls, follow the trail straight ahead and down Ramona Creek. It's a gentle 1.6-mile descent, featuring several log crossings of the creek, with views of rock walls on the right. See if you can spot a little section of "underground" creek as well. After 1.9 miles you hit the PCT; turn left, pass a horse trail, cross Ramona Creek in 0.5 mile, rejoin the trail you came in on, cross the Sandy River again, and turn right to head back to the car. It gets a little weird in here, so make sure you have a map.

• •

GPS TRAILHEAD COORDINATES N45° 23.220' W121° 49.905'

DIRECTIONS From Portland, take US 26 to Zigzag. Turn left onto Lolo Pass Road, 0.6 mile past milepost 41. Go 4.2 miles and turn right onto FR 1825, 0.1 mile past a sign for Mount Hood National Forest and marked CAMPGROUNDS AND TRAILHEADS. Stay right at 0.7 mile, cross a bridge, and continue another 1.7 miles to turn left onto Spur Road 100, which leads 0.3 mile to the trailhead. (This intersection is occasionally without signs, so trust your odometer.) Going right at this last fork would take you 0.3 mile to Lost Creek Campground, which has water and restrooms.

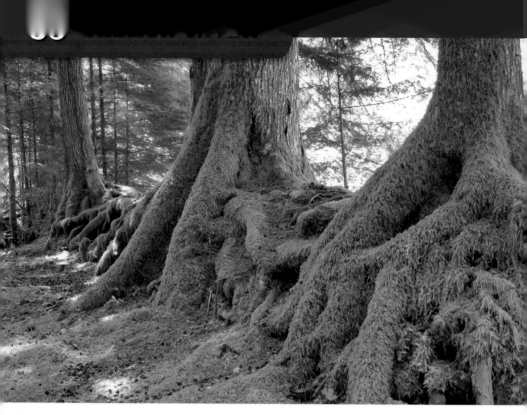

Three trees taking full advantage of a nurse log

THIS TRAIL CAN be thought of as having three sections: The upper and lower sections, described here, are easy to get to, and in the fall they host spawning salmon. The uppermost section, accessed by a different road near Trillium Lake, is less interesting and tougher to find; its only advantage is that hardly anybody hikes it. Hardier hikers can take an optional side trip to Devils Peak.

DESCRIPTION

Lower Section

This is Old Salmon River Trail #742A. From the roadside parking area (the first one you came to while driving in), you'll start out downhill through a forest of Douglas-firs and western red cedars. You'll be close to the river after 0.1 mile and follow it most of the way. (You'll also pass access to four other trailheads along the road, so be sure to remember where you left your car.) After two footbridges over side creeks, you come to the first of several trails leading down to the river. You'll pass two more small bridges and, after 0.4 mile, come to a campsite where a log sticks out over the river. It's perfectly sturdy, but be sure of your balance before you go out on it.

The best thing about this trail, other than its convenience and the river itself, is the nature of the old-growth forest. Look for nurse logs—fallen trees that are now

DISTANCE: 5.2-mile out-and-back for lower section, 6.6-mile out-and-back for upper section

DIFFICULTY: Easy all the way to the campsites in the upper section, moderate–strenuous beyond that

SCENERY: Old-growth forest, spawning salmon in spring and fall, canyon view at top

EXPOSURE: Shady all the way to the top, where there are exposed rocks

TRAFFIC: Heavy all summer long

TRAIL SURFACE: Packed dirt, with rocks and roots

HIKING TIME: 2 hours for lower section, 3.5 hours for upper section

ELEVATION CHANGE: 200' in lower section, 950' in upper section

SEASON: Year-round; gets snow in winter

BEST TIME: October for the colors and salmon

BACKPACKING OPTIONS: Nice sites in the upper section

DRIVING DISTANCE: 50 miles (1 hour, 15 minutes) from Pioneer Courthouse Square

ACCESS: Northwest Forest Pass required (see page 14)

MAPS: USFS *Salmon-Huckleberry Wilderness*

WHEELCHAIR ACCESS: No

FACILITIES: Usually an outhouse at the upper trailhead; water and restrooms at Green Canyon Campground

CONTACT: Zigzag Ranger District, 503-622-3191, www.fs.usda.gov/mthood

LOCATION: Salmon River Trail on East Salmon River Road, 5 miles south of Welches, OR

COMMENTS: The Salmon River, which starts on the slopes of Timberline Ski Area, is the only river in the lower 48 states that is classified as a Wild and Scenic River from its headwaters to its mouth. To see its headwaters and ford it where you can skip across, do the Barlow Pass or Timberline Lodge trip, pages 160 and 204, respectively.

the home of new trees. Just past the campsite with the suspended log, you'll climb a set of steps, at the top of which is a massive western red cedar. You can't miss it—it's right next to the trail and about 10 feet thick at its base. At about the 1-mile mark, look for a hollowed-out cedar stump with a new tree growing from it; just past it is the biggest Douglas-fir (about 8 feet in diameter) on this stretch of the trail.

At about the 1.5-mile mark, you'll come to the first of two sections where the trail briefly joins the road. Take the second trail back into the woods; the first trail is used by anglers and dead-ends at the river. Continue 50 yards and look for three large trees—two firs and a cedar—that are almost bonded together. Just past here, where a downed tree lies along the bank, I came across several spawning salmon on a late-September hike. They were in the shallows just a few feet from shore. The fish will actually go several miles farther upstream; if you hike the upper section of this trail in the fall, you'll get more chances to see them.

There are two more highlights to this trail. One is a cedar tree so large that a hollowed-out area in its base is big enough to be called a cave. The other is a nurse log, cut into three pieces for trail-construction purposes, that is now host to no fewer than eight saplings.

When you've hiked a little more than 2 miles, you'll come to Green Canyon Campground, which has an outhouse and water. Then, after a second section on

Salmon River

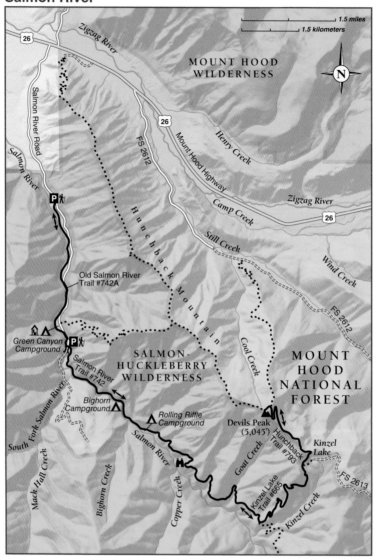

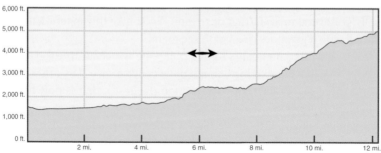

the roadside, you'll briefly drop back into the woods before emerging at the upper trailhead, where the road crosses the river.

Upper Section

Now for Salmon River Trail #742. From the trailhead at the bridge, walk upstream through a forest replete with massive Douglas-firs. Just less than 0.5 mile up, you'll pass a deep pool, where anglers often gather. A short distance past this, when you get another view of the river from about 40 feet above it, look (in September and October) for dark shapes swirling about in the pools. Those are salmon: the black-gray ones are chinook, and the less-often-seen gold ones are coho. Consider that they have spent their lives in the ocean and have swum some 75 miles up the Columbia River, about 41 miles up the Sandy, then about 20 miles up the Salmon.

At 1.5 miles, pass Bighorn Camp; then at the 2-mile mark, reach Rolling Riffle Camp, where a trail to the right leads to a little falls and deep pool. Beyond you'll pass the wilderness boundary and embark on your only real climb of the day, picking up nearly 600 feet in 1.3 miles on your way to an overlook of Salmon River Canyon. Go as far as the rock outcrop for the best view. Be very careful, and don't try any of the trails heading down toward the river—you might descend faster than intended.

Devils Peak Option

That scenic view is your recommended turnaround, as you're now 3.3 miles from the upper trailhead, but the trail goes another 10.8 miles upstream to a road near Trillium Lake. If you're feeling industrious, put in the big climb to the lookout tower at Devils Peak. Just continue 2.3 miles up Salmon River Trail #742, then turn left to climb Kinzel Lake Trail #665, following it 2.3 miles (and 1,600 feet) up to Hunchback Trail #793, which leads 1.6 miles (and another 700 feet) up to the 5,045-foot lookout. If you started at the bridge, you're looking at 9.8 miles one-way with a climb of 3,400 feet. You have other options for getting up there, but this one would be good as part of an overnight trip.

NEARBY ACTIVITIES

Start your day with French toast at the Zigzag Inn, 0.1 mile east of Salmon River Road (70162 US 26, Welches, OR; 503-622-4779; zigzaginn.com).

• •

GPS TRAILHEAD COORDINATES N45° 18.646' W121° 56.615'

DIRECTIONS Take US 26 from Portland, driving 36 miles east of I-205. Turn right on Salmon River Road. Continue 2.7 miles to reach the lower trailhead, just beyond the sign for Mount Hood National Forest, or drive 4.9 miles to the upper trailhead, at a bridge over the river.

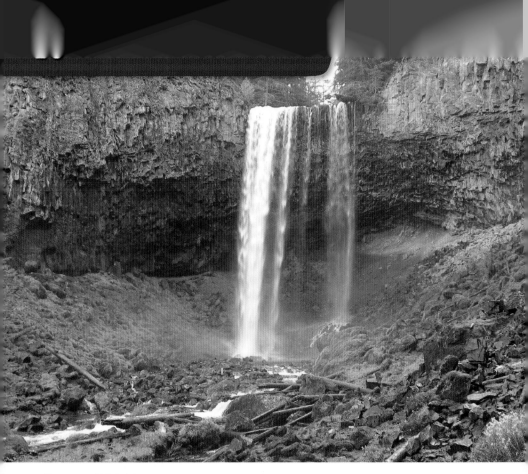

Tamanawas Falls in late summer

THIS IS A classic waterfall in a dramatic setting at the end of an easy, beautiful hike that's perfectly suited for a family outing. *Tamanawas* (pronounced ta-MAH-na-was) is a Chinook word for a friendly guardian spirit, and it's an appropriate name for this pleasant hike.

DESCRIPTION

There is an interesting history of nature versus trail in this little canyon. When I first moved to Oregon in 1996, the trail crossed the creek because years before, a massive rockslide had wiped out one side of the canyon. Then a flood in 2000 wiped out those two trail bridges, but it didn't keep folks away. Officially the trail was closed that entire summer, but Oregonians displayed their typical respect for the government by hiking the "closed" trail in such numbers that the U.S. Forest Service acquiesced and made the new, hiker-created trail—across the massive rockslide—the official one. The Forest Service hasn't rebuilt the bridges, so the trail you hike today is what the locals came up with in 2000, across a big rockslide. Then another slide came down here in 2016; see Comments in box above.

DISTANCE & CONFIGURATION: 3.4-mile out-and-back

DIFFICULTY: Easy

SCENERY: Two mountain streams, plunging waterfall

EXPOSURE: Shady all the way, then open at the end

TRAFFIC: Heavy on summer weekends, moderate otherwise

TRAIL SURFACE: Packed dirt and rocks

HIKING TIME: 2.5 hours

ELEVATION CHANGE: 590'

SEASON: June–November

BEST TIME: July–September

BACKPACKING OPTIONS: None

DRIVING DISTANCE: 75 miles (1 hour, 40 minutes) from Pioneer Courthouse Square

ACCESS: Northwest Forest Pass required (see page 14)

MAPS: Green Trails *Map 462 (Mount Hood)*, USFS *Mount Hood Wilderness*, USGS *Dog River*

WHEELCHAIR ACCESS: No

FACILITIES: None at trailhead; water and restrooms 0.5 mile south on OR 35, at Sherwood Campground

CONTACT: Hood River Ranger District, 541-352-6002, www.fs.usda.gov/mthood

LOCATION: Tamanawas Falls Trailhead on OR 35, 11 miles south of Parkdale, OR

COMMENTS: In October 2016 a very large rockslide came down onto this trail, just before the falls. This has happened before, in 2000, and a new trail—really just a way through the slide— was created by hikers. But this one is bigger, and as of press time, more than a year later, the U.S. Forest Service had not even made an announcement on their website about it. People have been climbing over it, but I wouldn't recommend it with kids. For the latest, check with the Forest Service or the trip reports forum at oregonhikers.org.

From the trailhead, walk right and cross the East Fork Hood River on a one-log bridge with handrails. Note the milky color of the river; that's silt from glaciers up on the mountain. At the far end of the bridge, join East Fork Trail #650, and follow it to the right, where it parallels the road 0.5 mile. Ignore the mileage on that sign, by the way—you're 1.6 miles from the falls, not 2.

At 0.7 mile, you'll leave East Fork Trail and cross Cold Spring Creek on Tamanawas Falls Trail #650A. Now enjoy a lovely stretch right along the creek, passing numerous cascades, creekside picnic areas, and forest features, and in 0.7 mile come to that rockslide area, where Tamanawas Tie Trail #650B splits off to the right. This is an interesting option if you are looking for a rather epic and solitary hike. Trail #650B climbs out of this canyon and in 0.5 mile connects to Elk Meadows Trail #645. Turn left here, and the trail follows Cold Spring Creek all the way to its source, about 7 miles up at Elk Meadows (see Hike 33, page 169). This section of trail doesn't get much maintenance, and it goes through a 2006 burn, but you have a better chance of seeing deer and elk than other people. Sadly, much of this was targeted for a timber sale as of press time, so who knows what the conditions will be.

Back at the junction of #650A and #650B, at the rockslide, the original Tamanawas Falls Trail dropped here to cross the creek; the new route goes slightly left to cross the rockslide where hikers made their way in 2000 (and at the far end of which the

Tamanawas Falls

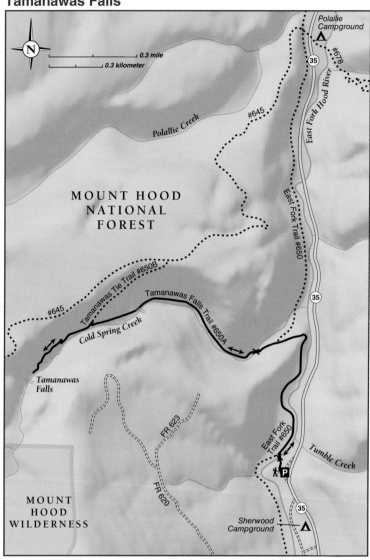

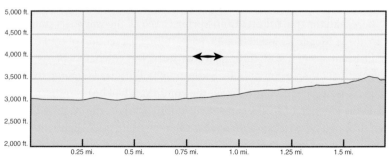

2016 slide came down.) The path winds through the boulders, and from the far side it's about 0.2 mile to the falls.

What makes this falls so special is that even in late summer there's plenty of water coming over it, and it's rimmed by basalt walls, many of which are pink because pieces have so recently fallen into the chasm. For this reason, take care if you want to go nearer (or even behind) the falls, as you'll be walking on wet rocks with no official trail and with cliffs above you—cliffs that provide ample evidence that rocks could come crashing down at any time. These are just little reminders from Mother Nature that we are, after all, just visitors in her world.

One other feature to note: a few of the trees around the falls are western larches, which you might not know unless you're here in late October and they've turned their brilliant shade of gold. Assuming it isn't raining too hard, it's a lovely time to visit.

NEARBY ACTIVITIES

Drive 7.5 miles north of the trailhead on OR 35, then turn left to visit the Hutson Museum (4697 Baseline Road, Parkdale, OR; 541-352-6806; tinyurl.com/hutson museum), which features local history, Indian artifacts, and memorabilia of the early settlers. Open April–October.

• •

GPS TRAILHEAD COORDINATES N45° 23.831' W121° 34.305'

DIRECTIONS Take US 26 from Portland, driving 51 miles east of I-205. Turn north (left) on OR 35, following signs for Hood River. Drive 15 miles on OR 35; 0.2 mile past Sherwood Campground, park at the trailhead, on the left. It's the same amount of time, though 13 miles longer, to get here by taking I-84 to Hood River and driving south on OR 35.

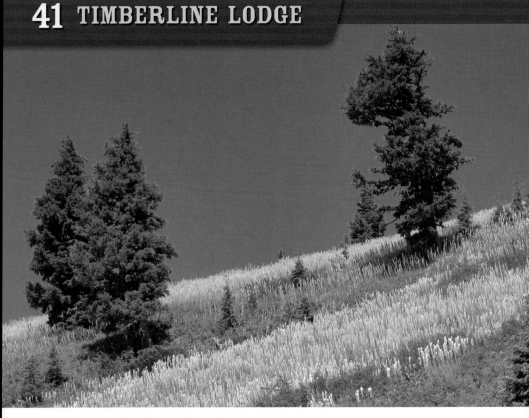

Peak beargrass on the trail to Paradise Park

IF YOU SPEND just one summer day in the Portland area, you should spend it at Timberline Lodge. If you go on only one summer hike, you should go to Paradise Park in August or early September. But fear not—if you aren't up for a 13-mile loop, shorter options abound at this spectacular mountain palace.

DESCRIPTION

Timberline Lodge was built in 1937 by the Works Progress Administration and dedicated by President Franklin D. Roosevelt the same day that he dedicated Bonneville Dam. But as astounding as the interior is, it's the setting that beckons one to spend time here. Only a few peaks in Oregon rise above it, and with few trees around, the views are amazing, especially to the summit of Mount Hood—the highest point in the state—3 miles away, and to Mount Jefferson, 45 miles south. In August, wildflowers bloom everywhere.

White River Canyon Overlook

Let's start with the shortest hike. Follow a sign to the right of the lodge, pointing you to the Pacific Crest Trail (PCT). You'll walk uphill a couple hundred yards, perhaps wondering why you're suddenly breathing heavily: it's because you're now at

DISTANCE & CONFIGURATION: 13-mile balloon loop to Paradise Park, 4.8-mile out-and-back to Zigzag Canyon overlook, 2.2-mile out-and-back or loop to Silcox Hut, 0.6-mile out-and-back to White River Canyon

DIFFICULTY: Easy to White River Overlook or Zigzag Canyon Overlook, moderate to Silcox Hut, strenuous to Paradise Park

SCENERY: Flower-filled meadows, deep canyons, waterfalls, glaciers

EXPOSURE: Both shady and open

TRAFFIC: Heavy all summer long

TRAIL SURFACE: Dirt, rock, pavement, sand

HIKING TIME: 30 minutes–7 hours

ELEVATION CHANGE: 2,300' to Paradise Park, virtually none to White River Overlook, 1,065' to Silcox Hut, 400' to Zigzag Canyon Overlook

SEASON: July–October

BEST TIME: August and September

BACKPACKING OPTIONS: Good sites in Paradise Park

DRIVING DISTANCE: 64 miles (1 hour, 30 minutes) from Pioneer Courthouse Square

ACCESS: Oregon Sno-Park Permit required November 1–April 30

MAPS: Green Trails *Map 462 (Mount Hood)*, USFS *Mount Hood Wilderness*

WHEELCHAIR ACCESS: A few patches of (steep) road around the lodge

FACILITIES: Full services at Timberline Lodge

CONTACT: Zigzag Ranger District, 503-622-3191, www.fs.usda.gov/mthood

LOCATION: Timberline Lodge Trailheads at end of Timberline Highway, 6 miles northeast of Government Camp, OR

COMMENTS: No matter what the weather looks like, bring warm clothing for this hike.

6,000 feet elevation. At the PCT, turn right and walk 0.3 mile to the White River Canyon Overlook (you'll have to skip over a couple of small creeks along the way).

If you'd like to do a one-way hike with a car shuttle, this trail is also the top of the Barlow Pass trip (Hike 31, page 160).

Silcox Hut

For our next-toughest destination, start in the parking lot, walk up a set of steps, and turn right after 20 yards, following signs for Mountaineer Loop Trail #798. Stay straight when you cross the PCT/Timberline Trail, and after passing the water tower join a road to the hut. Timberline Lodge rents this hut out to groups of 12 or more during the winter. And in the summer, you can ride the Magic Mile chairlift up here then walk down. If you're not a big spender, there's a bench to sit on outside.

Follow Mountaineer Loop Trail west by crossing under the chairlift and looking for a service road headed downhill. When it bends left, look for a trail headed down again. It drops to the PCT/Timberline Trail 1 mile west of the lodge, in forest broken up by flowered meadows. Turn left and walk to the lodge. If that's all too confusing, just walk up and down the road. Or take the chairlift up and walk down.

Zigzag Canyon Overlook

Enough with the preliminaries: let's head for Zigzag Canyon and Paradise Park. From the lodge, follow the PCT/Timberline Trail left; it will cross under two chairlifts and then descend into the woods. Hike 0.8 mile, ignoring Mountaineer

Timberline Lodge

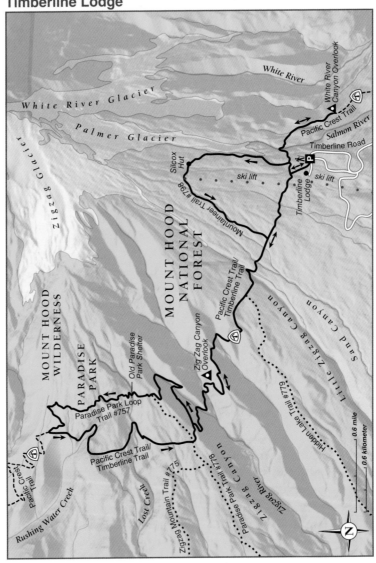

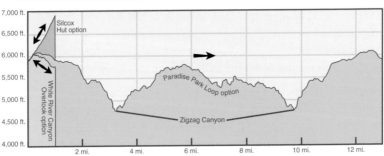

Loop Trail on the right. Continue 1.4 miles, going through Little Zigzag Canyon and passing Hidden Lake Trail #779 to the left, leading to Hidden Lake 3 miles below. Keep truckin' through meadows and forests, past flowers and little springs. The best of these are around 2 miles out from the trailhead, the farthest with a cool view of Mt. Hood Skibowl and Tom, Dick, and Harry Mountain, described in the Mirror Lake profile (Hike 37, page 188).

At 2.4 miles, you'll find yourself standing at the edge of a massive gash in the hillside, with Mount Hood rising to your right. This is Zigzag Canyon. If you've had enough at this point, head back and you'll have done a 4.8-mile out-and-back trip. But for the real prize of this part of the mountain, keep going.

Paradise Park

You may have noticed on a map that Paradise Park is actually below Timberline Lodge, making it seem pretty easy. But what you need to know, standing at Zigzag Overlook, is that in the next 3 miles, while crossing Zigzag Canyon and climbing up to Paradise Park, you'll descend 800 feet and then climb 1,000 feet. Just believe that it's worth it, and press on.

Down at the bottom of the hill, you'll have to hop across the Zigzag River—look for the waterfall just upstream—and, 0.7 mile up the other side, take the first right, onto Paradise Park Loop Trail #757. Then, yes, keep climbing toward Paradise Park. (You can also stay on the PCT/Timberline Trail for 2.1 miles to the lower end of our loop, and you'll save yourself several hundred feet of climbing but still see some great waterfalls.)

As you head up Paradise Park Loop Trail, things start to get really spectacular. The number and variety of flowers in this area—lupines, daisies, lilies, and bushy-looking pasqueflowers—and, of course, the plump sweetness of huckleberries in late summer make it a prime destination. Another big flower highlight is the bear-grass show in July. Hike 1 mile (gaining 700 feet) to reach Paradise Park Trail #778 coming in from the left; you can take it 0.6 mile down to the PCT and shorten your walk by 3.8 miles. But those 3.8 miles are fairly flat and very beautiful, so keep going. But first you might want to wander up and off-trail here; there are a few social trails leading into the high country, ultimately headed for Mississippi Head. You'll see a few of these trails as we go.

Staying on Paradise Park Loop Trail #757, in 0.2 mile you'll cross the first of several forks of Lost Creek, spy an amazing campsite on a ledge above it, and 0.1 mile later come to the site of the old Paradise Park Shelter, one of several built in the 1930s for people hiking the Timberline Trail.

The trail turns right just before the shelter foundation and starts a long, wonderfully flat traverse through über-scenic Paradise Park. After 1.2 miles of paradise, you'll descend into the forest again, where your trail intersects the PCT/Timberline Trail; this area provides great views down Sandy River Canyon.

(Turning right here leads down 3 miles to the Sandy River and the Ramona Falls hike, for a killer car-shuttle hike.)

Turn left instead, onto the PCT/Timberline Trail, and start back toward the lodge. After an easy 0.5 mile, you'll pass under a waterfall on Rushing Water Creek; below you are an amazing slot canyon and a view down into Sandy River Canyon. Hike another 0.5 mile, descending now, to return to Lost Creek. Look for a trail that leads uphill just after the crossing; it first passes a little double waterfall, then a magical, hidden cove with yet another waterfall—they're everywhere. It's not hard to find campsites in this area, either.

Another 0.7 mile brings you to the lower end of Paradise Park Trail #778, where a horse corral and its smell will encourage you to keep moving. The descent is steeper now, and in 0.4 mile you'll return to the junction where your loop started, Paradise Park Loop Trail #757. Follow the PCT back down into the canyon and, well, hate to tell you, but from here—with 9.5 miles under your belt—you have 3.5 miles to go, gaining 1,100 feet, and you've seen it all before.

But hey, it was worth it, right? Besides, you have Timberline Lodge to enjoy now. And you deserve it.

NEARBY ACTIVITIES

Though it's crowded, spend some time exploring Timberline Lodge (503-272-3311, timberlinelodge.com). Watch the film *The Builders of Timberline* to hear the story of how artists and artisans came together during the Depression to create this masterwork.

* *

GPS TRAILHEAD COORDINATES N45° 19.841' W121° 42.551'

DIRECTIONS Take US 26 from Portland, driving 48 miles east of I-205. Turn left onto the well-marked Timberline Highway, 0.3 mile past the rest area at Government Camp. Follow Timberline Highway 6 winding miles to the parking lot.

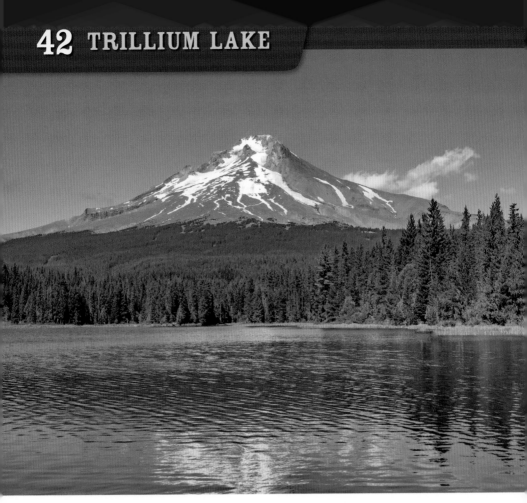

This view of Mount Hood makes Trillium Lake a popular destination all year.

A PRIME PLACE to take the kids or to stretch your legs after driving up from Portland, Trillium Lake is a tiny body of water with a friendly scene and an impressive and popular view of Mount Hood. In addition to some short, easy hikes, you'll have opportunities to fish, boat, or picnic—or just lie around, catch some rays, and watch the ducks.

DESCRIPTION

Most outdoorsy Portlanders know Trillium Lake as a cross-country-skiing area, famed for the terror felt by many beginners on the long hill you'll drive down from US 26. But in the summer the lake is a beautiful, peaceful place to get a taste of what the Mount Hood area has to offer. And if you have kids along, they can swim, fish, and paddle in the lake all day.

By the way, the lake isn't natural. The dam you'll start on was built in 1960, submerging a sprawling, marshy meadow; you'll get a sense of what it was like on this

DISTANCE & CONFIGURATION: 1.9-mile loop

DIFFICULTY: Easy

SCENERY: Marshes, lake, birds, forest

EXPOSURE: Shady, except when crossing the dam

TRAFFIC: Heavy all summer long, moderate when school is in session, moderate–heavy in winter, as well

TRAIL SURFACE: Packed dirt, boardwalk, pavement

HIKING TIME: 1.5 hours

ELEVATION CHANGE: Essentially none

SEASON: June–October

BEST TIME: August and September

BACKPACKING OPTIONS: None

DRIVING DISTANCE: 60 miles (1 hour, 20 minutes) from Pioneer Courthouse Square

ACCESS: Northwest Forest Pass required (see page 14); $5/vehicle/day without pass. Oregon Sno-Park Permit required November 1–April 30.

MAPS: Green Trails *Map 462 (Mount Hood)*, USFS *Mount Hood Wilderness*

WHEELCHAIR ACCESS: The trail was built to be barrier-free, with boardwalk and finely compacted rock.

FACILITIES: Restrooms in day-use area near dam; water at campground

LOCATION: Trillium Lake Day Use/Picnic Area on Forest Service Road (FR) 2656 (Trillium Lake Road), 4 miles south of Government Camp, OR

CONTACT: Zigzag Ranger District, 503-622-3191, www.fs.usda.gov/mthood

hike. To hike around the lake, start at the day-use area, just before the road crosses the dam at the lake's southern end. Stop here and take the picture of Mount Hood that so many others have taken. In case you're wondering, that square area of snow high up on the mountain is Palmer Glacier, the scene of summer-long skiing and snowboarding at Timberline Ski Area. Walk along the road atop the dam, perhaps ask how the fishing is, and, at the far end of the dam, follow Trillium Lake Trail #761 to the right, into the woods.

On the first part of the trail, you won't be right by the lake because the shore on that side is marshy and covered with tall grass. So you'll have to enjoy the forest. At 0.6 mile, a short boardwalk heads right, providing a glimpse of the shoreline. At 0.8 mile, a campsite on the right affords access to a relatively private lakeshore spot. Beyond this point, the trail becomes a boardwalk that traverses a marshy area thick with vegetation. It will seem like you're swimming through the wildflowers late in the summer.

As you round the northern end of the lake, you'll pass from marsh to meadow, with a view of a corner of the lake that's covered with lily pads; follow a side path to check it out. You'll come to a junction with the Trillium Lake Bike Trail on the left, but stay right. Then, coming back to the more crowded eastern shore, you'll find numerous beaches for the kids to romp on or for you to sunbathe on. At 1.7 miles— just 0.2 mile from where you started, going the other way—there's a boat ramp and another parking lot. Just beyond that is a dock you can walk out onto (it has rails, so you don't have to worry about the kids) and maybe even jump off for a swim. I was out there late one summer, with the sun setting and a few pink-hued clouds hanging

Trillium Lake

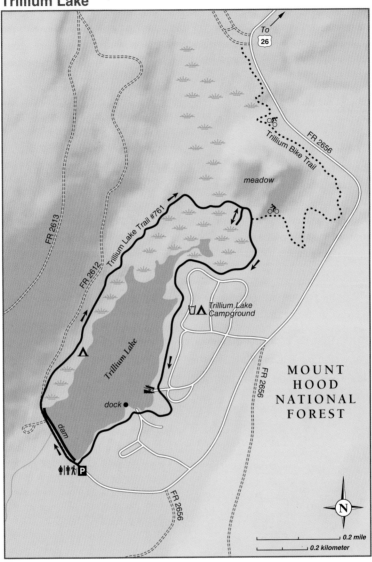

around Mount Hood across the way, and some grown-ups on the dock were talking about the stock market and housing prices. Some people just don't get it.

When you drive out, go past the lake for a piece of Oregon history. Head across the dam and drive 1 mile on the unpaved road; turn right and go 0.5 mile; and then make another right and park immediately on the right, near a white picket fence. That's a pioneer-era graveyard. Across the road is Summit Prairie, where Barlow Road travelers rested the day before tackling the infamous Laurel Hill.

By the way, this is a popular place in the winter, as well. You'll have to park up at US 26 and walk down, but you can also get here on winter trails from Government Camp. Skiing or snowshoeing out onto the frozen lake is something everybody should do. Parking is on US 26, either in the lot at the top of Trillium Lake Road (just walk down the main trail behind the gate) or in the Mazamas lot next to the big Oregon Department of Transportation equipment yard (look for signs marking the trail).

NEARBY ACTIVITIES

You must stop at some point at the Huckleberry Inn in Government Camp (call 503-272-3325 or visit huckleberry-inn.com for directions and a map). They have huckleberry pies, pancakes, milkshakes, and ice cream, and they serve pretty good cheeseburgers, too. And giant donuts. And they have a legendary mound of butter. I'm serious. I love that place.

* *

GPS TRAILHEAD COORDINATES N45° 15.992' W121° 44.483'

DIRECTIONS Take US 26 from Portland, driving 49 miles east of I-205. Turn right onto FR 2656 at a sign for Trillium Lake. At the bottom of the hill, proceed straight ahead for the day-use areas. The hiking trail, as described here, starts in the second day-use area you come to.

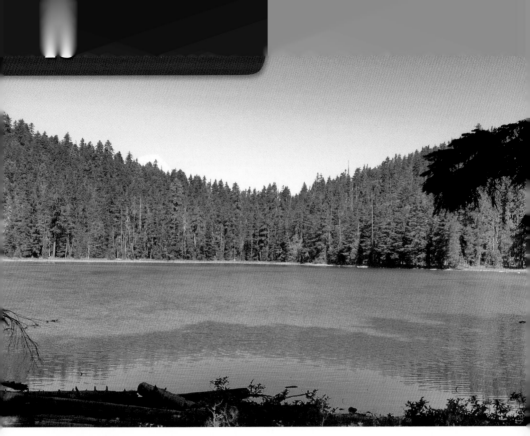

Lower Twin Lake

WHETHER YOU'RE A day hiker or an overnighter, you won't find much of a challenge here: the total elevation gain averages less than 200 feet per mile, making this an easy-to-reach, easy-to-hike introduction to the Pacific Crest Trail (PCT) and the world of mountain lakes.

DESCRIPTION

For long-distance hikers on the PCT, the Twin Lakes are a diversion used mainly for water or camping—and even then they're often ignored. Long-distance hikers passing through these parts are just a few miles from both a US highway and Timberline Lodge, so there's not much here for them.

In fact, this trail was originally part of the Oregon Skyline Trail, and later the PCT, but the PCT was moved up the hill when the lakes started becoming overused.

What's here now are two lovely lakes and a viewpoint, all within easy reach. You can simply hike in to a lakeside campsite with only 4 round-trip miles of hiking and in half a day see all the sights this area has to offer. Another suggestion before we get started: consider combining this with the hike from Barlow Pass to Timberline Lodge (Hike 31, page 160); by adding a car shuttle, you have a one-way hike of just under 10 miles that winds up high on the slopes of Mount Hood.

DISTANCE & CONFIGURATION: 4-mile out-and-back to Lower Twin Lake, 9.4-mile balloon loop to both lakes and Palmateer Point

DIFFICULTY: Moderate

SCENERY: Two mountain lakes, old-growth forest, nice view of Mount Hood

EXPOSURE: Shady all the way, except at viewpoint

TRAFFIC: Heavy on summer and winter weekends, light otherwise

TRAIL SURFACE: Packed dirt, with rocks and roots

HIKING TIME: 2 hours to Lower Twin Lake, 6 hours to see it all

ELEVATION CHANGE: 1,360' to just the lakes, 1,935' to include Palmateer

SEASON: June–October or winter

BEST TIME: August and September for hiking

BACKPACKING OPTIONS: Sites at both lakes

DRIVING DISTANCE: 63 miles (1 hour, 30 minutes) from Pioneer Courthouse Square

ACCESS: Northwest Forest Pass required (see page 14) May 1–October 31, Oregon Sno-Park Permit required otherwise

MAPS: Green Trails *Map 462 (Mount Hood)*, USFS *Mount Hood Wilderness*

WHEELCHAIR ACCESS: No

FACILITIES: Restrooms at trailhead; water at nearby Frog Lake Campground

CONTACT: Hood River Ranger District, 541-352-6002, www.fs.usda.gov/mthood

LOCATION: Twin Lakes Hiking Trail on US 26, 7 miles southeast of Government Camp, OR

COMMENTS: This hike is also a popular snowshoeing and Nordic-skiing trip.

One more thing: I did this hike once in mid-August in the midst of a monarch butterfly migration. If you find yourself at the center of this, it's astonishing—hundreds of butterflies fluttering around you, seemingly oblivious to your presence. The migration is fascinating because the butterflies are born in California, fly to Oregon, lay eggs, and die; the ones born in Oregon then fly to Washington, lay eggs, and die; and those monarchs fly to Canada, lay eggs, and die. Some of the ones born in Canada then return to California, to the same trees their "ancestors" used, often flying 100 miles in a day. Unreal.

At the parking lot at Frog Lake Sno-Park, head for the west end of the lot and walk into the woods near a hiker sign. You'll see a picnic table and garbage can here, along with two outhouses nearby—all to keep the place up to Northwest Forest Pass code. Go 100 feet and turn right to take the PCT; you'll notice some evidence of the annual snowfall here, such as the height of the sign on your right and that of the blue-diamond marker on a nice hemlock on the trail. That's all related to winter sports; this trail is wildly popular with the ski and snowshoe crowds for its easy access and excellent grade.

You'll appreciate that grade as you head uphill on a highway of a trail, wide enough for two people to walk shoulder-to-shoulder and of such a mellow steepness (gaining 500 feet in 1.5 miles) that you'll hardly notice it—especially if the abundant huckleberries are ripe.

When you reach the beginning of Twin Lakes Trail #495, turn right on it, and you'll soon descend a hill and spy Lower Twin Lake through the trees on your right.

Twin Lakes

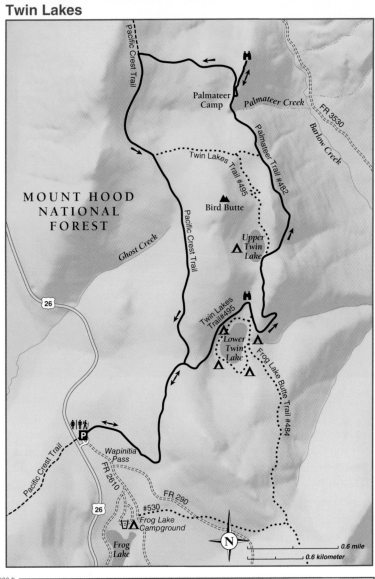

MOUNT HOOD
NATIONAL
FOREST

Pacific Crest Trail

Palmateer
Camp

Palmateer Creek

FR 3530

Barlow Creek

Palmateer Trail #482

Twin Lakes Trail #495

Bird Butte

Ghost Creek

Upper
Twin
Lake

26

Twin Lakes
Trail #495

Lower
Twin
Lake

Frog Lake Butte Trail #484

Wapinitia
Pass

Pacific Crest Trail

FR 2610

26

FR 290

#530

Frog Lake
Campground

Frog
Lake

N

0.6 mile

0.6 kilometer

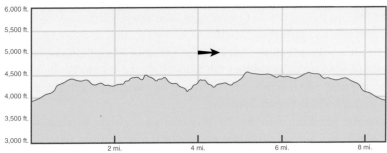

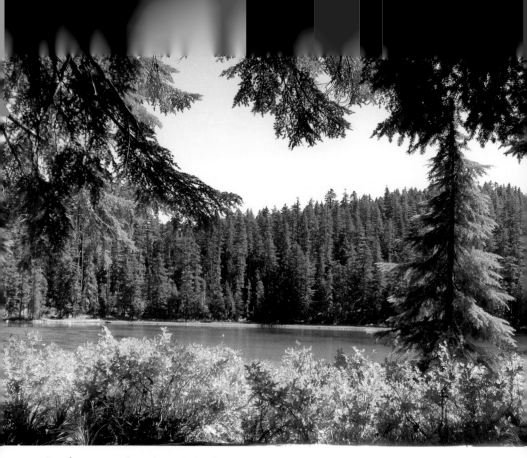

One of many campsites at Lower Twin Lake

You'll also see a social trail or two plunging down the hillside to the shore, but don't use them—you'll add to erosion, and the main trail goes to the same place. After a total of 2 miles (including a short stretch past the lake, up a drainage), you'll arrive at a junction with Frog Lake Butte Trail #484 at the northeast shore of the lake. You'll find enough camping for a village here, and practically nothing alive on the ground, but there's also a trail that goes all the way around the lake, leading to other camp-sites along the way.

To head for Upper Twin Lake and the rest of the hike, stay on Twin Lakes Trail #495. You'll round a bend, climb briefly, and in 0.7 mile come to a rocky area with a view (on the left) back down to Lower Twin in its steep-sided, forested bowl. Hike another 0.25 mile to reach Upper Twin and its own round-the-lake trail. The better campsites are on the left shore, but there is a view of Mount Hood from the east (right) shore. And if you're making the loop, that's the way to go anyway. Upper Twin, by the way, gets less use, but that might be because it's smaller, much more shallow, and not well suited to swimming.

Along the lakeshore, you'll come to a trail on the right marked PALMATEER VIEW. Great name, huh? Sounds like a pirate or something, but alas, it's the name of a sheepherder from pioneer days. This is Palmateer Trail #482—turn right here and you'll descend to the headwater of Palmateer Creek (which may be dry for your visit), then climb briefly to a large meadow called Palmateer Camp. From here, a moderately steep trail on the right leads 0.3 mile to the viewpoint.

This view gives you a rare perspective on Mount Hood, from the southeast, and the local stretch of the PCT. Climbing behind the ridge on your left, the PCT drops off its end to Barlow Pass, then climbs to Timberline Lodge, the gray roof of which is visible from your viewpoint.

You're also looking straight across (to the north) at Barlow Butte, where meadows unfold on the side facing you; there is a 2-mile trail up it from Barlow Pass. The drainage between you and the butte is that of Barlow Creek, traced by the historic Barlow Road, which was an overland portion of the Oregon Trail used by people who didn't want to risk their lives on the Columbia River. You can still drive this road all the way to The Dalles if your car has some clearance; access it just off OR 35, at the trailhead to the Barlow Pass trip.

Descending from the viewpoint, turn right on Palmateer Trail #482 at Palmateer Camp, and in 0.7 mile—after keeping straight at the junction for Devils Half Acre—you'll be back at the PCT. Barlow Pass is 1.2 miles to the right, but to return to the car, turn left. You'll pass Twin Lakes Trail #495 twice in an up-and-down, forested 4-mile walk back to the trailhead. Pick some more huckleberries while you're at it.

. . . .

GPS TRAILHEAD COORDINATES N45° 13.757' W121° 41.982'

DIRECTIONS Take US 26 from Portland, driving 55 miles east of I-205 to reach Frog Lake Sno-Park; it's 2 miles past the Chevron station, which you cannot possibly miss. The trailhead is in the left corner as you enter, and the parking spots to the left of it will be in the shade all day.

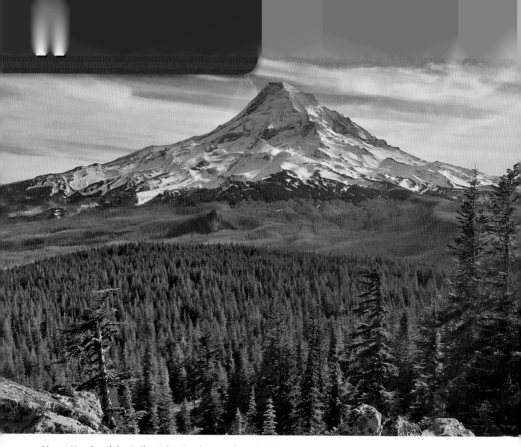

Mount Hood and the Dollar Lake Fire damage from Owl Point

THIS FAIRLY EASY trail to several flower-filled bowls at the treeline on Mount Hood is more than worth the long drive to the trailhead. Since 2011, however, it has a whole new character, as several miles of it burned intensely that summer, giving us all a rare chance to watch a forest regrow.

DESCRIPTION

The 2011 Dollar Lake Fire ravaged the north side of Mount Hood. Often, the effects of fires are overstated, but this was complete devastation. On this hike you'll walk through the burn, and the experience is fascinating. You'll also see how the forest is recovering. All you have to do is climb slightly for a couple of miles and you're in (unburned) wildflower heaven.

From the trailhead, go 0.2 mile to a sign and wilderness registration at Vista Ridge Trail #626, where the burn area starts. To the left is your first hiking option, which I suggest if you don't feel like climbing much but want a great view.

Owl Point (4 miles round-trip, 500'; full route not shown on map)

To your left is a section of trail that for years was unmaintained, becoming essentially a "lost" trail. But in 2007, dedicated volunteers from oregonhikers.org cleared 178 logs

DISTANCE & CONFIGURATION: Balloon loop with options of 4–11 miles

DIFFICULTY: Moderate, with one tricky river crossing

SCENERY: Mountain streams, rocks, glaciers, meadows, flowers, results of a 2011 forest fire

EXPOSURE: In a burned forest for a couple of miles, then in and out of healthy forest and meadows

TRAFFIC: Heavy on summer weekends, moderate otherwise

TRAIL SURFACE: Packed dirt, roots, rocks, ash

HIKING TIME: 3–6 hours

ELEVATION CHANGE: 500' to Owl Point, 1,560' to Cairn Basin, 1,790' to Elk Cove

SEASON: July–October

BEST TIME: August and September

BACKPACKING OPTIONS: Plentiful

DRIVING DISTANCE: 77 miles (2 hours, 10 minutes) from Pioneer Courthouse Square

ACCESS: No fees or permits required

MAPS: Green Trails *Map 462 (Mount Hood)*, USFS *Mount Hood Wilderness*

WHEELCHAIR ACCESS: No

FACILITIES: None at trailhead; closest services at Zigzag Mountain Cafe (70171 E. US 26, Rhododendron, OR; 503-622-7681)

LOCATION: Vista Ridge Trailhead at end of Forest Service Road (FR) 1650, 28 miles northeast of Welches, OR

CONTACT: Hood River Ranger District, 541-352-6002, www.fs.usda.gov/mthood

from the trail and restored this 2-mile section to Owl Point. This event was also a primary factor in the forming of a nonprofit group called Trailkeepers of Oregon. The path, now official again, is called Old Vista Ridge Trail #626A, and it offers great views and a rare opportunity for solitude on Mount Hood.

The first 0.5 mile is a bit steep, gaining 300 feet, and offers a prefire forest experience. Things then level off, and when you've gone 0.8 mile look for a couple of viewpoints to the right. Each reveals the alpine slopes of Mount Hood, the burned forest below that, the Clear Branch drainage, and Owl Point, which is the big rocky area on the left. Beyond it, you can see Bald Mountain in the Hood River Valley.

After reaching the top of the ridge, you'll start back downhill and pass through a meadow. This will be wet at times and require some route-finding to keep your feet dry. Just past it, a trail leads right about 500 feet to The Rockpile, which offers an amazing view of Hood—almost as nice as the one you're headed for.

Just 0.1 mile farther on the main trail, Old Vista Ridge Trail intersects Owl Point Trail, a 0.1-mile spur to a viewpoint named for the great horned owls that nest in the area. The path climbs briefly through forest then emerges to follow the edge of a large talus slope along a 500-foot cairn-marked route.

Off to the right as you face Hood, look for burned Vista Ridge approaching the mountain. The big hill right in front of Hood is Barrett Spur, which you can hike to. The next big open spot to the left is Elk Cove. The forested ridge off the far left is Stranahan Ridge, on which are Cloud Cap Saddle and the Cloud Cap Inn.

Be sure to sign the "summit" register, and then you might as well head back. Old Vista Ridge Trail continues another 1.2 miles past more viewpoints and on to Perry

Vista Ridge

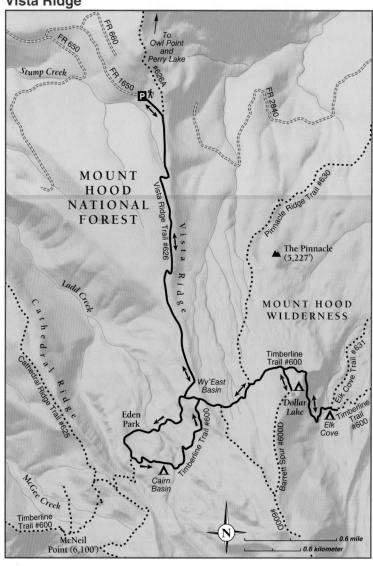

Map labels:
- FR 650
- FR 660
- FR 1650
- #626A
- To Owl Point and Perry Lake
- Stump Creek
- P
- FR 2840
- MOUNT HOOD NATIONAL FOREST
- Vista Ridge Trail #626
- Pinnacle Ridge Trail #630
- The Pinnacle (5,227')
- Vista Ridge
- Ladd Creek
- Cathedral Ridge
- Cathedral Ridge Trail #625
- MOUNT HOOD WILDERNESS
- Timberline Trail #600
- Elk Cove Trail #631
- Wy'East Basin
- Dollar Lake
- Timberline Trail #600
- Eden Park
- Elk Cove
- Timberline Trail #600
- Barrett Spur #600D
- Cairn Basin
- McGee Creek
- #600D
- Timberline Trail #600
- McNeil Point (6,100')
- N
- 0.6 mile
- 0.6 kilometer

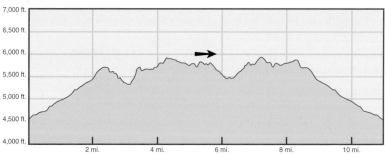

Elevation profile: 7,000 ft. / 6,500 ft. / 6,000 ft. / 5,500 ft. / 5,000 ft. / 4,500 ft. / 4,000 ft.
Distance markers: 2 mi. / 4 mi. / 6 mi. / 8 mi. / 10 mi.

Lake (more of a pond, really), but because this involves rougher trail and another 500 feet of elevation gain, and because Owl Point is the local highlight, you could probably skip this section.

Vista Ridge Trail to Eden Park, Cairn Basin, and Wy'East Basin (4.8 miles one-way, 1,560')

Back at the wilderness kiosk, turn right and head toward Mount Hood—and into the burn. In 2012 this whole area was black trunks and ash. By 2017 it was lush with fireweed and saplings. Nature rocks. You also have views all around, which wasn't the case before the fire. The trail gets just a bit steeper after a couple of miles, and 2.5 miles from the kiosk, you'll arrive at Eden Park Trail. Congratulations! You've now climbed the biggest hill of your day, 1,200 feet—wasn't much, was it?

Turn right toward Eden Park, and you'll briefly plunge downhill and then start heading around to the left, crossing babbling brooks and admiring abundant flowers. After just under a mile of this, you'll cross Ladd Creek, where logs have usually been placed to make a bridge. A quarter mile on, you'll be in Eden Park, which might be the loveliest mountain meadow you've seen—so far. To preserve the fragile landscape, stay on the trails.

To continue to Cairn Basin, cross Eden Park and follow the trail through the trees as it turns toward Mount Hood. It will climb a small hill, with a view back down to Eden Park, then pass through a notch and arrive 0.2 mile ahead at campsites in Cairn Basin. Here you can turn right on Timberline Trail #600 to connect with the McNeil Point trip (Hike 36, page 184), which is just 0.3 mile and a tricky creek crossing away. Or you can go left on Timberline Trail, following a sign for Elk Cove. Doing that, at the far end of the campsites, you'll wade or jump Ladd Creek again—this crossing might be a bit too deep and swift in the early summer—and after that it's basically a flat mile to Wy'East Basin.

Wy'East Basin to Elk Cove (2.4 miles round-trip, 300')

When you arrive in Wy'East Basin, your car is 3 miles to your left (go 0.3 mile to Vista Ridge Trail #626, and follow it out the way you came) and Elk Cove is to your right. It's easy and beautiful, so go for it. Just 1.2 flat miles away, Elk Cove is the most spectacular of these destinations. Here, you'll find wildflowers throughout August, huckleberries late in the month, and reddish-orange mountain ash in October.

As you head back on Timberline Trail #600, about a quarter mile from Elk Cove, keep an eye out for a side trail leading up to Dollar Lake. It's unsigned but follows a draw uphill in an area of short trees and a tiny stream that's more of a wet spot in the trail. If you get back as far as Pinnacle Ridge Trail #630, you've missed it by about 5 minutes. Dollar Lake—so named because it's almost perfectly round, like a silver dollar—offers nice campsites, and as you'll see, the 2011 Dollar Lake Fire didn't burn the area around the lake.

Barrett Spur Addition (up to 3.6 miles round-trip and 1,500')

Here's one final challenging, off-route option. Barrett Spur is the massive ridge on the left side of Mount Hood when seen from Portland. You can get to a little over 7,000 feet on it, using a social trail that starts from Wy'East Basin. There's nothing official about it, so all I can say is stick with it and be careful. On the way back down, look for a junction that will lead you to Dollar Lake.

• •

GPS TRAILHEAD COORDINATES N45° 26.531' W121° 43.554'

DIRECTIONS From Portland, take US 26 to Zigzag; turn left on Lolo Pass Road. Drive 10.7 miles and take the second right at Lolo Pass, onto FR 18, signed for Lost Lake. (If you're using Google Maps, it may tell you to go straight at the pass; don't.) After 5.5 miles of gravel, you'll be back on pavement, and 5 miles beyond that—having driven a total of 10.5 miles on FR 18—make a hairpin right to take the paved FR 16. (A sign here points to Vista Ridge Trail #626. You can also get to this intersection by way of Hood River; it's longer but smoother.) Go 5.4 miles and turn right at a large intersection onto FR 1650, which quickly becomes a good gravel road. The trailhead is 3.6 miles ahead, at the end of the road. Note that twice during this stretch, you'll need to stay left and uphill on the bigger of two roads.

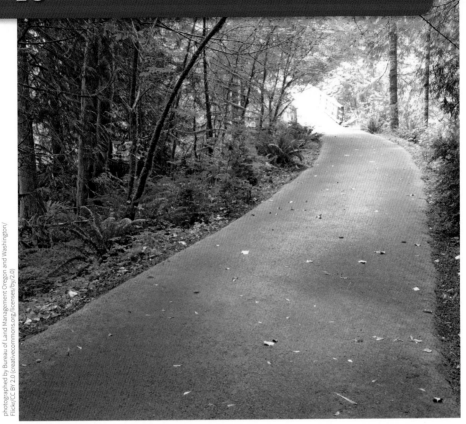

photographed by Bureau of Land Management Oregon and Washington/Flickr/CC BY 2.0 (creativecommons.org/licenses/by/2.0)

Both loops of this hike are wheelchair traversable.

AS MUCH AN educational experience as a hiking one, this hike offers a glimpse into the Pacific Northwest world of birds, fish, plants, and water. The crown jewel of Wildwood is its underwater-viewing structure, especially when various species of salmon and trout are returning to the area to spawn. Oh, and there's a huge climb option, as well.

DESCRIPTION

The 33-mile-long Salmon River is the only river in the lower 48 states that is classified as a National Wild and Scenic River from its headwaters to its mouth—in this case, from Mount Hood to the Sandy River, 3 miles below Wildwood. As far from the sea as it is, the river still gets several runs each year of anadromous fish—fish that are born in freshwater, go to the ocean, and then return to the freshwater of their birth to spawn and die. Although salmon are the most famous of these—and this bend of the Salmon River does get runs of salmon—steelhead do the same thing. Moreover, native trout inhabit this stretch of the river.

DISTANCE & CONFIGURATION: Two loops totaling 1.75 miles; 10.6-mile out-and-back to Huckleberry Mountain

DIFFICULTY: Easy for loops, strenuous to Huckleberry Mountain

SCENERY: Wetlands, meadows, streams, big-time summit viewpoint

EXPOSURE: Alternately shady and open on loops, sunny on mountain hike

TRAFFIC: Moderate–heavy on summer weekends, light otherwise

TRAIL SURFACE: Gravel, pavement, boardwalk (loops), packed dirt (hike to mountain)

HIKING TIME: 2.5 hours for the two loops, 6 hours for Huckleberry Mountain

ELEVATION: Virtually none for lower loops, 4,300' to Huckleberry Mountain

SEASON: Year-round; see note in the directions, below, about winter parking. The trail up the mountain is generally snow-free June–October.

BEST TIME: Late summer and fall

BACKPACKING OPTIONS: None in the park. If you're spending the night up in the wilderness, tell park staff which car is yours.

DRIVING DISTANCE: 43 miles (1 hour) from Pioneer Courthouse Square

ACCESS: $5/vehicle/day. Note that even during the season, the gate is locked between sunset and 8 a.m. In winter, when the gate is closed, park to the left of it and walk 0.5 mile up the road to the trailhead.

MAPS: Free maps in parking-area kiosk

WHEELCHAIR ACCESS: Both lower loops

FACILITIES: At parking area

LOCATION: 65670 US 26, Welches, OR

CONTACT: Bureau of Land Management, Salem District, 503-622-3696, blm.gov/visit/wildwood -recreation-site

To sample this natural wonderland, hike two loop trails: the 1-mile Wetland Boardwalk Trail and the 0.75-mile Cascade Streamwatch Trail. To take Wetland Boardwalk Trail, start to the left of the parking-lot kiosk, where you'll find restrooms and free maps. You'll cross a 190-foot-long wooden bridge over the Salmon River, where in fall and winter you just might see coho salmon and steelhead spawning below. Once over the bridge, follow the signs onto the boardwalk. You'll visit several lookouts affording views of various parts of the wetland: a cattail marsh, an overgrown beaver dam, an area filled with skunk cabbage, and a wetland stream. At each lookout, a notebook-style informative display describes the area's wildlife. And if you're quiet and go in the morning, there's a good chance you'll even see some wildlife. Be sure to take the gravel Return Trail back to the parking lot, if only to admire the size of some 90-year-old stumps.

Cascade Streamwatch Trail starts at the same kiosk and takes you on a tour of the world of an anadromous fish. In fact, to navigate the trail, you just follow the metal fish in the pavement. Along this trail, you'll visit an overlook of the river, a three-dimensional model of the Mount Hood area, several great picnic areas with grills, and then the fantastic underwater-viewing structure. Here, you can see tiny fish most of the year and try to identify them using the chart on the wall. From late October to mid-December, you might even catch a glimpse of an adult salmon. You have a better chance of seeing bigger spawning fish a little later on the trail, when it drops to the riverside. Look for winter steelhead in January, spring chinook salmon

Wildwood Recreation Site

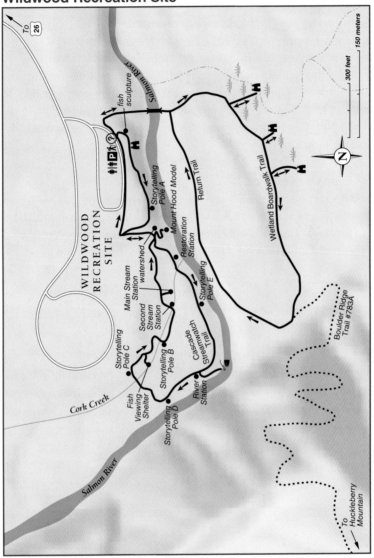

in March and April, summer steelhead in May, and coho and fall chinook from late September to mid-November. In case you're wondering, the Salmon River is closed to salmon fishing—you can fish for native trout at limited times, but it's all catch-and-release, with artificial lures only.

If it's exercise and a view you're after, take Boulder Ridge Trail #783A up to Huckleberry Mountain—and I do mean up: it climbs 4,300 feet in 5.1 miles to a tremendous viewpoint. Starting at the southwest end of Wetland Boardwalk Trail,

225

you'll climb a series of switchbacks for just under 2 miles to reach a spot with a view of Mount Hood. From here, it's a slightly less severe grade. Another 0.5 mile of climbing puts you at another view from a saddle; from there you'll put in 2 more miles to another saddle then make a right onto Plaza Trail, heading 1 mile to the summit.

Important note: On the way down, make absolutely sure you take the same Boulder Ridge trail. Not only will going down the Plaza Trail put you in the wrong place; it will put you at a private-property line, and you'll have to come all the way back up to the junction.

NEARBY ACTIVITIES

Wildwood Recreation Site is a full-service, 600-acre recreation area, with picnic areas for rent (some can be reserved) in addition to ball fields, basketball courts, horseshoe pits, and a play area. There is also a completely flat nature trail that visits the ruins of an old mill. For rental information, call 877-444-6777 or visit recreation.gov.

• •

GPS TRAILHEAD COORDINATES N45° 21.009' W121° 59.523'

DIRECTIONS Take US 26 from Portland, driving 33 miles east of I-205; turn right at a large sign reading CASCADE STREAMWATCH, 0.5 mile past the Mount Hood RV Village. Drive 0.1 mile past the trailhead sign to the parking area for both trails. The road is gated from the weekend after Thanksgiving until the third Monday in March. During that time, you'll have to park at the gate (no charge) and walk in; restrooms in the park are left open.

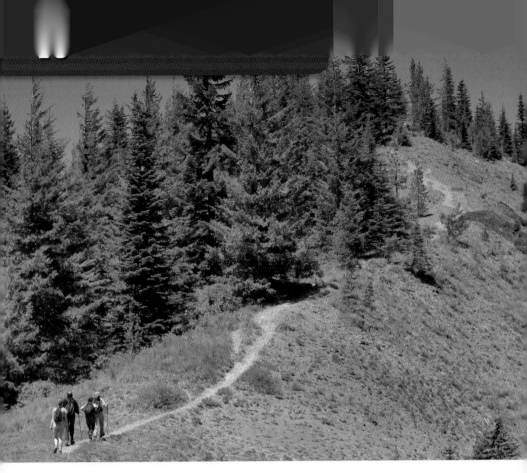

Heading up the final ridge to Zigzag Mountain

THIS IS REALLY three hikes in one: a cool, shady amble along a creek; a moderate climb to a beautiful lake with a view of Mount Hood; and a strenuous climb to an old lookout site, with an even better view of Mount Hood.

DESCRIPTION

Burnt Lake Trail #772 starts in an area that burned in 1904 and 1906; look for charred stumps here and there for what remains of that old forest. Now it's all cool, moist, and shady as you wind your way up through a young forest, with Burnt Lake Creek off to your right and Lost Creek to your left. If that name sounds familiar, it's because there are enough things called "Lost" in Oregon (not to mention things called "Salmon," "Elk," and "Huckleberry") to fill a whole hiking book.

Walk 0.25 mile and, just past a big cedar on the right, the forest gets a little more interesting. At just under 0.5 mile, an unmarked trail to the left leads to a clifftop view toward the main stem of Lost Creek. On the main trail, you'll get your first glimpse of actual water around 1 mile out, and at just under 2 miles you'll hop across a tiny creek.

DISTANCE & CONFIGURATION: 4.6-mile out-and-back for falls, 6.8-mile out-and-back for lake, 9.4-mile out-and-back for mountain

DIFFICULTY: Easy along creek, moderate to lake, strenuous to mountain

SCENERY: Shady creekside forest, lovely mountain lake, spectacular summit view

EXPOSURE: Some ridgetop walking near summit

TRAFFIC: Heavy on summer weekends, moderate otherwise

TRAIL SURFACE: Packed dirt, some rocks

HIKING TIME: 4 hours to lake, 6 hours to do it all

ELEVATION: 1,420' to lake, 2,300' to peak

SEASON: June–October, though there will be some snow higher up in early summer

BEST TIME: August and September

BACKPACKING OPTIONS: Great sites at lake

DRIVING DISTANCE: 54 miles (1 hour, 20 minutes) from Pioneer Courthouse Square

ACCESS: Northwest Forest Pass required (see page 14)

MAPS: Green Trails *Map 461 (Government Camp)*

WHEELCHAIR ACCESS: No

FACILITIES: None at the trailhead—stop in Zigzag on the way.

LOCATION: Burnt Lake Trailhead at end of Muddy Fork Road, 10 miles northeast of Welches, OR

CONTACT: Zigzag Ranger District, 503-622-3191, www.fs.usda.gov/mthood

Continue climbing ever so gently 0.5 mile, past some old burned-out snags, and look for a trail dipping left to a picnic site by a Lost Creek Falls. This is a good place to turn around—2.3 miles out—if you're tired or you have little kids in tow.

Soon you'll make a switchback to the right and climb 1 mile, passing several small creeks, some of them in open areas that offer views back along the valley you've been coming up. You'll see Mount Hood over your right shoulder, but the real views start just after you cross Burnt Lake's outlet creek and arrive at the shores of this local wonder.

You'll immediately realize that lots of folks come up here; even if it's not crowded when you arrive, you'll notice trails leading all over the place. If you're camping, you must stick to designated spots and refrain from making wood fires. If you're just up here for the day, linger a bit, explore the trail around the lake, take a swim, and soak in the rays and the views of Hood. Turn back here, and you have a 6.8-mile day.

To reach the lookout, another 1.3 miles and 800 feet up, continue right on the trail as it leads away from the lake, following a pointer toward Zigzag Mountain Trail #775. Cross a marshy area, then switchback up and out of the lake basin, intersecting Zigzag Mountain Trail after 0.8 mile. Turn right here, and it's quite a steep 0.25 mile climb to a viewpoint of Mount Hood where rhododendrons surround you. After the trail levels, continue straight through another junction and push up the steep, final 0.3 mile to the rocky summit.

From the top, your view runs from two-humped Mount Rainier in the north to Mount Jefferson in the south, with Olallie Butte just left of it. Left of Mount Hood, between it and Mount Adams, look for an open stretch alongside a ridge, bisected by a trail—that's Bald Mountain and a section of Timberline Trail, which you can visit

Zigzag Mountain

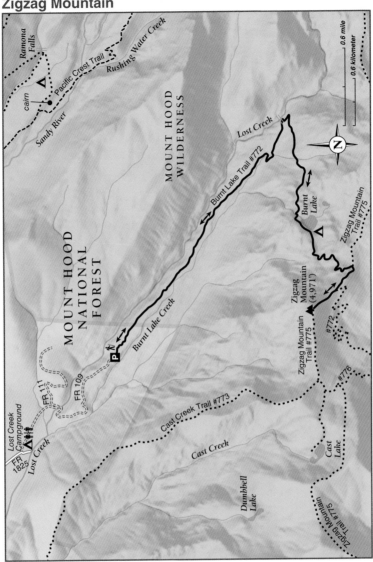

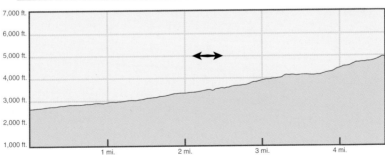

on the McNeil Point trip (Hike 36, page 184). The valley below is that of the Muddy Fork Sandy River, which starts at Sandy Glacier, clearly visible from here, left of the summit. To the right, beyond Zigzag Glacier, you can see dramatic Zigzag Canyon, which you can visit on the Timberline Lodge trip (Hike 41, page 204), and beyond that are two buildings that are part of Timberline Lodge, alongside Palmer Glacier.

So it's a two-creek, one-lake, four-volcano, three-glacier day, and yet you have still more trails to explore. The trail you took to the summit, Zigzag Mountain Trail, continues west over the summit toward Cast Lake and a veritable noodle bowl of trails, including the continuation of Burnt Lake Trail #772, which you left behind at the junction just below this summit. So you could make a loop out of all that, or even head for the lookout atop the west end of Zigzag Mountain—if, for some reason, what you've already done isn't enough. Or, instead of going back down to the lake, stick with Zigzag Mountain Trail for 3.7 up-and-down miles to Paradise Park, connecting with Hike 41. There's a day hike for ya!

• •

GPS TRAILHEAD COORDINATES N45° 22.332' W121° 49.328'

DIRECTIONS Take US 26 from Portland, driving 36 miles east of I-205 to Zigzag. Turn left (north) onto Lolo Pass Road, which is 0.6 mile past milepost 41. Go 4.2 miles and turn right on Forest Service Road (FR) 1825, which is 0.1 mile past a sign for Mount Hood National Forest and is marked CAMPGROUNDS AND TRAILHEADS. Stay right at 0.7 mile, cross a bridge, and, 2 miles later, just past Lost Creek Campground, go straight at a junction onto gravel FR 109, continuing 1.3 miles to the trailhead.

The "Champagne tower" of Ramona Falls (Hike 38, page 192)

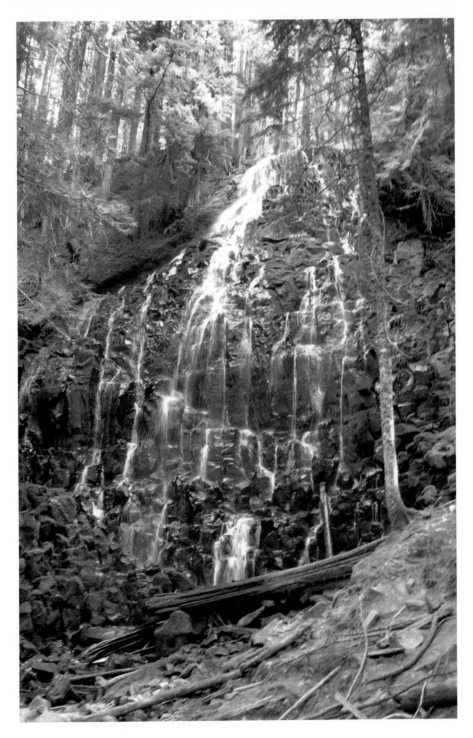

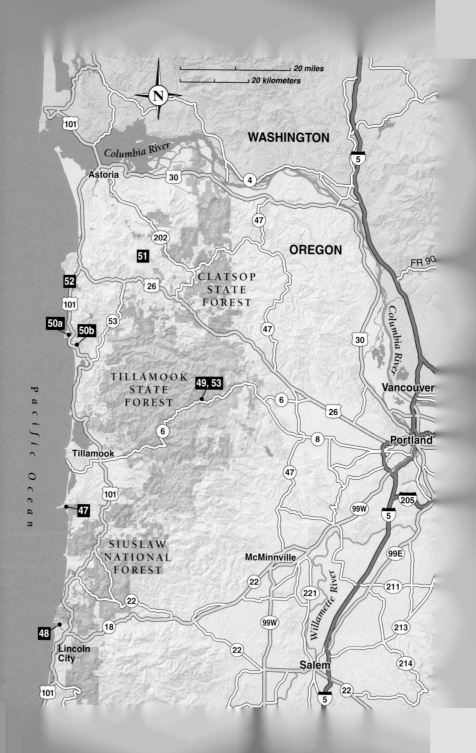

THE COAST AND COAST RANGE

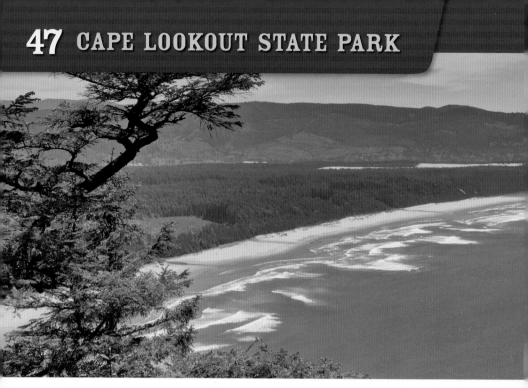

South Beach from the Cape Trail

THIS PARK OFFERS everything you'd want from the Oregon coast: old-growth forest; secluded beaches; clifftop views; and wildlife on land, wing, and water. You've got three options from the trailhead.

DESCRIPTION

When you park at this trailhead, you'll have three options to choose from, and it's all downhill from here. Of course, you'll have to come back uphill to get to your car, but even the 800-foot climb from the beach is so well graded, you'll hardly be winded when it's done. (On our elevation profile for this hike, I've included the beach route and the cape route.)

Cape Trail

Start with the best of the three trails. Taking the trail behind the sign at the far end of the lot, continue straight when you get to a junction 100 yards ahead. After a few minutes in younger forest, you'll be hiking through that rarest of treats: a coastal old-growth forest. Some nice Sitka spruces and hemlocks grow here, and the whole thing is as peaceful as can be. Look also for interesting forest features like a split stump, nurse logs with new trees growing on them, and widow-makers hanging over your head. This trail also manages to stay muddy in places year-round.

At 0.5 mile out, the trail dips down among some giant hemlock trees, and at 0.6 mile you'll come to a plaque honoring the flight crew of a B-17 bomber that

DISTANCE & CONFIGURATION: 4.8-mile out-and-back to end of cape, 3.6-mile out-and-back to South Beach, 4.6-mile out-and-back to picnic area, with combinations available

DIFFICULTY: Moderate

SCENERY: Old-growth forest, high cliffs, whales

EXPOSURE: Some pretty extreme clifftop walking without rails

TRAFFIC: Moderate–heavy

TRAIL SURFACE: Gravel, dirt, mud

HIKING TIME: 3 hours to end of cape, 2.5 hours to South Beach, 3 hours to picnic area

ELEVATION CHANGE: 800' to cape, 1,000' up from day-use area, 840' to beach

SEASON: Year-round, with mud and storms in winter and spring

BEST TIME: July–September for weather, March and April for whales

BACKPACKING OPTIONS: None

DRIVING DISTANCE: 82 miles (1 hour, 45 minutes) from Pioneer Courthouse Square

ACCESS: No fees or permits required at trailhead, but parking in day-use area is $5/day.

MAPS: USGS *Sand Lake*; free brochure at main park area and on park website

WHEELCHAIR ACCESS: No

FACILITIES: Portable restroom at trailhead May–September; restrooms, showers, and water at campground

CONTACT: 503-842-4981, tinyurl.com/capelook

LOCATION: Cape Lookout State Park, 13000 Whiskey Creek Road, Tillamook, OR

COMMENTS: The park gets an average of 90 inches of rain annually, compared with Portland's 37.5 inches—you've been warned.

crashed into the cape just to the west in 1943. After another 0.5 mile, you'll get a view north; look for the three rocks just off Cape Meares and the town of Oceanside. You can make out an arch in the middle rock—in fact, all three have such arches, and they're called the Three Arch Rocks. I also spotted a whale below this section once. When you get to some moderately nerve-wracking drop-offs on the left, along with inspiring views south, you're almost done.

At the tip of the cape, you're looking 270 degrees around and 400 feet straight down at the crashing sea. There's a protective cable at the end of the cape, but in other places you'll be right at the top of a cliff. On a calm day—which is rare in a place that gets around 90 inches of rain per year—it's not uncommon to see seals or sea lions below.

But the main attraction is the gray whales. Thousands of them make the trip each year from the Bering Sea in Alaska to Baja California in Mexico, a swim of some 6,000 miles. In late December and early January, when they go south, they tend to be farther out. But in March and April, they're on their way back north with newborn calves, so they go slower and stay closer to shore. At these times of year, bring binoculars (and rain gear); you might see dozens of whales in a day. For the best viewing, go early in the day, when the sun will be behind you as you look west.

South Beach Trail

At the junction very near the parking lot, heading downhill puts you on the trail to South Beach. Avoid the temptation to take any of the various cutoff trails, as they add

Cape Lookout State Park

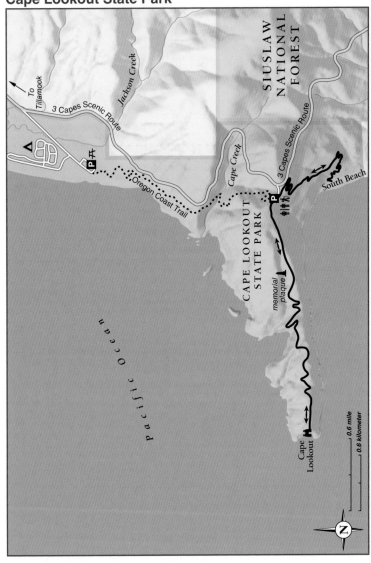

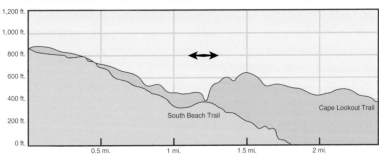

to erosion. If the 1.5-mile, 800-foot descent seems a little tedious (like when the beach looks as though it's just right there below you but you're walking more sideways than down), just know that you'll be thankful for this easier grade on your way back up.

You can also hike down the beach, which extends 4 miles south to Sand Lake, but eventually you'll get into an area where cars are allowed, which sort of detracts from the wilderness feeling. The tide pools are to the right.

North Trail

The last option from the trailhead is across the lot, going north on the Oregon Coast Trail. It's 2.3 miles, all downhill, to the picnic area and the nature trail, which are by the campground. On the way, you'll pass a couple of viewpoints, a bouncy little bridge, and some massive trees—one of which I could walk through, and I'm 6-foot-1. You will also probably have the trail largely to yourself.

If you have two cars, leave one at the upper trailhead and then start down at the day-use area. Go up and out to the cape, and maybe down to the beach as well, then end your day at the upper trailhead. Or start above and finish with a downhill—up to you, of course.

NEARBY ACTIVITIES

Take advantage of Tillamook's tourist stops, most notably the collection of airplanes at the Tillamook Air Museum (6030 Hangar Road, Tillamook, OR; 503-842-1130; tillamookair.com). Two cheese factories are to the north. The Tillamook Cheese Factory (4175 US 101 N, Tillamook, OR; 503-815-1300; tillamook.com) is the best known; for slightly more exotic choices, as well as wine tastings and a petting zoo, visit the Blue Heron French Cheese Company (2001 Blue Heron Dr., Tillamook, OR; 503-842-8281; blueheronoregon.com).

* *

GPS TRAILHEAD COORDINATES
Cape Trailhead N45° 20.484' W123° 58.470',
Day-Use Area N45° 21.635' W123° 58.168'

DIRECTIONS From Portland, take US 26 to OR 6; bear left, following a sign for Tillamook. Drive 51 miles to Tillamook and continue straight through the intersection with US 101. You'll be following signs for Cape Lookout State Park and the 3 Capes Scenic Route. After crossing US 101, go two blocks and turn left on Stillwell Avenue. Drive two more blocks and turn right on Third Street. Drive 4.5 miles and turn left onto Whiskey Creek Road. After 5.2 miles, you'll pass the state-park campground and day-use area; this is where you find the lower trailhead. The upper trailhead is 2.7 miles past the campground, on the right.

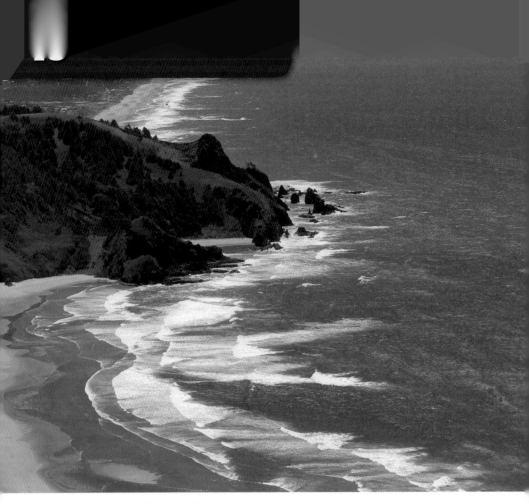

View down to the beach from Cascade Head

IMAGINE STANDING HIGH atop a windswept, flower-covered meadow, with the sea and the coast spread out below you and not a tree to block the view. Or imagine peeking into a hidden cove where sea lions bark, a waterfall plunges, and waves crash. Well, you don't have to imagine either scene: you can go to Cascade Head.

DESCRIPTION

Harts Cove Trail

At the start, you might think you've got it made, because it's all downhill and steep—it loses about 500 feet in the first 0.5 mile. Too bad you have to walk back up at the end of the hike. The forest here is a young one of mostly Sitka spruce; notice that only the tops of the trees are green. That's because these lower portions don't get any sun. Notice also the large stumps; there's one right on the side of the trail that you can get on top of and measure for yourself.

DISTANCE & CONFIGURATION: 5.4-mile out-and-back to Harts Cove; 2.5- or 3.2-mile out-and-back to Cascade Head Preserve

DIFFICULTY: Moderate, plus an easy option after July 15

SCENERY: Old-growth forest, waterfalls, sea cliffs, wildflowers, wildlife

EXPOSURE: In forest at first, then meadows

TRAFFIC: Heavy on summer weekends, moderate otherwise

TRAIL SURFACE: Packed dirt, some roots

HIKING TIME: 3 hours to Harts Cove, 1–2.5 hours for preserve

ELEVATION CHANGE: 1,000' for Harts Cove, 200' or 1,170' for Cascade Head

SEASON: The road to the Harts Cove Trailhead and upper Cascade Head Preserve Trailhead is open July 16–December 31. The lower Cascade Head Preserve Trailhead at Knight Park is open year-round.

BEST TIME: July–September

BACKPACKING OPTIONS: No camping allowed

DRIVING DISTANCE: 86 miles (2 hours) from Pioneer Courthouse Square

ACCESS: No fees or permits required

MAPS: USGS *Neskowin*

WHEELCHAIR ACCESS: No

FACILITIES: Outhouse at Knight Park, but no facilities at upper trailheads and no drinkable water on the trail

CONTACT: The Nature Conservancy, 503-802-8100, tinyurl.com/cascadeheadpreserve; Hebo Ranger District, 503-392-5100, www.fs.usda.gov/siuslaw

LOCATION: Knight County Park, 3 miles northwest of Otis, OR

COMMENTS: Dogs are prohibited on both trails at Cascade Head Preserve.

After 0.7 mile you cross Cliff Creek and enter a different world. Here you can find out what a Sitka spruce looks like after about 300 years. You'll probably also hear what hundreds of sea lions sound like—they're to the left, and you might get to see some later. Now the hiking gets flatter as you go out to the end of the ridge to a bench with a view of Harts Cove. Wrap back around to the right, through the drainage of Chitwood Creek. Half a mile past the bench, walk under a massive blown-down spruce and then out into the meadows atop the bluff—yet another world.

It's important to stay on the trails here; the area is fragile. If you come in July or August, you'll be part of a landscape that looks like it was lifted from the upper reaches of Mount Hood, with goldenrod, lupine, Indian paintbrush, and violets in abundance. Follow the trail that heads for the trees on the left; there's a wonderful spot to sit, with a front-row view into Harts Cove. The waterfall you see is on Chitwood Creek, which you just crossed. As for the louder-than-ever sea lions, they are mostly around the point to the south, but if you have binoculars you might be able to see some of them lounging on rocks or the far beach.

There's no real beach to access here, but you can get close to the water. From the trees, walk west and keep left. Look for a steep trail, almost a slide in spots, that you can descend to the rocky shore. This rock, and all of Cascade Head in fact, is lava that flowed from hundreds of miles inland. If you make your way to the right 100 yards

Cascade Head

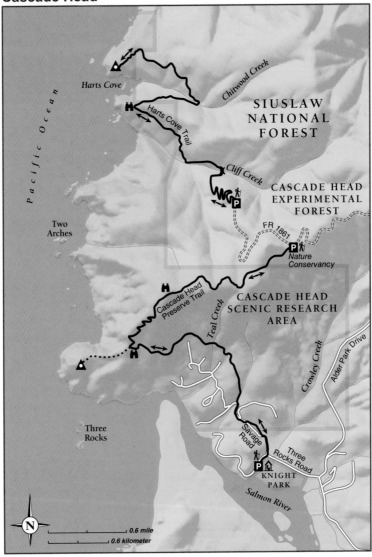

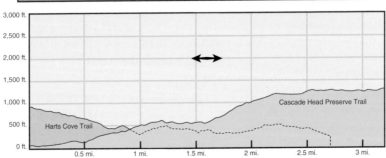

or so on the rock, you'll have a fabulous view of the headland; Cape Kiwanda to the north; and, farther off, Cape Lookout.

Cascade Head Preserve

If it's after July 15; the upper road is open; and you want an easy, flat, 2.5-mile round-trip hike, start up here. The trail, actually an old roadbed, traverses a young and unexciting forest to the main-attraction meadow. After that first viewpoint, there's another 0.5 mile farther down.

My advice is to start down below. It's a better, more scenic walk, and effort always makes one more appreciative. From the parking lot at Knight Park, start near the interpretive sign; you'll spot the trailhead directly across Three Rocks Road. The first 0.5-mile stretch crosses private property, switching from boardwalks to trail and occasionally right along the road, so make sure you stay on the path.

Finally heading into the woods from the original trailhead, the trail starts steeply, over steps and roots, then mellows after 0.2 mile, where a massive spruce guards the path. Enjoy coastal scenery—spruces and ferns, skunk cabbage and devil's club, and a small meadow filled with foxglove—as you cross several small streams on boardwalks and continue climbing, now on a more moderate grade. When you reach a junction less than a mile out, keep left, and in a few moments you'll reach a sign telling you you're entering Siuslaw National Forest property. At 1.4 miles, you'll come to a registration station and donation box for The Nature Conservancy.

At this point, you'll probably have been hearing the ocean for a while, and at 1.5 miles you'll finally emerge from the tunnel of vegetation to see the Pacific and the mouth of the Salmon River some 600 feet below. The trail is flat and wonderful for 0.25 mile—look for elk on the bluffs and bald eagles in the sky. At a switchback to the right, the path starts to climb more steeply.

In summer, you'll climb through waist-high flowers, with birds chirping, swallows swooping, butterflies fluttering, and bumblebees buzzing. From any of the switch-backs, wander out, carefully, toward the cliff edge to peer north; you might spot sea lions below. When you see a sign reading DANGER: HAZARDOUS CLIFFS, you've gone 2 miles and gained 1,000 feet. Only 0.25 mile and a couple hundred feet to the top! The spot where the upper trail emerges from the woods is 0.3 mile past the summit.

As you take it all in from the top of the hill, consider this: back in the 1960s, this meadow was slated to become a housing development, but conservation-minded folks banded together, bought it, and donated it to The Nature Conservancy. Now also designated as a United Nations Biosphere Reserve, it's protected as the home of the Oregon silverspot butterfly, whose caterpillar eats only a rare violet that lives in these meadows. That's why Forest Service Road (FR) 1861 and the upper part of the trail are closed January 1–July 15. The silverspots emerge in late August and hang out here for about a month.

NEARBY ACTIVITIES

Back on OR 18, a mile before you reached US 101, you passed through the town of Otis. It's the home of an Oregon coast tradition, the Otis Cafe (1259 Salmon River Highway; 541-994-2813; otiscafe.com), where you'll find 28 seats, a line outside, and the biggest portions this side of a logging camp. Famous for its sourdough pancakes, German potatoes, and whole-wheat molasses toast, the café also makes wonderful pies.

• •

GPS TRAILHEAD COORDINATES
Cascade Head Preserve (Lower Trailhead) N45° 2.506' W123° 59.556'
Cascade Head Preserve (Upper Trailhead) N45° 3.641' W123° 59.305'
Harts Cove Trailhead N45° 3.893' W123° 59.723'

DIRECTIONS Your first target is the intersection of OR 18 and 22, near the town of Willamina. You can get there by taking I-5 south to Salem and following OR 22 or by taking OR 99W through Sherwood and Newberg. In normal traffic it's the same amount of time either way. From that intersection, you're now on OR 22/18; head west 25 miles and turn right on US 101. For the lower, year-round trailhead to Cascade Head Preserve, go 1.2 miles north and turn left on Three Rocks Road. Go 2.4 miles, turn left, and park at Knight Park. To reach the trailhead, follow a trail along the road behind the information sign.

For the two upper trailheads, drive 3.8 miles north of OR 18 on US 101 and turn left onto unsigned FR 1861, just before the top of a hill. Stay left at 2.4 miles, still on FR 1861. The upper Cascade Head Preserve Trailhead is 0.8 mile past this turn, on the left. The Harts Cove Trailhead is at the end of the road, 1 mile ahead.

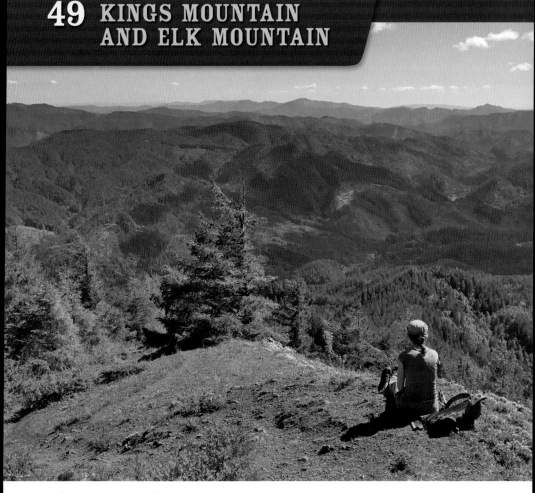

Taking in the view atop Kings Mountain

I'VE LAID OUT four options: a steep hike up Kings Mountain, a *really* steep scramble up Elk Mountain, a killer loop that includes both, and a more casual (though lengthy) trip along Elk Creek. With a campground at one trailhead, why not spend the night and do a couple of hikes?

DESCRIPTION

All these hikes are in Tillamook State Forest, which has a fascinating story behind it. In August 1933, a fire started in Gales Creek Canyon. The temperatures had been in the 90s for weeks, and humidity was at an all-time low. The fire started as a fairly standard conflagration, but a hot, dry wind came in from the east, and in less than 24 hours, the 40,000-acre blaze turned into a 240,000-acre nightmare. This "explosion" threw up a mushroom cloud 40 miles wide that rained 2 feet of debris on a 30-mile stretch of the Oregon coast.

DISTANCE & CONFIGURATION: Loop and out-and-back options of 5.2–13.4 miles

DIFFICULTY: Moderate–strenuous

SCENERY: Second-growth forest, regrowth after fires, wildflower meadows, panoramas on top

EXPOSURE: Shady on the way up, open on top; some dangerous sections up above, especially if it's wet

TRAFFIC: Moderate on summer weekends, light otherwise

TRAIL SURFACE: Packed dirt, with some rock; sheer rock and steep scrambles on Elk Mountain

HIKING TIME: 3.5 hours to Kings Mountain, 8 hours for either loop

ELEVATION CHANGE: 2,500' for Kings Mountain, 2,080' for Elk Mountain, 3,700' for the traverse

SEASON: Year-round, but there will often be snow on top in winter. Recent rains make some slopes very slippery.

BEST TIME: May and June for wildflowers and cool(er) temperatures

BACKPACKING OPTIONS: None

DRIVING DISTANCE: 45 miles (1 hour) from Pioneer Courthouse Square

ACCESS: No fees or permits required

MAPS: USGS *Jordan Creek*. The State of Oregon also has a downloadable map; click "Grab a Map" at tinyurl.com/tsfhikes.

WHEELCHAIR ACCESS: No

FACILITIES: Restrooms and water at Elk Creek Campground; vault toilet at Kings Mountain Trailhead

CONTACT: Tillamook State Forest, 503-357-2191, tillamookstateforest.blogspot.com

LOCATION: Elk Creek Campground or Kings Mountain Trailhead on OR 6, 12 miles west of Glenwood, OR

COMMENTS: Because of the mountain terrain, avoid these hikes if it's been raining hard or there's snow on the ground.

A major fire burned every six years until 1951, by which time 355,000 acres and enough timber for more than a million large homes had been destroyed. Logging came to a halt; wildlife was decimated; rivers were choked with sediment and debris; and, most importantly for the forest, seed cones were annihilated, meaning that the forest wouldn't grow back on its own. Eventually, more than 72 million seedlings were hand-planted, and in 1973 what had been known as the Tillamook Burn was renamed Tillamook State Forest.

These hikes offer you a chance to explore one or two of the highest points in the forest and to have a look at how the place has recovered. Keep an eye out for charred logs, for example, and remember that 80 years ago most of this area was bare.

Kings Mountain Trail (5.2 miles out-and-back; strenuous)

This hike gives you the most reward for your effort. It's a tough climb, but it's not as hard as Elk Mountain. From the Kings Mountain Trailhead on OR 6, set out through a forest of alder and incredible sword ferns, with Dog Creek off to your right. At 0.1 mile, you'll see, but not take, Wilson River Trail on your right (Hike 53, page 261). It's the return portion of a killer loop described later.

Around 1 mile, things get nasty-steep; the next mile gains about 1,300 feet, compared to 800 in the first mile. When your trail makes a sharp right, look for a small trail to the left leading to a peak called Kings Jr. Go a few feet out there for your first real

Kings Mountain and Elk Mountain

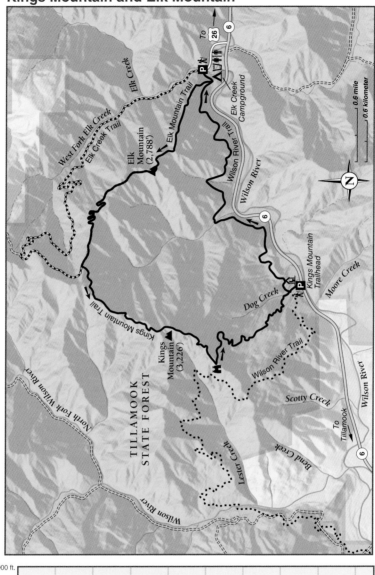

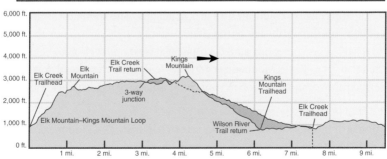

view north. Lester Creek, below you, flows into the Wilson River to your left; Kings Mountain rises directly behind you, higher than the rocky peak you can see from here.

The last 0.6 mile of this hike gains about 900 feet, so take your time. If you're here in May or June, you'll have no doubt it's worth it when you walk past a picnic table (thanks to Troop 299 from Tigard) and out into the meadows, which in early summer are filled with flowers. The summit is now just 0.3 mile ahead, marked by a sign. The view stretches from the ocean to the Cascades. Be sure to sign the trail register, one of the few in Oregon.

If you want to do both peaks, I strongly suggest starting with Elk Mountain (profiled below) and coming back this way.

Elk Mountain Trail (3-mile out-and-back; strenuous)

This is the steepest, roughest trail in this book. It climbs 1,900 feet in 1.5 miles, making it considerably steeper than Dog Mountain (Hike 6, page 44). If you ascend this trail, don't come back down it—do the traverse and return on Kings Mountain Trail or the easier Elk Creek Trail.

From the trailhead at Elk Creek, head up Wilson River Trail 0.2 mile, then take off up Elk Mountain Trail. There's an immediate big step; get used to it. Along the next 1.5 miles, you'll get some views and some spring-summer flowers, but mainly there's a whole lot of up. You'll pass a sign on a tree indicating 2,500 feet elevation, which is nice except that then the trail starts back down. The real summit, at 2,788 feet, has a register placed by the Mazamas, who maintain the trails in this area. If you face Wilson River on the summit, Kings Mountain is to your right.

My advice is to continue on the trail toward Kings Mountain; it dives steeply off the summit and becomes rocky and brushy in places; then it goes up and down and all around for a mile until it enters an old roadbed. After another mile you pop out onto a ridge with views south and a three-way trail junction (200 feet higher than your peak) with the Kings Mountain and Elk Creek Trails.

Elk Mountain–Kings Mountain Loop
(11.2 miles, 7.5 miles with shuttle; very strenuous)

This traverse means business. The high point is 3,205 feet above sea level, and you started at 900 feet . . . but the total elevation gain is 3,700 feet. Even in dry weather, the 1.3-mile ridgetop traverse could stir up a fear of heights. The spookiest section is along the top of cliffs on the north side of the ridge, where snow lingers later than in other places. In recent years somebody added a rope on at least one section to help with traction. When you get to Kings Mountain at 4.9 miles, enjoy the view, head down the steep trail described above, and then hop in your car or hike back to Elk Creek Trailhead.

Elk Creek Trail (4 miles one-way; moderate)

This option is of interest mostly as a safer return trip from Elk Mountain. To do that, it's easy to follow from the three-way junction described above.

If you're looking for a hike to do with the kids, start at the Elk Creek Trailhead. Ascending, walk along the main creek, which has a steelhead run (river otters have reportedly been seen here). Several side trails offer access to the water. At 0.5 mile you come to the confluence of Elk Creek and its West Fork; head up the West Fork 1 mile before starting your climb out of the canyon. After 2.5 miles of gradual uphill walking, arrive at the junction with Elk Mountain Trail.

• •

GPS TRAILHEAD COORDINATES
Elk Creek Trailhead N45° 36.618' W123° 27.999'
Kings Mountain Trailhead N45° 35.814' W123° 30.378'

DIRECTIONS Take US 26 from Portland to OR 6; bear left, following a sign for Tillamook. To start at Elk Mountain, go 23 miles to Elk Creek Campground, on the right just past milepost 28. The road is gated in winter, but it's only 0.3 mile to the trailhead, just beyond the campground. For Kings Mountain, continue 3 more miles on OR 6 to the trailhead, on the right just before milepost 25.

Early summer flowers and views from Kings Mountain

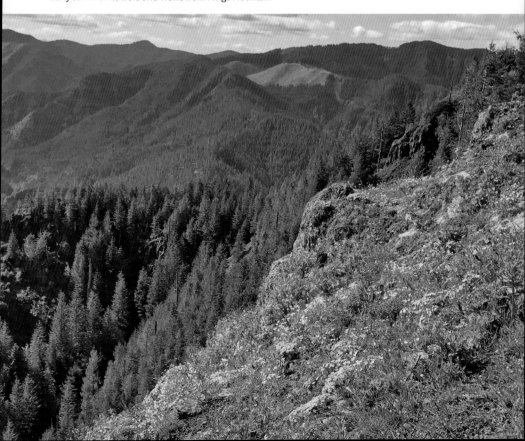

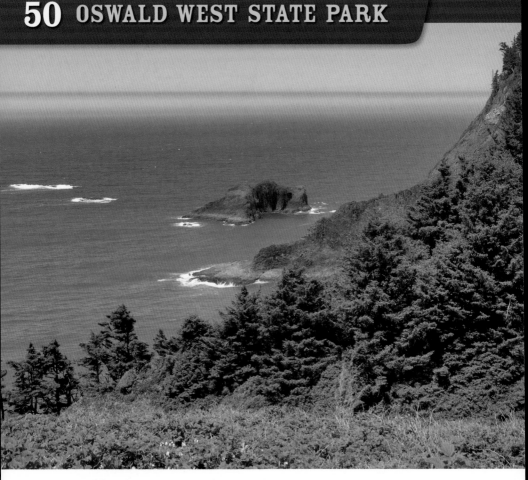

Looking north from the Oregon Coast Trail on Cape Falcon

THIS POPULAR PARK includes two of the best hikes on the northern Oregon coast: a nearly flat stroll through old-growth forest to a clifftop ocean view, and a vigorous hike to a peak with a grand panorama.

DESCRIPTION

Cape Falcon

About five steps from the parking lot, you find yourself in a rare old-growth coastal forest, walking a wide, mostly flat path with Short Sand Creek down on your left. Cruise 0.5 mile to a junction with the Oregon Coast Trail, which here dips down to the left 0.3 mile to Short Sand Beach. Cape Falcon is to your right. Straight ahead is a view of Smugglers Cove.

Turn right, cross a small creek, and after 0.8 mile, where the trail makes a sharp left, look to your right for a downed tree, which left a large, disfigured stump. Some

DISTANCE & CONFIGURATION: 6-mile out-and-back to Cape Falcon, 2.5- to 9-mile out-and-back to Neahkahnie Mountain

DIFFICULTY: Easy to Cape Falcon, strenuous to Neahkahnie Mountain

SCENERY: Old-growth forest, waterfalls, several clifftop vistas of the sea

EXPOSURE: Shady, with clifftops at the cape and a rocky scramble at the mountain summit

TRAFFIC: Heavy all summer, especially on weekends; moderate otherwise

TRAIL SURFACE: Packed dirt, with some gravel; brief rock-scrambling on Neahkahnie

HIKING TIME: 3 hours to Cape Falcon, up to 5 hours for Neahkahnie Mountain

ELEVATION CHANGE: 160' to Cape Falcon, 840' or 1,450' to Neahkahnie Mountain

SEASON: Year-round, but wet in winter

BEST TIME: Whenever it's not raining

BACKPACKING OPTIONS: None

DRIVING DISTANCE: 91 miles (1 hour, 50 minutes) from Pioneer Courthouse Square

ACCESS: No fees or permits required

MAPS: USGS *Arch Cape;* Oregon State Parks also has a downloadable map online; click "Brochures" at the website below.

WHEELCHAIR ACCESS: No

FACILITIES: Restrooms and drinking water near second parking area off US 101

LOCATION: Cape Falcon Trailhead on US 101, 4.5 miles south of Arch Cape, OR

CONTACT: 503-368-3575, oregonstateparks.org/park_195.php

more-imaginative hiking friends of mine dubbed this stump "The Throne of the Forest King." Assume the throne to survey your kingdom, which includes a nice little grove of Sitka spruce and hemlock.

Half a mile past that, ignore a trail that plunges to the left. On the main trail, just after a footbridge over a creek, a brushy path to the left leads 100 feet to a view of a tiny hidden waterfall. If you take this trail left another 100 yards or so, often having to nearly crawl through the brush, you find yourself at the top of an even larger falls that goes right down to the ocean.

A short distance later, back on the main trail, you'll start out toward the end of Cape Falcon itself. You'll get views back into Smugglers Cove and up to Neahkahnie Mountain then descend through the trees once more to a junction. The Oregon Coast Trail continues to the right. For the end of the cape, turn left and walk about 0.2 mile through a near tunnel somebody hacked through the salal. Out at the end, you'll be atop an unrailed 200-foot cliff, with the sea below and Falcon Rock out in front of you. There are good picnicking spots under the trees. In late May and early June, the grassy bluffs here are awash in Indian paintbrush and irises. Look for seals and sea lions below. Make sure to get up to the very top of the hill to see the views north.

Back at the junction, walk left a bit to add more scenery to your day. This is the Oregon Coast Trail, which stretches (in one form or another) from California to the Columbia River. In this next mile or so, you'll get three more views of the Pacific Ocean.

Oswald West State Park

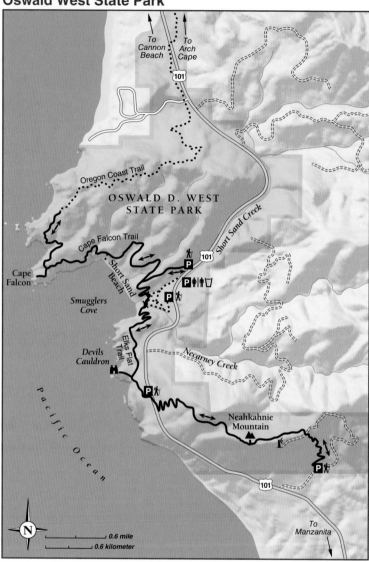

To
Cannon
Beach

To
Arch
Cape

101

Oregon Coast Trail

OSWALD D. WEST
STATE PARK

Short Sand Creek

Cape Falcon Trail

Cape
Falcon

Short Sand Beach

Smugglers
Cove

101

Elks Flat Trail

Devils
Cauldron

Necarney Creek

Neahkahnie
Mountain

P a c i f i c   O c e a n

N

0.6 mile

0.6 kilometer

To
Manzanita

101

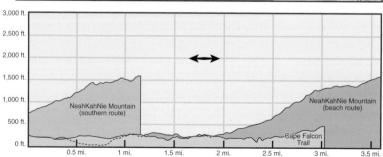

3,000 ft.

2,500 ft.

2,000 ft.

1,500 ft.

1,000 ft.

500 ft.

0 ft.

NeahKahNie Mountain
(southern route)

NeahKahNie Mountain
(beach route)

Cape Falcon
Trail

0.5 mi.　1 mi.　1.5 mi.　2 mi.　2.5 mi.　3 mi.　3.5 mi.

250

Perhaps all these trailheads have you confused. Well, don't be. It's really very simple. Neahkahnie Mountain has a killer view from 1,600 feet above the ocean, and you have two easy options for getting there: The shortest is a 2.5-mile round-trip from the southernmost trailhead, gaining 850 feet; a slightly longer option starts at the "middle trailhead" on US 101 and gains 1,450 feet in 2.5 miles. My favorite longer option starts at the beach and offers more to see as it gains 1,700 feet in 4 miles. With two cars, you could start down by the beach, go over the mountain, come out at the southern trailhead, and put in only 5.5 miles one-way.

First, the shortest option, starting at the southernmost trailhead: Switchback up through open areas filled with tasty red thimbleberries in late summer, and after 1 mile cross a road and climb gradually another 0.5 mile. Right where you pop out into the open, after you cross to the west side of the ridgeline, you'll see a little trail heading up and to your right—that's the summit trail. It's a little rocky scramble, nothing intense.

For the beach option, which is the longest and most scenic route, start at the west-side parking lot for Oswald West State Park. Walk 0.1 mile down the trail, among some awesome Sitka spruces, toward Short Sand Beach to reach a junction offering a choice between beach and campground; choose beach. Walk 0.1 mile, turn left at another junction, and cross a wonderfully bouncy suspension bridge over Necarney Creek. Take a few minutes to explore the lovely beach, which has nice tide pools on the left.

On the Elk Flats Trail toward Neahkahnie Mountain, you'll climb a ridge covered with fantastic trees. When you come out into the open, in a meadow more than 200 feet above the sea, you'll have gone 1.5 miles since leaving your car. Just ahead you'll see two trails splitting off to the right. Ignore the first one you come to. The second leads to a clifftop viewpoint among the trees, looking down at Devils Cauldron. And don't wander around in these meadows. I know a guy who fell into a 15-foot hole here and had to be pulled out with a rope.

At the top of the meadows, you will reach a parking area on US 101; this is where the "middle option" for climbing Neahkahnie begins. From this lot, cross the highway, and climb 0.6 mile in the open before reentering the forest. At this point, you're about 1,000 feet above sea level. You'll climb gradually after this, even dropping at times, and when you come around a corner and hear the ocean again, you have a mile to walk and 300 feet to gain. Eventually you'll be back in the open and see a small, rocky trail heading up to the left; that leads 100 feet up to the viewpoint.

From the viewpoint on Neahkahnie (not actually the summit, but good enough), you can see all the way south to Cape Meares; look for Three Arch Rocks offshore. If it's a really clear day, you might make out Cape Lookout, south of Cape Meares. The beach town seemingly at your feet is Manzanita, and the body of water beyond it is

Nehalem Bay. During the invasion-scare days of World War II, the Coast Guard had a lookout up here, while soldiers patrolled the beaches on horseback and blimps from Tillamook cruised offshore.

If you can, time your arrival on the summit for just before sundown. It's quite a show from up here, and even at dusk you'll have no problem getting back to your car, especially if you came the short way. Just bring a light.

One final suggestion: you can, with a car shuttle, start at Arch Cape and follow the Oregon Coast Trail to any of these other trailheads. If you start there, visit Cape Falcon and Short Sands Beach, then go over Neahkahnie to the south side; that would be an awesome 11.8-mile one-way tour. The Arch Cape Trailhead is off Shingle Mill Lane; look for a wooden post, and don't block anyone's driveway.

NEARBY ACTIVITIES

I have a soft spot for the family-operated Ecola Seafoods Restaurant & Market (503-436-9130; ecolaseafoods.com), located at (208 N. Spruce St. in Cannon Beach, 11 miles north of the Cape Falcon Trailhead. I feel strongly that they serve the best clam chowder around.

• •

GPS TRAILHEAD COORDINATES
Cape Falcon Trailhead N45° 45.787' W123° 57.580',
West Parking Area (beach option) N45° 45.595' W123° 57.562',
South Trailhead N45° 44.448' W123° 56.0752'

DIRECTIONS Take US 26 from Portland and turn south on US 101. The Cape Falcon Trailhead is 14 miles ahead, on the right. The restrooms are at the West Parking Area, 0.1 mile ahead on the left. The middle trailhead and parking area on US 101 is 1.2 miles up on the right. For the South Trailhead to Neahkahnie, drive 2 miles past the restrooms and turn left onto a gravel road by a brown hiker sign. The trailhead is 0.4 mile up, on the left.

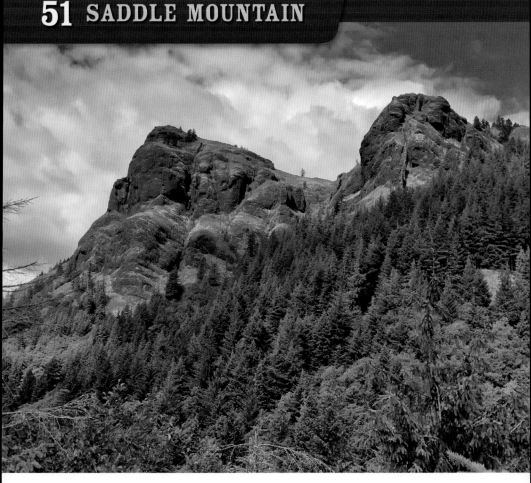

The one view of Saddle Mountain you get in the park

THE HIGHEST POINT in northwest Oregon, Saddle Mountain is also one of the most popular hiking trails in the state. Traversing flower-filled meadows unparalleled in this part of the state, it affords a view from the top that stretches from the ocean to the mouth of the Columbia to the Cascades.

DESCRIPTION

Saddle Mountain just doesn't seem to belong in its surroundings. It's the highest point in this part of the state, but the hills around it aren't even close. It doesn't even resemble them, with its two-headed, rocky summit of "pillow lava," which looks like that because it erupted underwater, millions of years ago when this area was the sea-floor. When you get on top of Saddle Mountain, you might think you're on Mount Hood, with the faraway views and abundant wildflowers. Of course, as crowded as it gets on summer weekends, you might think you're in a city park right after quitting

DISTANCE & CONFIGURATION: 5.2-mile out-and-back

DIFFICULTY: Strenuous

SCENERY: Deep forest, wildflowers, panoramic view

EXPOSURE: In the forest, then out in the open on top; occasionally steep on some loose rocks and metal fencing—slippery if there's been rain or snow

TRAFFIC: Very heavy on summer weekends, heavy on other summer days, moderate otherwise

TRAIL SURFACE: Packed dirt with rocks, then just rocks and metal grating

HIKING TIME: 3.5 hours

ELEVATION CHANGE: 1,600'

SEASON: Year-round but does get snow in winter

BEST TIME: June and July for the flowers

BACKPACKING OPTIONS: None on trail; campground at trailhead open March–October

DRIVING DISTANCE: 71 miles (1 hour, 40 minutes) from Pioneer Courthouse Square

ACCESS: No fees or permits required

MAPS: USGS *Saddle Mountain;* Oregon State Parks has a downloadable map; click "Brochures" at tinyurl.com/saddlehike.

WHEELCHAIR ACCESS: No

FACILITIES: Restrooms at trailhead; closed November–February

LOCATION: Saddle Mountain Trailhead at end of Saddle Mountain State Park Road, 16 miles west of Elsie, OR

CONTACT: Saddle Mountain State Natural Area, 503-368-5943, tinyurl.com/saddlemountain

time on a weekday. Regardless, it's a great hike, so start early in the morning and get there before everybody else, or go later and maybe catch a sunset over the ocean.

When you get out of your car, you might be a little intimidated as you look up at the mountain. You might even see some speck-sized people up there. The good news is you'll be up there soon enough; the bad news is that's not the summit.

Things start out mellow, in a young forest filled with big old stumps—relics of logging in the 1920s and fires in the 1930s. After you've hiked 0.2 mile, you'll see a side trail to the right, which leads 0.1 mile to a great view of all of Saddle Mountain—the only one in the park, oddly enough. At 0.7 mile, you'll pass through an area where storms took down a bunch of trees. Then you'll start climbing, gaining about 1,100 feet in the next 1.4 miles, and occasionally walking on a combination of rocks and metal grating, called gabion, put in for traction. You'll also start to catch glimpses of the rocky world you're headed for, and you'll pass a picnic table in an unlikely spot. Somebody even put in mileage markers on this trail. When you clear out of the forest, you'll be at 2,900 feet, just 300 feet below the summit.

Now you're out in the serious flower meadows. Several rare species grow here, such as Saddle Mountain saxifrage and Saddle Mountain bitter cress—species that survived the last ice age on these slopes. Stay on the trail and on the footbridges, and remember that it's illegal to pick the flowers. You'll descend briefly and cross the saddle—this is the point you can see from the car, which is now visible, if very small, on your left. You'll also see some of the former trail construction projects in here, like two somewhat random sets of stairs. Eventually you'll turn back up and climb the last,

Saddle Mountain

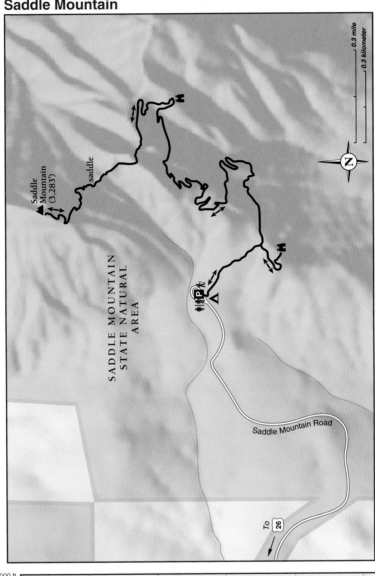

Saddle Mountain (3,283')

saddle

SADDLE MOUNTAIN STATE NATURAL AREA

Saddle Mountain Road

To 26

0.3 mile
0.3 kilometer

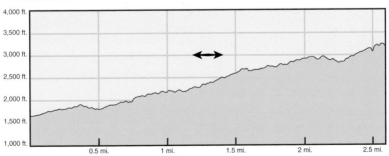

4,000 ft.
3,500 ft.
3,000 ft.
2,500 ft.
2,000 ft.
1,500 ft.
1,000 ft.

0.5 mi.   1 mi.   1.5 mi.   2 mi.   2.5 mi.

steep scramble to the summit, in places with handrails to hold onto. Be grateful for the gabion; this all used to be really interesting on wet days when it was just a trail.

On a clear day, you can see from the volcanoes of the Cascades to the Pacific and to the mouth of the Columbia, just beyond Astoria to the north. See if you can spot the Astoria Tower. On a (rare) really clear day, you can make out the mountains of the Olympic Peninsula beyond that. I also once spotted Saddle Mountain from Chinidere Mountain in the Columbia River Gorge, at the top of the Herman Creek hike (Hike 8, page 53). Needless to say, I've never managed to pick out Chinidere from Saddle Mountain.

NEARBY ACTIVITIES

You no doubt noticed Camp 18 (42362 OR 26, Elsie, OR 97138; 503-755-1818; camp 18restaurant.com) a few miles before the turnoff from US 26—and how could you not? It might look like a logging museum, and it is, but it's also a restaurant with famously filling portions and log decorations. As one newspaper story put it, "You can throw on one serious feedbag." It's not a bad way to prepare for (or recover from) an assault on Saddle Mountain. Be sure to check out the old photos, and ask for a table by the bird feeder.

• •

GPS TRAILHEAD COORDINATES N45° 57.767' W123° 41.391'

DIRECTIONS Take US 26 from Portland, traveling 63 miles west of I-405, and turn right at a sign for Saddle Mountain State Park. The trailhead is 7 miles ahead, at the end of Saddle Mountain Road.

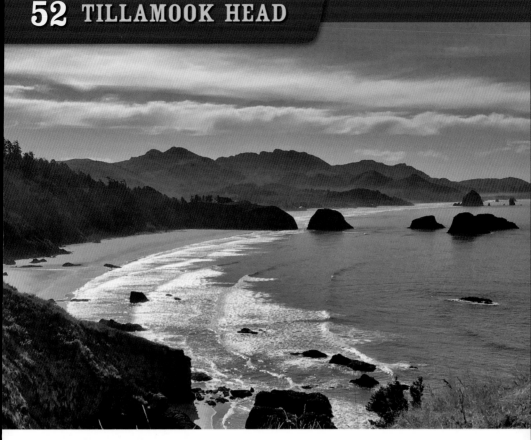

Crescent Beach from the Ecola State Park picnic area

IF IT'S BEACH scenery you're after, this is your hike. Ecola State Park is a gorgeous place, with forested trails connecting scenic beaches and hilltop viewpoints. And if you're up for it, do a one-way shuttle over Tillamook Head—maybe even from just outside Cannon Beach all the way to Seaside.

DESCRIPTION

First, a little history. On January 7, 1806, William Clark was on his way to see a beached whale the natives had told him about. He and 12 others, including Sacagawea, went over Tillamook Head (he humbly named it Clark's Mountain) on a trail that forms the basis of the modern-day path. Clark wrote of the view, "From this point I beheld the grandest and most pleasing prospects which my eyes ever surveyed." He also said the coast had "a most romantic appearance." From his description, it's pretty certain that the exact piece of land he stood on washed into the sea decades ago, but you can still experience pretty much the same view.

And if you're wondering about the name Ecola, it comes from the local Indians' word for whale, not anything to do with the deadly bacteria that sounds similar.

257

DISTANCE & CONFIGURATION: 3-mile out-and-back or 12-mile point-to-point

DIFFICULTY: Easy–moderate

SCENERY: Beaches, headlands, lush forests, seabirds, creeks

EXPOSURE: In and out of the sun, with occasional clifftop viewpoints

TRAFFIC: Heavy in some areas on summer weekends, light–moderate otherwise

TRAIL SURFACE: Dirt, rocks, roots, mud

HIKING TIME: 2–7 hours

ELEVATION CHANGE: 700'–1,350'

SEASON: Year-round, but super muddy in winter

BEST TIME: March and April for whales, any clear day otherwise

BACKPACKING OPTIONS: One site with shelters 1.5 miles up from Indian Beach.

DRIVING DISTANCE: 79 miles (1 hour, 30 minutes) from Pioneer Courthouse Square

ACCESS: $5 day-use for parking at Ecola State Park

MAPS: Ecola State Park has a downloadable map; click "Brochures" at tinyurl.com/ecolahikes

WHEELCHAIR ACCESS: No

FACILITIES: Restrooms at state park trailheads; none on northern end

CONTACT: Ecola State Park, tinyurl.com/ecolasp, 503-436-2844

LOCATION: Ecola State Park on Ecola Park Road in Cannon Beach, OR

COMMENTS: In 2017 the trail from Ecola Beach Day Use Area to Indian Beach was closed due to storm damage; repair work was being planned, but check with the park before you try to hike that section.

Now for the hiking: if you're just up for an out-and-back, you should stay on the Cannon Beach (south) side of Tillamook Head. The only reason to hike the north half is if you're doing the point-to-point with a car shuttle (or using public transit to get around). So I will describe this from south to north, with the best section—if you want to walk only a few hours—being up from Indian Beach 2.5 miles to Clark's Point of View.

If you want to do the point-to-point, it is best to start at Ecola Beach Day-Use Area—if the trail from there to Indian Beach has reopened (see Comments in box above). From there, you can explore south 1.8 miles to Crescent Beach before starting north. In its easy 1.5 miles, this trail never gets far from the view, and at a couple of points it's right at the edge of the cliff—though with fences. When you get to Indian Beach, a favorite with surfers, go left and wander down to the sand for a bit.

To hike the section north of Indian Beach, which is a bit tougher than the section south of it, take the left trail just beyond the restroom (The right trail, marked Clatsop Loop, is a boring road walk to the same place.) You'll pass another view or two, but you'll also go through muddy patches. After 1.5 miles you'll come to an old road and a campsite called Hiker's Camp. Turn left for a World War II–era bunker that housed radar equipment and, just past that, an ocean view from more than 700 feet up. The lighthouse out there—which, no matter what it looks like, is a full mile from the coast—was built in 1881 but decommissioned in 1957. It was known as Terrible Tilly by the unfortunate souls who used to live out there and maintain the light (imagine the weather they had to endure). Strangely enough, in 1980 it was

Tillamook Head

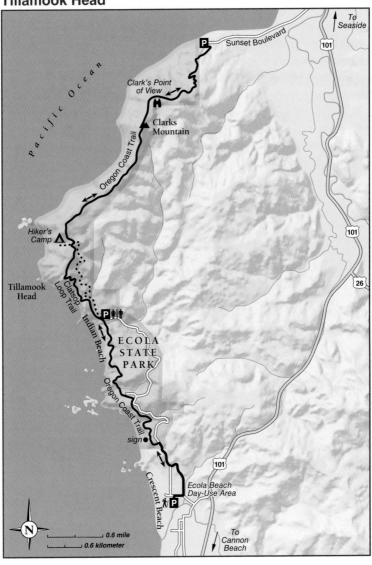

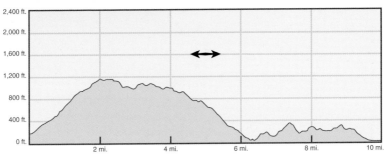

bought and converted into a columbarium, a repository for the ashes of cremated bodies. That ended in 1999, so for now it's just an old lighthouse.

Back up the road, turn left for more forest and more views. Half a mile up from the campsite and after some switchback climbing, you'll come to a series of viewpoints out to the left, one of which is officially known as Clark's Point of View. Trouble is, a sign marking the spot tends to disappear, presumably tossed into the sea by yahoos. Unless you have a car at the Seaside end, turn back here.

To do the town-to-town walk, stash a car at the northern trailhead, which is labeled "Tillamook Head" on Google Maps and is at the end of Sunset Boulevard. Then start at one of the trailheads on the south side.

• •

GPS TRAILHEAD COORDINATES
Ecola Point N45° 42.272' W123° 24.667'
Northern Trailhead N45° 44.994' W123° 39.137'

DIRECTIONS From Portland, take US 26 west 76 miles to US 101. For the suggested trailheads in Ecola State Park, turn south on US 101 and after 2.9 miles take the exit for Fir Street. Continue 0.1 mile, turn right onto E Fifth Street; after another 0.1 mile turn right into Ecola State Park. The pay booth is 1.5 miles ahead, adjacent to Ecola Point parking. Indian Beach is another 1.5 miles up the main road.

To leave a car at the northern trailhead in Seaside, go north on US 101 for 3 miles and turn left onto Avenue U. Take the next left, S Edgewood Street, and follow it 1.3 miles to the trailhead. The road will change names to Ocean Vista Drive and Sunset Boulevard, but just continue straight.

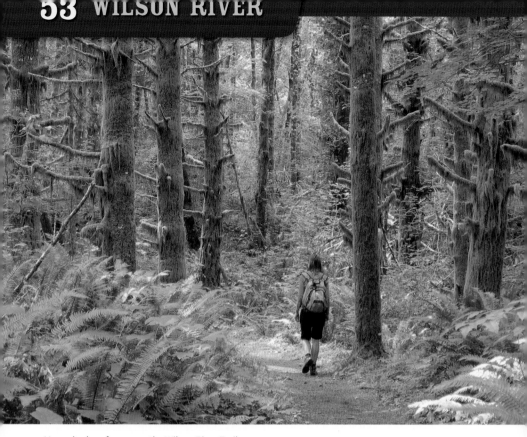

Many shades of green on the Wilson River Trail

THIS TRAIL EXPLORES the canyon of the Wilson River, where salmon and steelhead come to spawn. For many years it was known to nonanglers as "that river along Highway 6 on your way to Tillamook," but with a trail and a forest educational center now in place, plus a healthy forest making a comeback after catastrophic fires, the Wilson is a destination all its own.

DESCRIPTION

This is a year-round hike that's close to Portland and offers something for everybody: steep hills, flat sections, solitude, picnic areas, forests, views, you name it. There's a good chance that the Kings–Jones or Footbridge–Keenig section will have snow in winter, but otherwise it should be open. Come in spring for flowers and maximum water flow, or in October for amazing fall colors and migrating fish.

If you want to do the whole nearly 21-mile hike at once, stash a car at Keenig Creek, start your hike at Elk Creek, and know that you'll have my respect and admiration, for whatever it's worth. Otherwise, pick a section. I advise a car shuttle—it's easy to work out, and it means you don't have to backtrack.

DISTANCE & CONFIGURATION: 3.5- to 7.4-mile out-and-back or point-to-point, or 20.6-mile point-to-point

DIFFICULTY: Easy–strenuous; it's up to you.

SCENERY: Second-growth forest, river, occasional views from up high

EXPOSURE: In forest the whole way

TRAFFIC: Moderate on summer weekends, light otherwise

TRAIL SURFACE: Packed dirt, some rocks

HIKING TIME: Varies for each section; 12 hours for the whole thing

ELEVATION CHANGE: Varies by section; 3,950' for the whole thing

SEASON: Year-round, but might get snow in winter, especially the Kings Mountain–to–Jones Creek section

BEST TIME: March and April for flowers, October for fall colors

BACKPACKING OPTIONS: None

DRIVING DISTANCE: About 50 miles (1 hour) from Pioneer Courthouse Square, depending on which trailhead you choose

ACCESS: No fees or permits required

MAPS: Free brochures available from Tillamook State Forest, or click "Grab a Map" at tinyurl.com/tsfhikes.

WHEELCHAIR ACCESS: Only around Tillamook Forest Center (see Nearby Activities)

FACILITIES: At Elk Creek and Jones Creek Campgrounds, both closed in winter

LOCATION: Easternmost trailhead is Elk Creek Campground on OR 6, 12 miles west of Glenwood, OR

CONTACT: Tillamook State Forest, 503-357-2191, tillamookstateforest.blogspot.com

Elk Creek to Kings Mountain (3.7 miles, 550')

This hike is most often done as part of the formidable Elk and Kings Mountains loop (Hike 49, page 243), but it's a nice forest stroll on its own, with the highlight being a series of meadows just 0.5 mile from the Kings Mountain Trailhead.

From the Elk Creek Trailhead, you'll ascend a steep 0.2 mile to reach the even steeper Elk Mountain Trail. Continue on Wilson River Trail, and the grade will let up a bit before the path becomes a long, mostly flat traverse. At 2 miles, descend to a bridge over Dog Creek. The next mile is more of the same, until you descend to the meadows at 3.2 miles. Try to get here in the morning or late afternoon, and if you're quiet you might see some elk. Another 0.5 mile brings you to Kings Mountain Trail, where you can turn left and descend 0.1 mile to that trailhead. Or keep going.

Kings Mountain to Jones Creek (7.4 miles, 1,500')

This is the toughest, highest, and most scenic section. It also never visits the Wilson River, because private land along the river necessitates a big climb up the slopes of Kings Mountain.

Leaving Kings Mountain Trail, turn left 0.1 mile up from Kings Mountain trailhead. You first cross a jeep track with a sign reading KINGS MT. JR. and then climb 1,200 feet in 1.5 miles on a steady grade. Just before the hilltop is a nice lunch spot, a trailside log where some old roadbeds intersect.

Next you'll start downhill, crossing lots of tiny creeks in the Lester Creek drainage. Around 3 miles, you'll come to the Lester Creek Pinnacles, a big rock formation

Wilson River

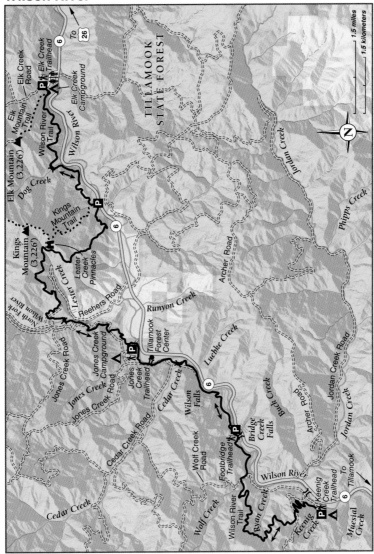

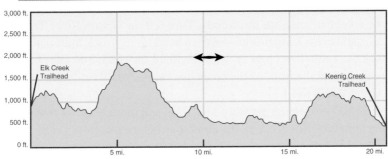

with a tree growing atop it. Here you'll find two good viewpoints and a chance to head out (carefully) to the rock itself.

Half a mile later, hike down steeply and, at 4 miles total, traverse a tiny meadow where several more old roads intersect. Keep moseying along, drop through a particularly lush area with a sea of sword ferns, and at 5.5 miles cross the North Fork Wilson River on a large, scenic bridge. At the far end are a picnic table and a side trail leading down to the river.

Follow the path downstream, and after 100 yards pass Lester Creek Falls across the Wilson, which is adorned with a bright-orange NO TRESPASSING sign. Over the next 1.9 miles, you'll cross two roads and a small ridge then pop out at Jones Creek Trailhead.

Jones Creek to Footbridge (3.5 miles, 300')

This is the most popular section, owing to its ease of access, lack of big hills, and proximity to the river. The Jones Creek area has a campground nearby and a series of picnic sites along the first stretch of the trail. After 0.3 mile, you'll reach a big bridge leading over to Tillamook Forest Center, which has exhibits about the forest and its history (see Nearby Activities, opposite page). The trail stays on the north side of the river, occasionally on roads, and after a mile crosses Cedar Creek on a one-log bridge over a deep pool that looks like a good place for a dip.

Just past the bridge, keep left to avoid power lines, and at 1.3 miles look for a social trail leading down to a rocky area along the river. A quarter-mile ahead is a better trail to a sandier beach. Soon after, you'll climb about 1 mile to pass the 100-foot Wilson Falls, which may seem overrated if it hasn't rained lately.

The last 1.5 miles of this section traces a fern-filled bowl then makes a long, gradual descent to the trail over to Footbridge Trailhead. Even if you intend to keep going, it's worth a trip down to the river here. There's a huge logjam; a swimming hole with a rock outcropping and a swing rigged from a log; and the footbridge itself, which crosses the Wilson at a deep, placid pool in a small gorge. To get to the trailhead from here, turn left at the far end of the bridge, and walk 100 (protected) yards along the shoulder of the highway.

Footbridge to Keenig Creek (6.1 miles, 535')

This is a lonesome stretch with another big hill. If you're starting at Footbridge, walk up the road from the parking lot, cross the bridge, and follow the trail across the creekbed and into the woods. Turn left on Wilson River Trail. In the first mile, you'll cross a log bridge and then head up to a rock bluff with views of the Wilson. At 1 mile, you join Wolf Creek Road for about 500 feet; head right, up the road, to find the trail. At the creek just below, you'll find a log bench for a break—which you'll need.

After Wolf Creek, things get steep for a mile, and then the grade relents a bit. A few creeks and waterfalls break up the monotony before you cross a ridge at 2 miles to start a 3-mile traverse in and out of side canyons.

When you hit Cedar Butte Road, it's only 1.5 downhill miles through switchbacks and a recent clear-cut. Not much to see, but by this time you're probably just ready to be done.

NEARBY ACTIVITIES

Tillamook Forest Center (tillamookforestcenter.org) is open in spring and fall, Wednesday–Sunday, 10 a.m.–4 p.m.; summer hours are 10 a.m.–5 p.m. daily; closed in winter. Admission and programs are free. Remember, though, if you park here and go hiking, your car will be stuck if you don't return before the gates are locked at closing time.

• •

GPS TRAILHEAD COORDINATES
Elk Mountain Trailhead N45° 36.619' W123° 27.998'
Keenig Creek Trailhead N45° 32.605' W123° 36.733'

DIRECTIONS Take US 26 from Portland and bear west on OR 6, following a sign for Tillamook. The trailheads are all along the right side of the highway. For Elk Mountain, go 23 miles to Elk Creek Campground, just past milepost 28; the trailhead is 100 yards past the campground. Kings Mountain Trailhead is 3 miles farther along. Jones Creek Trailhead is in a day-use area between mileposts 22 and 23; head for the campground, then turn left just after a bridge. Footbridge Trailhead is a parking area on the right at milepost 20. For Keenig Creek Trailhead, go 2 miles past Footbridge, turn right on Cedar Butte Road, cross the bridge, and immediately turn left. The trailhead is 0.2 mile ahead, on the right.

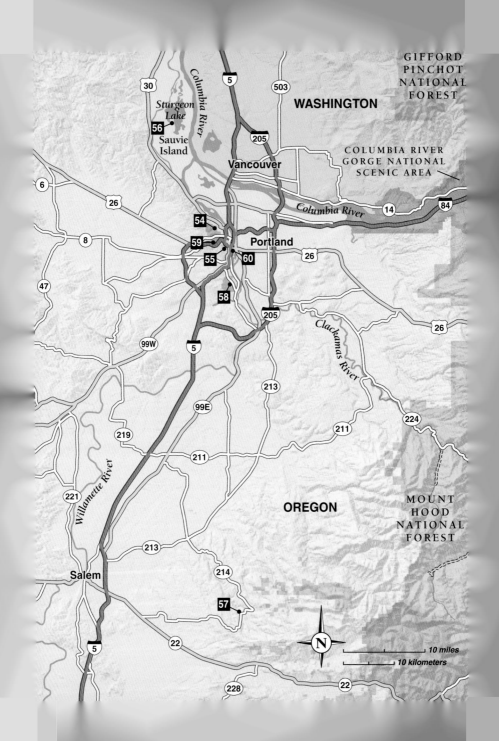

PORTLAND AND THE WILLAMETTE VALLEY

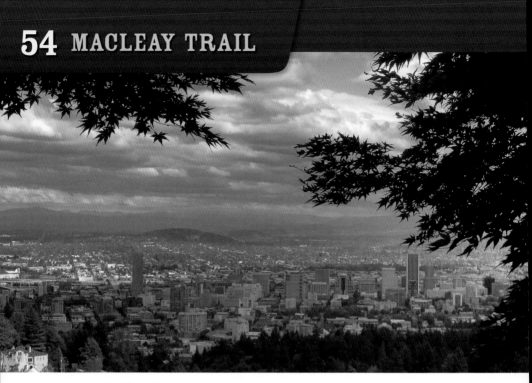

Downtown Portland from the lawn at Pittock Mansion

ON THE EASIER trip to the Audubon Society, you'll see two monumental trees and enjoy close-up views of caged wildlife. If you put in a little more effort, you'll get that and some history with a great view and another monumental tree. You can even connect this with another hike.

DESCRIPTION

First, if the headquarters of the No Ivy League at the trailhead is open, look inside. As of 2013, the project had cleared more than 100 acres of English ivy and saved some 30,000 trees in Forest Park from the invasive vine. In this building the crews house some of their trophies—ivy roots bigger than you can imagine. Gawk, get some water, and head up the trail. What you're walking up here is Balch Creek, named for Danford Balch, who once owned this land and was the first man in Portland to be tried and hanged for murder. Small as it is, the creek was the original water supply for the city of Portland. And if that doesn't amaze you, consider that in 1987 the Oregon Department of Fish and Game discovered a native population of cutthroat trout living in this tiny stream. Balch Creek is one of only two year-round streams in all of Forest Park. Check some of the deeper pools, and you just may see some of the quite small fish. Please keep your dog on a leash and out of the water.

This land, by the way, was sold by the Balch family and eventually wound up being donated to the city by a prominent Scottish merchant in town named Donald Macleay—apparently because he was tired of paying taxes on it. One of the

DISTANCE & CONFIGURATION: 2.6-mile out-and-back to Upper Macleay Park and Audubon Society, 4.5-mile out-and-back to Pittock Mansion

DIFFICULTY: Easy to Upper Macleay Park and Audubon Society, moderate to Pittock Mansion

SCENERY: Quiet woods, predatory birds (in cages), three must-see trees

EXPOSURE: Shady all the way except at road crossing

TRAFFIC: Moderate on the trail weekdays, heavy on weekends and at mansion

TRAIL SURFACE: Packed dirt, some gravel, short paved section

HIKING TIME: 1 hour for Audubon Society, 2.5 hours for Pittock Mansion

ELEVATION CHANGE: 440' to Upper Macleay Park, 880' to Pittock Mansion

SEASON: Year-round, 5 a.m.–10 p.m. daily

BEST TIME: Any clear day for the view

BACKPACKING OPTIONS: None

DRIVING DISTANCE: 3 miles (10 minutes) from Pioneer Courthouse Square

ACCESS: No fees or permits required

MAPS: Forest Park maps at Audubon Society

WHEELCHAIR ACCESS: Lower 0.25 mile is paved; mansion area is entirely accessible.

FACILITIES: Water and restrooms at trailhead, Audubon Society, and mansion

LOCATION: Lower Macleay Park at end of NW Upshur Street in Portland

CONTACT: Portland Parks and Recreation, 503-823-7529, tinyurl.com/macleaypark

conditions of Macleay's gift was that the paths be wide enough for hospital patients to be wheeled through in the summertime.

The path is still wide and now adorned with rails, bridges, benches, and stumps to sit on while admiring the creek. At 0.8 mile, look for a Douglas-fir on your left that is marked with a plaque identifying it as a Portland Heritage Tree, one of some 300 such trees around town to be forever protected from the saw. This one happens to be the tallest tree in the city—last measured at 242 feet in 1997—and is thought to be the tallest in any major US city.

At 0.9 mile, you'll join the 30-mile Wildwood Trail at the Stone House, built by the Works Progress Administration during the 1930s; it was a restroom until the early 1960s, when a storm destroyed its pipes by uprooting numerous trees. In fact, legend has it that the building is also the scene of nocturnal battles between the ghosts of Danford Balch and his victim, Mortimer Stump, a neighbor who had eloped with Balch's teenage daughter. (If there's a better Old Portland name than "Mortimer Stump," I want to know what it is.)

Stay straight (upstream) on Wildwood Trail, and in the next 0.5 mile you'll cross the creek and climb to Upper Macleay Park. Whether you're headed for Pittock Mansion or not, make a right here and walk 100 yards to the Portland Audubon Society. They rehabilitate injured owls and hawks here, and you can view the caged birds for no charge; they also have an extensive collection of mounted animals and an excellent gift shop and bookstore. Three loop trails explore sanctuaries from here; free maps of those and all of Forest Park are available at the gift shop. Particularly worth visiting is a shelter overlooking a pond, just below the headquarters. You can impress

Macleay Trail

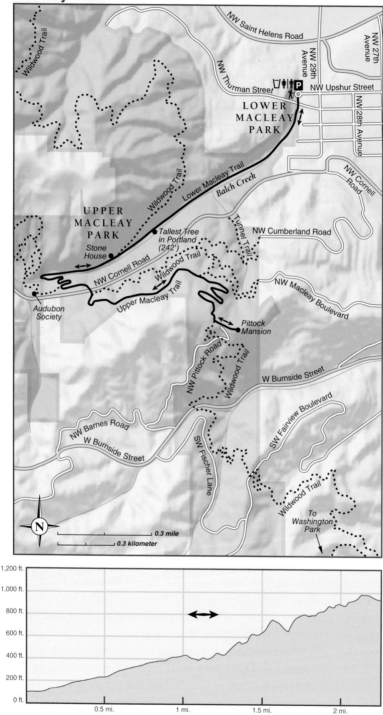

your friends by telling them that the massive sequoia beside the parking lot is actually less than 100 years old. They grow quickly at first.

To do a hike of just 2.6 miles, head back to the car. To add another 2.3 miles and just over 400 feet in elevation, stay on Wildwood Trail by walking along Macleay Park's parking lot, crossing busy NW Cornell Road at a crosswalk, and reentering the forest. After 100 yards, turn right on Upper Macleay Trail. This trail climbs about 0.2 mile then flattens. At 0.5 mile, you'll find a wooden bench with a cool pattern on it. Just past that, rejoin Wildwood Trail, turning right and uphill for the final 0.6 mile to the Pittock Mansion parking lot.

The home (see Nearby Activities, below) is to your left. Wander out to the front yard to enjoy the roses and a view of city and mountains, and admire another spectacular tree: a European white birch that offers shade to two benches with great views.

If you took the bus, you don't have to walk back down the trail. You can, instead, follow the paved path around the house, head down the driveway about 50 yards, and look for Wildwood Trail heading down and to the left. It dives down 0.6 mile to W Burnside Street. Cross it (carefully), walk up the road to the right about 200 feet, and take bus 20 (Burnside/Stark) downtown. (As of 2017, plans were afoot to finally build a bridge here, and more than $350,000 had been raised by the Portland Parks Foundation. Check tinyurl.com/westburnbridge for the latest on construction plans.)

From Burnside, you can also continue on Wildwood Trail to connect with the Washington Park and Hoyt Arboretum hike (Hike 59, page 289). A flat 0.5 mile gets you to a junction with the Creek Trail, part of the Hoyt Arboretum hike. You can also just follow signs for 0.55 mile to the visitor center, and from there another 0.4 mile to the Washington Park MAX Station.

NEARBY ACTIVITIES

Pittock Mansion was built in 1914 by the owner-publisher of *The Oregonian;* his wife founded the Portland Rose Society. It is open for tours daily (3229 NW Pittock Drive, Portland, OR; 503-823-3623; pittockmansion.org).

• •

GPS TRAILHEAD COORDINATES N45° 32.151' W122° 42.751'

DIRECTIONS From SW Fourth Avenue downtown, drive 1.2 miles west on W Burnside Street and turn right onto NW 23rd Avenue. Go 0.8 mile and turn left onto NW Thurman Street. Go six blocks to NW 28th Avenue and turn right. Go one block, turn left onto NW Upshur Street, and follow it three blocks to the trailhead, at the end of the road. The trailhead can also be reached by TriMet: From downtown, take bus 15 (Belmont/NW 23rd), but make sure it's headed for NW Thurman Street and not Montgomery Park. Get off at Thurman and 29th, walk one block, and descend a flight of steps beside the bridge.

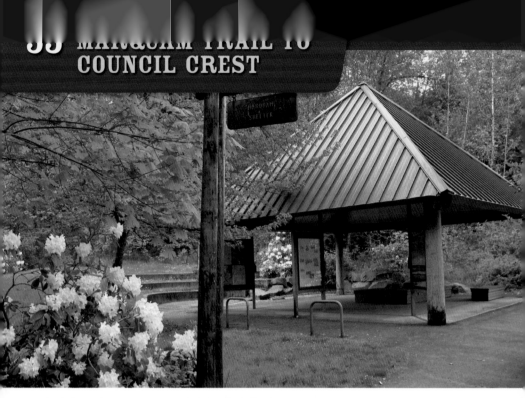

The shelter at Marquam Nature Park during rhododendron season

THIS PLEASANT TRAIL through a wooded gulch just minutes from downtown leads to the highest point in Portland: a park where you can take in a view of four volcanoes. What a city we live in!

DESCRIPTION

Council Crest got its name in 1898 when a group of visiting ministers met there after a 2-hour wagon drive. They assumed the American Indians must have held many a council there. It turns out they probably didn't, but the name stuck. In the early and mid-20th century, you could ride a trolley to the top and visit an amusement park. Today you can get here by car or bus, but the best way is to walk up Marquam Trail through the woods.

At the trailhead shelter, two signs lead you to Marquam Trail, a 7-mile stretch of the 40-Mile Loop that passes through Marquam Nature Park, running from Willamette Park to Washington Park. The Shelter Loop Trail is a 1.2-mile interpretive traverse that meets Marquam Trail and returns to the shelter. If you got a brochure and feel like adding the Shelter Loop Trail, take the path on the left that says 0.7 MILE instead of the one on the right that says 0.4 MILE. The Shelter Loop Trail leads you 0.3 mile up the creek to a junction. Turn right here; numbered signs along the way point out various local flora and fauna as you head 0.4 mile back to the right to reach Marquam Trail.

DISTANCE & CONFIGURATION: 3.7-mile out-and-back with side loop

DIFFICULTY: Easy on Nature Loop Trail, moderate to Council Crest

SCENERY: Woods, impressive homes, sweeping vista on top

EXPOSURE: Shady all the way up, open on top, a couple of street crossings

TRAFFIC: Heavy on weekends and weekday evenings, moderate otherwise

TRAIL SURFACE: Packed dirt, gravel

HIKING TIME: 2 hours

ELEVATION CHANGE: 820'

SEASON: Year-round, 5 a.m.–midnight daily

BEST TIME: Any clear day

BACKPACKING OPTIONS: None

DRIVING DISTANCE: 1 mile (5 minutes) from Pioneer Courthouse Square

ACCESS: No fees or permits required

MAPS: Available at trailhead and at tinyurl.com /marquamtrailmap

WHEELCHAIR ACCESS: No

FACILITIES: Water at trailhead and at Council Crest

LOCATION: Marquam Nature Park on SW Marquam Street in Portland

CONTACT: Portland Parks and Recreation, 503-823-7529, tinyurl.com/marquamnaturepark; Friends of Marquam Nature Park, fmnp.org

Whichever way you went to start with, you'll get to this same junction. From here, if you don't feel like going up the hill, go down the Shelter Loop Trail, and walk 0.4 mile back to your car (this is the right-hand trail you skipped at the trailhead). But for the best view in town, continue up and follow the trail 0.5 mile up Marquam Gulch. Then make a left, following the signs to Council Crest. At this point the trail climbs a bit. Just before you cross the next road (SW Sherwood Drive), there's an extremely cool treehouse on your left. Oh, to be a kid in a neighborhood like this! Another 0.4 mile on, you'll cross SW Fairmount Boulevard and then continue uphill.

After crossing yet another road (Greenway Avenue), in an area planted decades ago with May-blooming rhododendrons, you'll walk uphill to reach the wide, open area atop Council Crest, where couples come to snuggle and kids come to throw a Frisbee. Rest a moment on the two benches there to admire the view of Mount Hood—and check out the dates inscribed here. The benches were dedicated to Frank and Nadia Munk, a couple who both made it to age 98, dying within a year of each other. Nadia, in whose dining room plans were made to save Marquam Gulch 40-plus years ago, was one of the park's cofounders. That group, which became Friends of Marquam Nature Park, stopped plans for apartments in the ravine and lobbied for multiple trailheads to make the area accessible as a retreat from the urban world.

Now climb to the stone circle at the top of the park. Plaques there point out the four volcanoes and give the native name for each. To the east you can see into the Columbia River Gorge. The view west goes out to Beaverton and, on a clear day, the Coast Range. Finally, for an odd little treat, find the small metal disc in the middle of this stone enclosure, stand on it facing Portland, and say, "Portland rocks."

Two more historical notes. The water tower above you used to be a 77-foot-tall wooden observatory in the amusement park. And the statue of the woman and

Marquam Trail to Council Crest

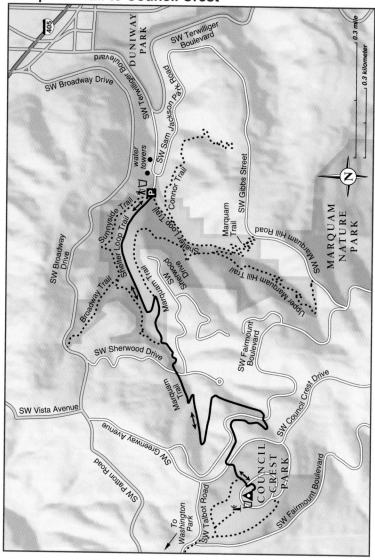

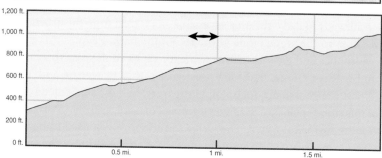

child playing was installed in 1956 and stolen one night in the 1980s. It turned up 10 years later in a drug house in town.

You can connect this trail to the Washington Park and Hoyt Arboretum trip (Hike 59, page 289) if you're up for something a little longer. To do so, as you start back down the trail take a left just after you enter the trees, turning north. This trail will traverse the hill briefly before descending to the right, eventually reaching the intersection of SW Talbot Road and Fairmount Boulevard. Walk down Talbot about 0.3 mile to the intersection with SW Patton Road. Turn right onto the sidewalk on the far side of Patton; 200 feet ahead you'll see a trail descending to the left. Follow it 0.8 mile through the forest until you reach an access road along US 26. Walk left 50 yards, cross the bridge over the expressway, and then look left for a trail going up the hill, into the trees again. This will lead you through a meadow, behind the World Forestry Center, and eventually, in 0.2 mile or so, to an intersection with Wildwood Trail. (This is also the end of Marquam Trail.) Turn right on Wildwood Trail, and in 0.1 mile you'll be at the parking lot; across that is the MAX station, where you can catch a train back to town if you don't want to keep hiking. You could also keep going on Wildwood—for another 30 miles or so.

To return from Council Crest, head 1.3 miles back down the trail, following signs for Marquam Shelter, and when you get to a junction pointing left 0.4 mile to Marquam Park, take it. That's the shorter route back to the car that you skipped earlier in favor of Shelter Loop Trail.

NEARBY ACTIVITIES

If it's Saturday, make it a great Portland day by hitting the Portland Farmers Market (503-241-0032, portlandfarmersmarket.org) at Portland State University, just a few blocks north of Marquam Nature Park and now open year-round. It runs 8:30 a.m.–2 p.m. April–October, and 9 a.m.–2 p.m. November–March, in the South Park Blocks.

· ·

GPS TRAILHEAD COORDINATES N45° 30.170' W122° 41.513'

DIRECTIONS From downtown Portland, drive south on Broadway Avenue. After it crosses I-405, take the second right onto SW Sixth Avenue, following the blue H signs leading to the hospital. (Don't take the right signed COUNCIL CREST.) Continue straight through three lights in the next 0.5 mile, passing two large concrete water towers on your right. When the road cuts back to the left, turn right on SW Marquam Street to enter a parking lot. You can also take TriMet bus 8 to the third light, SW Terwilliger Boulevard and Sam Jackson Park Road, and walk 200 yards up Sam Jackson Park Road to the trailhead.

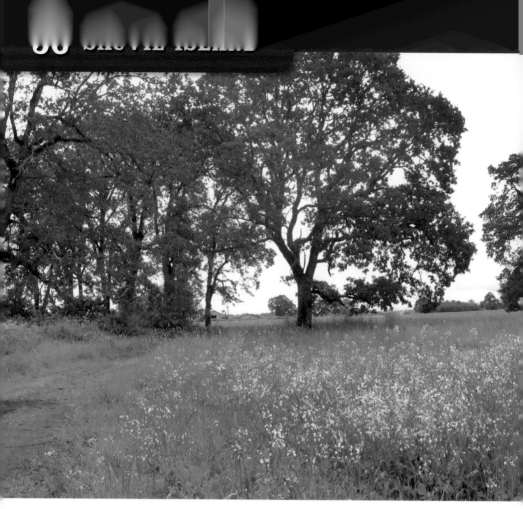

Summer flowers and greenery on the Oak Island Trail

TWO CASUAL STROLLS on the edge of the city offer a glimpse into the local world of wildlife—and into the past. Both are easy to reach and easy to do, and there's plenty more to experience on the island while you're there.

DESCRIPTION

Oak Island

Oak Island is actually a peninsula in a lake on an island in a river. It's also very much a stroll out in the country. You'll even pass crops. But even the crops are part of a plan by the Oregon Department of Fish and Wildlife to manage waterfowl in this area—and waterfowl is what Oak Island is all about.

Sauvie Island (named for Laurent Sauvé, a French Canadian employee of the Hudson's Bay Company) is a rest stop for migratory birds. At the peak of the fall migration, some 150,000 ducks and geese alight here, along with several thousand

DISTANCE & CONFIGURATION: 3-mile loop for Oak Island, 7-mile out-and-back for Warrior Rock

DIFFICULTY: Easy

SCENERY: Lakeshore, woods, meadows, beaches, birds

EXPOSURE: Mostly open for Oak Island, mostly wooded (but some on the beach) for Warrior Rock

TRAFFIC: Moderate on summer weekends, light otherwise

TRAIL SURFACE: Packed dirt, grass, some beach

HIKING TIME: 1 hour for Oak Island, 3 hours for Warrior Rock

ELEVATION CHANGE: Virtually none

SEASON: April 15–September 30 for Oak Island, year-round for Warrior Rock

BEST TIME: Mid-April–May for Oak Island, fall for Warrior Rock

BACKPACKING OPTIONS: None

DRIVING DISTANCE: 19 miles (45 minutes) for Oak Island, 26 miles (50 minutes) for Warrior Rock

ACCESS: Parking on the island is $7 per day or $22 for the season. Buy passes at Cracker Barrel Grocery (15005 NW Sauvie Island Road, Portland, OR 97231; 503-621-3960).

MAPS: USGS *St. Helens;* free map on-site and at tinyurl.com/oakislandtrailmap

WHEELCHAIR ACCESS: No

FACILITIES: Outhouse at each trailhead; nearest water at Cracker Barrel Grocery (see Directions, page 280)

LOCATION: At the end of NW Oak Island Road or Warrior Rock Lighthouse Point Trailhead at the end of Reeder Road on Sauvie Island in Portland

CONTACT: Sauvie Island Wildlife Area, 503-621-3488, tinyurl.com/sauvieislandwildlifearea

sandhill cranes. In all, about 250 species of birds spend time on the island each year, including bald eagles by the score in the winter. So if you were to go to Oak Island in the middle of a summer day, you might wonder what the big deal is. But if you come close to either opening or closing day, or early on a summer day when the animals haven't hidden from the heat yet, you might see a whole different world. Numerous songbirds also hang out here, in addition to ducks, geese, and even bald eagles that spend the whole summer.

From the trailhead, head around the gate and walk a few minutes on the trail/mowed roadway to a junction. Be sure to grab a guide from the box; it explains several signs around the trail. On the trail, go right, which takes you to a view of Sturgeon Lake, which at some times of year might be a long way off because it's so shallow. Turn left, hike 0.9 mile, and when the signed trail turns left follow another trail to the right, continuing 200 yards to The Narrows, a—you guessed it—narrow body of water that connects Sturgeon Lake to the east with Steelman Lake to the west. If it's clear, you'll see Mount St. Helens across the Columbia.

Continuing on the loop trail, you'll head back to the left and walk along a plowed area; Oregon Fish and Wildlife actually farms some 1,000 acres of its land on Sauvie Island as part of a cycle that brings alfalfa, corn, millet, and other foods to migratory birds in the winter and cattle in the summer.

Warrior Rock

In the fall of 1805, Meriwether Lewis and William Clark—while exploring the island that was the summer and fall home of the Multnomah Indians—camped on the

Sauvie Island

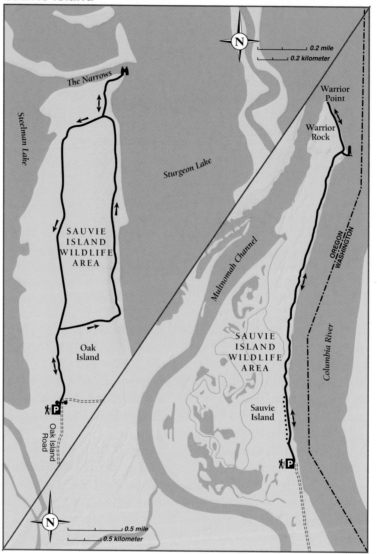

beach that's just beyond the parking area. If you would like to skip the beach entirely, walk over a low point in the fence at the southern end of the parking lot, then walk through the pasture, parallel to the river, to the trees. You'll find the road here.

To start on the beach, follow the trail out onto it, and stroll along, considering not only what it must have looked like in 1805 but also how quiet it is today. Look for animal tracks leading from the woods to the water; raccoons and deer are common here. But those critters move around mostly at night, and if the hunters and fishermen aren't out, you might have the place to yourself. In clear weather you might even make out the light on Warrior Rock, way downstream.

Walk the beach as far as you like; typically after 0.5 mile or so you'll need to bail, so look for a path to follow up into the woods. Up on the bluff, you'll encounter a trail that once served as a service road to the lighthouse. Follow it to the right, through a world of blackberry, oak, alder, and maple. After about 2.5 miles, at a point where the trail is right at the top of the bluff, look to the right for an old shipwreck on the beach. Just a few minutes later, you'll come to a large meadow; keep right 0.2 mile to the lighthouse.

Warrior Rock got its name when members of a 1792 English expedition up the Columbia (the party that named Mount Hood for the head of the English navy) found themselves surrounded on this rock by dozens of native warriors. They cleverly made peace and lived to tell the tale. The lighthouse, the smallest in Oregon, is maintained by the US Coast Guard. And speaking of ships, there's a decent chance you'll see an oceangoing vessel making its way roughly 70 river miles from Portland to the Pacific Ocean at Astoria.

Continue, if you'd like. A few minutes' walk up the beach, at the northwestern tip of Sauvie Island, you'll come to old pilings that no one seems able to explain. Leading theories are that it was a fish-processing plant, a boat works, or a loading dock for shipping milk from island dairies. Whatever it was, it offers a viewpoint of the town of St. Helens, which was founded in 1845. If you're wondering why the town and the nearby mountain are called St. Helens, well, the same English sailors who named Mount Hood and the Columbia River named the volcano for the English ambassador to Spain at the time, a certain Baron St. Helens. His real name was Alleyne FitzHerbert—thank goodness they chose his noble title.

Nothing like some useless trivia to contemplate while you're walking back to the car. Speaking of which, if you stay on the trail the whole way, you'll come to the cow pasture above the beach where you started. Just walk across it—careful where you step—to the fenced parking area and step over the low portion of the fence to your right, next to the hunters' check-in stand.

NEARBY ACTIVITIES

Many of the farms on Sauvie Island are "you pick 'em" operations, with treats such as berries, flowers, pumpkins, and corn mazes. You can't miss it. Stop and get a little something for dinner on your way home, if you don't get lost in a maze. Just beware that on October weekends (aka Halloween season) the traffic here is several levels beyond insane.

GPS TRAILHEAD COORDINATES N45° 42.846' W122° 49.247'

DIRECTIONS Take US 30 from Portland, driving 9 miles west of I-405. Turn right to cross Sauvie Island Bridge. Cracker Barrel Grocery (where you'll buy your parking pass) is on your left, on NW Sauvie Island Road, 0.1 mile beyond the bridge. Go 1.7 more miles on NW Sauvie Island Road and turn right on NW Reeder Road.

Oak Island: Drive 1.3 miles on NW Reeder Road, then turn left on NW Oak Island Road—although, since Reeder heads to the right here, it's more like continuing straight. After 3.1 miles you'll leave the pavement; stay straight, and the trailhead is 1.1 miles ahead, at the end of the road.

Warrior Rock: After 10 miles on NW Reeder Road, you'll leave the pavement and reach a series of parking areas for Welton Beach, just over the dike to your right. Past that is parking for Collins Beach—which happens to be clothing-optional but is blocked from the road by forest. At 2.3 miles after you leave the pavement, the road ends at the parking area for Warrior Rock.

Summer flowers and greenery on the Oak Island Trail

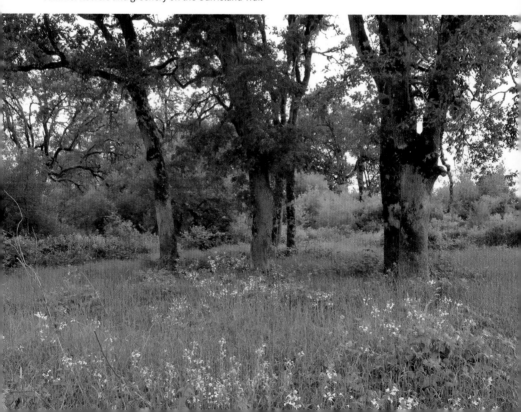

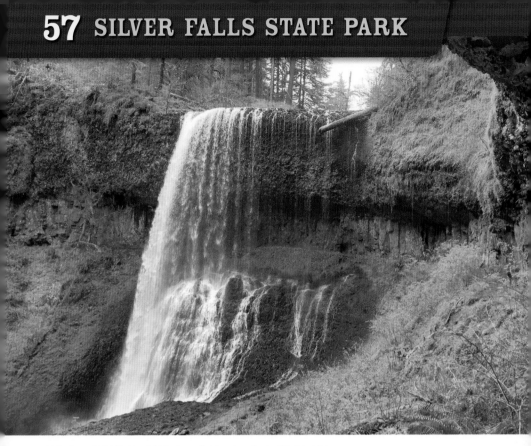

This view of Middle North Falls is available when the trail behind it is open.

IF IT'S WATERFALLS you're after, this easy loop—known as Trail of Ten Falls—is the hike of your dreams. You can also hike several shorter loops with views of one or more waterfalls.

DESCRIPTION

This is the crown jewel of the Oregon State Parks system. Unless it's a rainy weekday in the winter, you probably won't be alone here, but it hardly matters. It's one of the finest walks around. By the way, Silver Creek was named not for its color but for a pioneer named James Smith who settled here in the 1840s. He was known as "Silver" because it was said that he brought a bushel of silver dollars with him from back east.

Be sure to visit South Falls Lodge, which you will pass on the way from the parking lot to the hike. It was built of native stone and wood by the Civilian Conservation Corps (CCC) in 1941. Warm yourself by two massive fireplaces, enjoy photos of the park and some of the tools used by the CCC, and take advantage of that most modern of conveniences: a snack bar with an espresso stand. See if you can find Clark Gable, as well.

DISTANCE & CONFIGURATION: Loop of up to 7 miles

DIFFICULTY: Easy–moderate

SCENERY: Every type of waterfall, in a forested canyon

EXPOSURE: Shady all the way

TRAFFIC: Heavy spring, summer, and fall; light–moderate otherwise

TRAIL SURFACE: Pavement, gravel, dirt

HIKING TIME: Up to 4 hours

ELEVATION CHANGE: 1,300' for whole loop

SEASON: Year-round, but wet in winter and spring, with occasional snow or ice

BEST TIME: March and April for big water, September and October for fall colors

BACKPACKING OPTIONS: None

DRIVING DISTANCE: 61 miles (1 hour, 45 minutes) from Pioneer Courthouse Square

ACCESS: $5/vehicle/day. Annual State Parks pass is $30.

MAPS: Free maps in South Falls Lodge, at trailheads and online

WHEELCHAIR ACCESS: Much of the recommended loop is not accessible, but some falls are, as are many other trails. See the park map for details.

FACILITIES: Water, restrooms, snack bar, and gift shop at South Falls Trailhead

CONTACT: Silver Falls State Park, 503-873-8681, oregonstateparks.org

LOCATION: Silver Falls State Park, 20024 Silver Falls Highway SE, Sublimity, OR

COMMENTS: Dogs, even on a leash, are not allowed on Canyon Trail, described here. They are welcome (if leashed) on other trails in the park.

With your hot drink in hand, walk toward 177-foot South Falls, take in the view from the top, and contemplate the fact that in the 1920s a man named D. E. Geiser used to send old automobiles over the falls as a Fourth of July stunt. It's said that fishermen were pulling car parts out of the pool for decades. Now take the trail behind the sign. (*Note:* This is as far as dogs can go, even if they're leashed.) The trail will switchback down 0.2 mile then go behind South Falls. The cavelike setting was created over the millennia by water seeping through the rocks above, freezing and expanding, and then cracking away the rocks that now lie at your feet. Even in mid-summer, you'll get a little spray here; in winter or early spring, you may get soaked.

When the trail comes to a bridge 100 yards ahead, you can cross it to finish a 0.6-mile loop—your first opportunity to cut the hike short. Or walk 0.7 mile to the 93-foot Lower South Falls. Here the trail descends some steps, often wet even in summer, and passes behind the falls, a combination of curtain and cascade falls.

After another 0.2 mile, you'll come to your second chance to cut the loop short. Turn right and it's 1 mile along Maple Ridge Trail back to the lodge; continue straight and it's 1 mile to the 30-foot Lower North Falls. At this point you've left the South Fork of Silver Creek for the North Fork; the two combine downstream from here to form Silver Creek—this is why you're now walking upstream rather than down. Keep an eye out for deer and beaver, both of which live in the park. Humans left their mark too; on some of the big cedar stumps, you can still make out springboard slots, where loggers inserted boards to stand on as they cut the trees by hand.

Silver Falls State Park

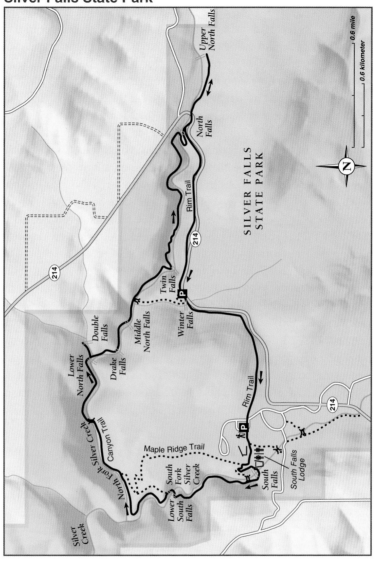

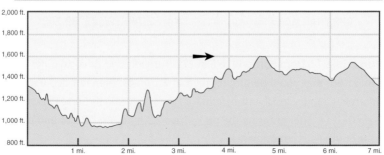

Just past Lower North Falls, make sure to go left for a 0.1-mile side trip to see Double Falls, at 178 feet. Its shallow splash pool, which you can get in if you like, almost always hosts a rainbow when the sun is out. Back on the main trail, you'll pass the 27-foot Drake Falls and 103-foot Middle North Falls (behind which is a small cave you can visit) in the next 0.4 mile. When you get to a bridge—the halfway point for the full loop—turn right for one last chance to cut the loop short. To do that, take this trail 0.3 mile to Winter Falls, then continue past it and up to a parking lot; turn right on Rim Trail and walk 1.2 miles back to the lodge to end your day at 4.2 miles.

If you ignore the bridge and continue straight, you'll walk 0.3 mile to reach the 31-foot Twin Falls, which has the hike's best picnic spot, at the creek's edge. Another 1.1 miles along (look for the rocks in the creek with ferns growing on top), you'll reach North Falls, which you'll see before you get there and which is probably the most spectacular falls in the park. Once again, the trail takes you behind the falls. Back there, look for the columns in the rock overhead, left when lava cooled around trees and then the trees rotted—15 million years ago.

After examining that, climb some steps, then head up along a railing with another view back down to North Falls. When you get to Rim Trail, on the right, go ahead and put in the flat 0.4-mile loop to Upper North Falls, a less visited 65-foot drop in an area with ample opportunity to rock-hop and explore.

On Rim Trail's 2.3-mile trip back to the lodge, you'll pass the top of Winter Falls—more of a damp spot in late summer and fall but worth descending to—and through pleasant forest where I have encountered deer on three occasions. Look for jaw-dropping, massive old trees in here. When you get to the picnic area, continue straight on a new trail, and you'll be back at the lodge in no time.

NEARBY ACTIVITIES

Just upstream from the South Falls parking area is an official swimming area in Silver Creek. The park also has campsites and cabins you can rent for the night; horses can be rented May–September.

• •

GPS TRAILHEAD COORDINATES N44° 52.769' W122° 39.268'

DIRECTIONS Take I-5 from Portland to Exit 271. Turn left and drive 14 miles on OR 214 to Silverton. Note that you'll be turning right at 2.7 miles, then left at 3.9 miles—both intersections have signs. In Silverton, follow signs for Silver Falls State Park, continuing 15 miles on OR 214. After entering the park, drive 2.3 miles on OR 214 and park on the right, at the South Falls parking area.

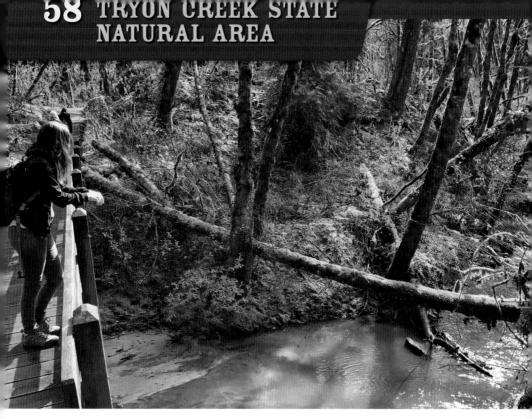

On High Bridge over Tryon Creek

TRYON CREEK, OREGON'S only state park in a major city, is the kind of place you want to visit over and over, just to see what's going on. Are the steelhead in? Are the trees wearing their fall colors yet? Are the trilliums in bloom? Are there any beavers around?

DESCRIPTION

Tryon Creek is named for Socrates Tryon, who homesteaded here in 1850. His family sold out in 1874 to Oregon Iron Company, which logged this area in the 1880s to provide fuel for its Lake Oswego foundry. Multnomah County started purchasing the land in 1969, and the park was dedicated in 1970. This process also led to the creation of Friends of Tryon Creek, which raised money to build the shelter, Nature Center, and other buildings.

What you see today is what's known as second-growth forest. But it's certainly not a second-class forest; some of those old tree trunks are amazing. This 670-acre park, in a ravine between Portland and Lake Oswego, hosts 50 species of birds, plus deer, beaver, fox, coyote, barred owl, and a winter steelhead-trout run, in addition to resident steelhead and cutthroat trout. In fact, whichever hike

285

DISTANCE & CONFIGURATION: 3-mile loop; 8 total miles of hiking trails in the park

DIFFICULTY: Easy

SCENERY: Woodsy ravine with creek, lots of wildflowers in spring

EXPOSURE: Shady

TRAFFIC: Heavy on weekends, moderate otherwise

TRAIL SURFACE: Packed dirt, gravel

HIKING TIME: 1 hour for recommended loop

ELEVATION CHANGE: 200'

SEASON: Year-round, 7 a.m.–sunset daily; Nature Center open 9 a.m.–4 p.m. daily

BEST TIME: April for the trillium bloom

BACKPACKING OPTIONS: None

DRIVING DISTANCE: 7 miles (20 minutes) from Pioneer Courthouse Square

ACCESS: No fees or permits required

MAPS: Free maps at Nature Center; click on "Brochures" at tinyurl.com/tryonsp.

WHEELCHAIR ACCESS: The 0.4-mile Trillium Trail offers two barrier-free loops.

FACILITIES: Water and restrooms at Nature Center

CONTACT: Tryon Creek State Natural Area, 503-636-9886, tinyurl.com/tryonsp

LOCATION: Tryon Creek State Natural Area on SW Terwilliger Boulevard, Portland

COMMENTS: The nonprofit Friends of Tryon Creek puts on numerous events in the park, from day camps to nighttime hikes to classes and lectures. To find out what's going on, call 503-636-4398 or visit tryonfriends.org.

you're doing, stop in at the Nature Center for the displays and schedule of ranger-led activities. They also typically have a board listing the various animals that have been seen in the park lately and where.

Numerous hiking options start at the Nature Center, so pick up a free map and make your own way, or call the park for a schedule of ranger-led hikes. For our suggested loop, when you come out of the Nature Center turn left, walk past Jackson Shelter, and start on Maple Ridge Trail. As the name implies, this area is home to many maples, which put on quite a yellow, red, and orange show in late October and early November. This also means that in winter and early spring, when the trees are without leaves, you'll be able to see through the forest more clearly, catching glimpses of the land formations, the creeks below, and perhaps animals.

Hike 0.2 mile, and reach a junction. As you can see on the park map, there is a network of trails up here on the level with the Nature Center, so stay left and wander around if you don't want to tackle any hills. Otherwise, take a right on Middle Creek Trail, and descend 0.2 mile. Turn right on the Lewis and Clark Trail, and follow it 0.25 mile to the very cool Terry Riley Bridge. This 48-foot span was built in 1998 by law students from Lewis and Clark College to honor a classmate who died of a heart attack. Come back and cross Tryon Creek at High Bridge. It's worth it to turn right here and explore the 0.4-mile North Creek Trail, if only to see the astonishing fields of summer-blooming impatiens (also known as jewelweed) and a few places to access the creek, one of them a deep pool at a bend.

Return to Middle Creek Trail and follow it 0.2 mile to an intersection with Cedar Trail. Follow this trail to the right as it crosses a horse trail (careful where

Tryon Creek State Natural Area

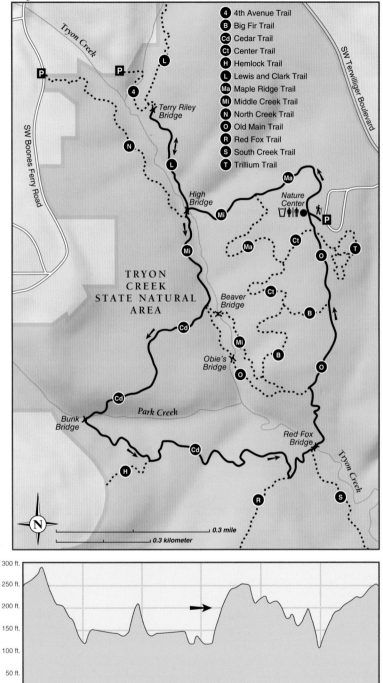

4 4th Avenue Trail
B Big Fir Trail
Cd Cedar Trail
Ct Center Trail
H Hemlock Trail
L Lewis and Clark Trail
Ma Maple Ridge Trail
Mi Middle Creek Trail
N North Creek Trail
O Old Main Trail
R Red Fox Trail
S South Creek Trail
T Trillium Trail

Tryon Creek

SW Terwilliger Boulevard

SW Boones Ferry Road

Terry Riley Bridge

High Bridge

TRYON CREEK STATE NATURAL AREA

Nature Center

Beaver Bridge

Obie's Bridge

Cedar Cd

Park Creek

Bunk Bridge

Red Fox Bridge

Tryon Creek

0.3 mile
0.3 kilometer

N

300 ft.
250 ft.
200 ft.
150 ft.
100 ft.
50 ft.
0 ft.

0.5 mi.   1 mi.   1.5 mi.   2 mi.   2.5 mi.   3 mi.

you step) and then climbs briefly into a more open forest. Keep an eye out for a downed cedar trunk on the right that has obviously been explored by many an adventuresome child.

Cedar Trail crosses Bunk Bridge after 0.4 mile then continues 0.5 mile to a junction with Red Fox Trail. Turn left here and cross Red Fox Bridge; if it's winter, keep an eye out for spawning steelhead. Climb briefly to Old Main Trail, then turn right and follow it back to the Nature Center.

NEARBY ACTIVITIES

The Original Pancake House (8601 SW 24th Ave., Portland, OR; 503-246-9007, originalpancakehouse.com), founded in 1953, isn't far away. This third-generation family business has spawned more than 120 franchises in 29 states (along with one location each in Japan and South Korea). Go there, get an apple pancake or a Dutch baby, and discover the joy of breakfast. It's cash-only, though.

* *

GPS TRAILHEAD COORDINATES N45° 26.495' W122° 40.542'

DIRECTIONS Take I-5 south from Portland, driving 3 miles to Exit 297 (Terwilliger/Bertha). Turn right at the end of the ramp, then take the first right on SW Terwilliger Boulevard. Stay on Terwilliger 2.5 miles; the main entrance to the park is on the right.

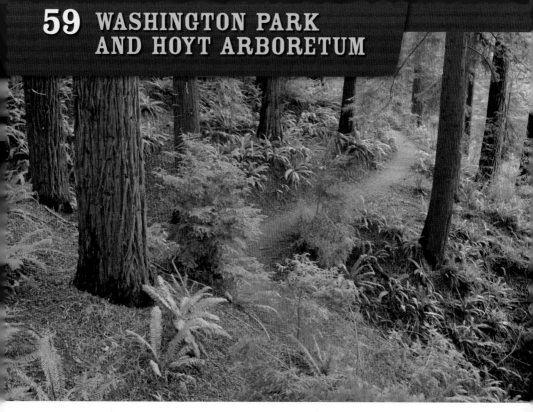

Looking down from the viewing platform in the Redwood Collection

A FAMILY COULD spend a weekend in Washington Park and never run out of things to do. The park has a zoo, a children's museum, the World Forestry Center, the Vietnam Veterans of Oregon Memorial, a world-class Japanese garden, the International Rose Test Garden, Hoyt Arboretum, and miles of hiking trails. TriMet runs a shuttle bus that connects it all. The loop described here is only a suggestion.

DESCRIPTION

This loop hike can be your base for exploring and an introduction to all that Washington Park has to offer. From a hiker's perspective, the heart of the park is Hoyt Arboretum, founded in 1928 on land that was completely clear-cut in the early 20th century. Stop at the visitor center (which is on this loop) for a helpful map.

Beginning your walk at the Vietnam Veterans of Oregon Memorial, follow the trail under and then across the bridge and through a circular series of memorials describing events at home and in Southeast Asia from 1959 to 1972. Follow the trail out of the memorial, and then turn left onto Wildwood Trail. (To your right is the beginning of this "wonder trail," which wanders some 30 miles through Washington and Forest Parks.)

DISTANCE & CONFIGURATION: 4-mile loop

DIFFICULTY: Easy

SCENERY: 1,400 species and varieties of plants, more than 5,000 labeled trees and shrubs

EXPOSURE: Shady, with the occasional open spot for city views

TRAFFIC: Heavy on weekends, moderate during the workday or bad weather

TRAIL SURFACE: Pavement, packed dirt, gravel

HIKING TIME: 2 hours for the recommended loop

SEASON: Year-round

BEST TIME: Spring for blooms, fall for colors

BACKPACKING OPTIONS: None

ELEVATION CHANGE: 300'

DRIVING DISTANCE: 2 miles (10 minutes) from Pioneer Courthouse Square

ACCESS: No fees to hike, but parking is $1.60/hour, up to $4/day October–March and $6.40/day April–September.

MAPS: Trail guide at visitor center

WHEELCHAIR ACCESS: Several barrier-free trails run through the area; ask at the Hoyt Arboretum Visitor Center.

FACILITIES: Water and restrooms at visitor center

LOCATION: Vietnam Veterans of Oregon Memorial at SW Knights Boulevard and S W Kingston Drive in Washington Park, Portland

CONTACT: Hoyt Arboretum, 503-865-8733, hoytarboretum.org

Stay on Wildwood Trail 0.4 mile as it circles right, crosses a road, and climbs a small hill to a viewpoint between two water towers. Look for Mount St. Helens and Mount Rainier, and then turn left on Holly Trail and walk 100 yards to the visitor center, where you'll find water, restrooms, really nice people, and a mountain of information. Return to the viewpoint, and turn left to continue on Wildwood Trail. In about 200 feet you'll come to Magnolia Trail on the left; take it 0.3 mile to the Winter Garden if you'd like to cut about 1.6 miles off your hike and stay in the arboretum. For a pleasant, woodsy stroll and access to other Washington Park attractions, stay on Wildwood Trail.

The wide, flat Wildwood Trail loops out 1.5 miles, with access along the way to the Hawthorne, Walnut, and Maple Trails—each touring a collection of those trees. At the 1.2-mile mark, you will have a view down to the right of the waterfall area of the Japanese garden; just after that, a trail on the right leads to the garden, the largest in the world outside Japan and a must-see. Just down a hill beyond that is the International Rose Test Garden, with more than 7,000 rosebushes in more than 550 varieties. Did I mention you could spend quite a while in Washington Park?

Back on Wildwood Trail, 0.3 mile past the Japanese Garden Trail, you enter Winter Garden and Beech Trail on the left. Stick with Wildwood, and 0.6 mile later, after passing a wonderful viewing platform, take a left on Redwood Trail to explore the sequoia collection. Shortly beyond that, you'll enter the redwood collection, which includes a specimen of the dawn redwood, which, until a few decades ago, was thought to be extinct.

Note: If you were to stay on Wildwood Trail here, you could add a 2.4-mile out-and-back trip to Pittock Mansion, which stands atop the Macleay Trail hike (Hike 54, page 268).

Washington Park and Hoyt Arboretum

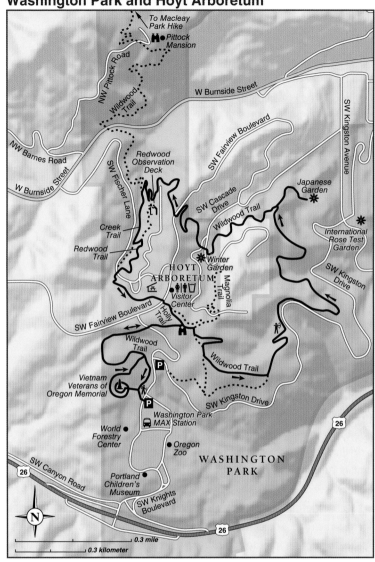

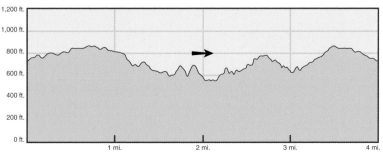

Back on Redwood Trail, when you come to a trail on the right marked TO CREEK TRAIL, take that, then go left on Creek Trail. It dead-ends at a road; pick up Redwood Trail again at the far side, and you'll pass through the larch collection and turn left on Fir Trail to reach Stevens Pavilion. Cross the road, and you're back at the visitor center. Turn right, take Holly Trail back to Wildwood Trail, turn right on it, and follow it 0.5 mile back to your car.

Or just get a map at the visitor center and explore on your own. As you'll see on the map, this loop is just a beginning.

NEARBY ACTIVITIES

The Portland Children's Museum (4015 SW Canyon Rd., Portland, OR 97221; 503-223-6500, portlandcm.org) features hands-on exhibits in a "center for creativity, designed for kids age 6 months through 12 years old." Kids can climb, swim, toss balls, act in a play, and even produce a movie.

· ·

GPS TRAILHEAD COORDINATES N45° 30.689' W122° 43.044'

DIRECTIONS The best way to get to this trailhead is to take MAX Light Rail. It takes you to the deepest transit station in North America—at 260 feet, the second-deepest in the world—which features artwork and displays on the geological history of the region. An elevator puts you right next to the World Forestry Center; turn right when you're facing the center, and the trailhead is across the road and about 100 yards uphill.

To drive here from downtown Portland, head west on US 26 and take Exit 72 (Zoo) after 1.3 miles. At the end of the ramp, turn right on SW Canyon Road. Then stay left (now on Knights Boulevard), circling the parking lot, and stay straight at the MAX station. Our trailhead is at the Vietnam Veterans of Oregon Memorial, 0.1 mile ahead on your left, with parking across the road. You can also park at the arboretum visitor center by continuing up Knights Road another minute and turning right onto Fairview Boulevard 0.1 mile.

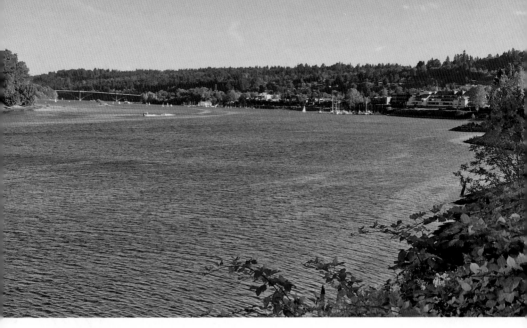

View south from the Greenway Trail, with Sellwood Bridge in the distance

TOUR CENTRAL PORTLAND and the Willamette River on a series of paved walkways. You can piece this one together on different days, mixing in tourist activities, or do it all in a pleasant day of wandering. It's a fine introduction to some of Portland's cooler elements, combining city access with peaceful natural spaces.

DESCRIPTION

I've broken this hike into several different sections, each with access points from the Portland Streetcar, MAX Light Rail, or TriMet Bus.

Portland Aerial Tram to Steel Bridge (2.4 miles)

South Access Portland Streetcar, SW Moody/Gibbs Stop (12760)

North Access MAX Light Rail, Old Town/Chinatown Station (8339)

From the Portland Streetcar stop (NS Line) at the base of the Portland Aerial Tram, walk north on SW Moody Avenue. You'll pass Tilikum Crossing bridge, one of many opportunities to make a shorter loop. But even if you're going all the way around, walk out to enjoy the view. At the far end is the Oregon Museum of Science and Industry (OMSI) and a streetcar/MAX stop. Otherwise, continue up Moody, passing under the Ross Island Bridge and soon coming to River Parkway, 0.8 mile north of the tram. Turn right on River Parkway and look for where the path resumes, at a

DISTANCE & CONFIGURATION: One-way, out-and-back, or big loop, with options of up to 12.2 miles

DIFFICULTY: Easy terrain, moderate difficulty depending on how far you go

SCENERY: City, river, forests, amusement park

EXPOSURE: In and out of the sun

TRAFFIC: Moderate–heavy

TRAIL SURFACE: Paved

HIKING TIME: 6 hours to do it all

ELEVATION CHANGE: Virtually none

SEASON: Year-round

BEST TIME: Anytime you want

BACKPACKING OPTIONS: None

DRIVING DISTANCE: None. See Description (starting on page 293) for transit access.

ACCESS: Parking fees or TriMet pass ($2.50 ages 18–64, $1 seniors 65+)

MAPS: Available from the Travel Portland visitor center (701 SW Sixth Ave., Portland, OR)

WHEELCHAIR ACCESS: Yes

FACILITIES: Several places along the way

CONTACT: Travel Portland, 503-275-8355, travelportland.com

LOCATION: Central Portland

COMMENTS: The South Waterfront area is still seeing some construction and might be a little different when you get there, but it will be much the same and easy to follow.

viewpoint under the I-5 Marquam Bridge. You'll be overlooking Poet's Beach, which offers river access and "inspired thoughts" engraved in stone. To the right, when this book was written, was a big open space, through which the path will go someday.

The next section of northbound trail reaches South Waterfront Garden in 0.3 mile; here you can walk down a dock with access to the river. The path continues through the RiverPlace neighborhood before coming onto the large (and often goose-filled) lawn in Tom McCall Waterfront Park. Just beyond is the Hawthorne Bridge, where you can find restrooms as well as stairs that access the bridge. Walk across the river to pick up another section of this walk on the other side.

Still on the west side, the path now enters a much-loved stretch of land. McCall Park was once a highway, but that was torn out to create a grassy, riverside expanse that's home to picnickers, disc tossers, and a series of festivals. You may also notice huge steel bollards; these secure ships during the annual Rose Festival, when McCall is filled with an amusement park. Along this stretch, you'll eventually arrive at the Burnside Bridge and the site of the Portland Saturday Market, which actually happens both weekend days from March through Christmas.

Just beyond the bridge is the Japanese Historical Plaza, whose cherry trees provide hope and color to rain-soaked locals in March. At the other end—1 mile north of the Hawthorne—you reach the Steel Bridge and the end of this section. The Old Town/Chinatown MAX Station is one block west, on NW Davis Street.

North of the Steel Bridge (1.4 miles round-trip)

South Access MAX Light Rail, Old Town/Chinatown Station (8339)

North Access Portland Streetcar, NW 10th/Northrup Stop (13604)

This flat and fairly quiet extension of the Willamette Greenway Trail is either an out-and-back for those doing the full loop or another exit that will lead you to the Pearl

Willamette River Greenway

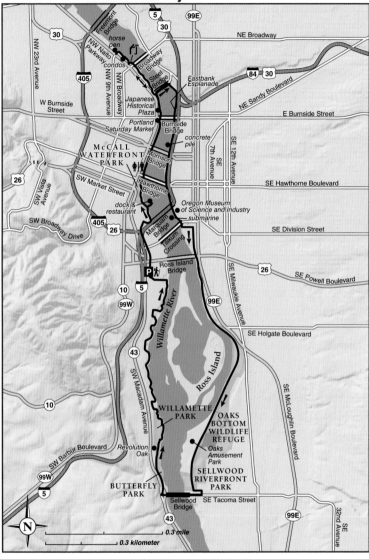

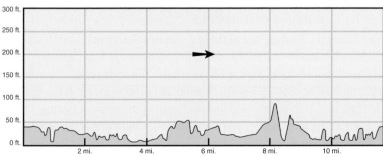

District. From the Steel Bridge, walk north across the railroad tracks, and look for a WILLAMETTE GREENWAY TRAIL sign leading right. Follow the path north, between condos and the river, and take note of the reminders that there's still a port in Portland: the grain elevators across the way and the seagoing vessels being serviced along the other side of the Willamette. Also look across the way for the arenas in the Rose Quarter.

The path soon turns to boardwalk and you pass under the Broadway Bridge then reach a viewing platform at the corner of the 1909 Albers Mill Building. Past that are much-more-modern condos with their fancy glass and water features. The trail ends at the corner of NW Ninth Avenue and Naito Parkway—at least it did at press time.

To reach Portland Streetcar Stop 13604, near Tanner Springs Park in the Pearl, walk across Naito Parkway and the railroad tracks on NW Ninth Avenue, walk one block, and turn right onto NW Northrup Street.

Steel Bridge to OMSI (1.5 miles)

North Access MAX Light Rail, Old Town/Chinatown Station (8339)
South Access Portland Streetcar, SE Water/OMSI Stop (13615)

Walk across the Steel Bridge, on either the upper or lower section. At the east end of the 890-foot walkway, turn right onto the Vera Katz Eastbank Esplanade. Enjoy the 280 trees and 43,695 shrubs (most native) planted along the trail, and in a few minutes come to the floating walkway. At 1,200 feet, it's the longest in the world. It's held in place by 65 pylons, each sunk 30 feet into the bottom of the river. Each section weighs 800,000 pounds, yet you can still feel it bobbing up and down. If you want to head back to the west side, you can do so on the Burnside Bridge via a staircase on the south side.

After passing under the Morrison Bridge (also accessible via a ramp), you'll see what looks like a strange rock formation; this is leftover concrete, dumped when the Morrison Bridge was being built. Just past the Hawthorne Bridge, which has a lookout point on the north side and access to cross back over the river, you'll come to OMSI. The path goes across the front of OMSI (past the submarine); a minute or two past that, you'll come to the east end of Tilikum Crossing, where the Streetcar/MAX stop is 50 yards to your left.

OMSI to Sellwood Bridge (3.9 miles)

North Access Portland Streetcar, SE Water/OMSI Stop (13615)
South Access TriMet Bus, SE 13th/Tacoma Stop (6709) or
　　　　　　　　Sellwood Riverfront Park

Pass under Tilikum Crossing, where there is some cool artwork, and then to the end of the Esplanade section at Caruthers Landing, where you'll get a viewpoint to the *Portland Spirit*'s home dock. Now walk away from the river on SE Caruthers Street for a block, then right onto SE Fourth Avenue. In two blocks, enter the Springwater Corridor Trail, a 21-mile former rail line that goes to the town of Boring.

Around the first mile marker you'll come to a series of grassy areas with benches and an art installation, as well as the Ross Island Sand and Gravel Company.

A third of a mile later, look for a trail leading right, into the woods; take it for a respite from the concrete and bikers. You'll wander 0.6 mile through cottonwood forest with several views of the river then rejoin the main path at an entrance for Oaks Bottom Wildlife Refuge. Here you can either stick with the main, paved path headed south or cross under the tracks into the refuge. There, make a couple of right turns, walking along a large pond and then cutting back over to this path.

Either way, you'll arrive at Oaks Amusement Park and, just past that, SE Spokane Street at Sellwood Riverfront Park. The Springwater Corridor Trail keeps going, and you can explore that way if you'd like. We'll go left on Spokane two blocks, right on SE Sixth Avenue, and right on SE Tacoma Street to head over Sellwood Bridge. Or left for a world of coffee shops, cafés, and antiques dealers in Sellwood.

Sellwood Bridge to OSHU Tram (2.9 miles)

South Access TriMet Bus, SE 13th/Tacoma Stop (6709) or
Sellwood Riverfront Park
North Access Portland Streetcar, SW Moody/Gibbs Stop (12760)

At the west end of the Sellwood Bridge, follow the path down, around, under the bridge, and back onto the Willamette River Greenway. (The obvious wooded area south of here is Powers Marine Park; when this was written it was still closed.) Heading north, you will pass Willamette Moorage Natural Area, where Stephens Creek actually has salmon and steelhead runs. Next up is Butterfly Park and then Willamette Park. Now you're back to an open riverside path, passing the Willamette Sailing Club and then reentering the world of condos. The 1.2 miles north of Willamette Park offer constant views of the river, and you'll pass benches, docks, and beaches.

After passing the River Forum office building on the left, you'll have to get around some private property by cutting through the office park, but the signs are easy to follow. (This area, the last gap in the trail, was slated for construction at press time, so it might connect through when you get there.) You'll arrive at SW Bancroft Street; turn right and walk a block to SW Bond Avenue. You can enjoy a brief riverside section by the Old Spaghetti Factory or head up Bond to SW Gaines and turn right to resume the riverside trail for a bit. After coming to a viewpoint of the Ross Island Bridge, turn west along SW Curry Street, and follow it three blocks to Moody. Turn right, and in two blocks you'll be at the base of the Portland Aerial Tram.

Or the entire above paragraph will have been replaced by a whole new section of riverside trail connecting to Poet's Beach.

· ·

GPS TRAILHEAD COORDINATES N45° 29.917' W122° 40.311'

DIRECTIONS See the public-transit access points for each section in the Description.

COLUMBIA SPORTSWEAR
columbia.com

Main Store
911 SW Broadway
Portland, OR 97201
503-226-6800

Outlet
1323 SE Tacoma St.
Portland, OR 97202
503-238-0118

THE MOUNTAIN SHOP
1510 NE 37th Ave.
Portland, OR 97232
503-288-6768
mountainshop.net

NEXT ADVENTURE (sells some used items)
426 SE Grand Ave.
Portland, OR 97214
503-233-0706
nextadventure.net

OREGON MOUNTAIN COMMUNITY
2975 NE Sandy Blvd.
Portland, OR 97232
503-227-1038
omcgear.com

PATAGONIA
907 NW Irving St.
Portland, OR 97209
503-525-2552
patagonia.com

REI
rei.com

Clackamas Town Center
12160 SE 82nd Ave.
Portland, OR 97086
503-659-1156

Hillsboro
2235 NW Allie Ave. (NW 194th Avenue
at Cornell Road)
Hillsboro, OR 97124
503-617-6072

Portland
1405 NW Johnson St.
Portland, OR 97209
503-221-1938

Tualatin
7410 SW Bridgeport Rd.
Portland, OR 97209
503-624-8600

APPENDIX B: Places to Buy Maps

GREEN TRAILS MAPS
greentrailsmaps.com

OREGON MOUNTAIN COMMUNITY
2975 NE Sandy Blvd.
Portland, OR 97232
503-227-1038
omcgear.com

REI
rei.com

Clackamas Town Center
12160 SE 82nd Ave.
Portland, OR 97086
503-659-1156

Hillsboro
2235 NW Allie Ave.
(NW 194th Avenue at Cornell Road)
Hillsboro, OR 97124
503-617-6072

Portland
1405 NW Johnson St.
Portland, OR 97209
503-221-1938

Tualatin
7410 SW Bridgeport Road
Portland, OR 97209
503-624-8600

BERGFREUNDE SKI CLUB

503-245-8543
bergfreunde.org

COLUMBIA RIVER VOLKSSPORT CLUB

walking4fun.org
Hikes scheduled at meetup.com
/walking-oregon-and-sw-washington
Facebook: tinyurl.com/
columbiavolkssport

FOREST PARK CONSERVANCY

210 NW 17th Ave., Ste. 201
Portland, OR 97209
503-223-5449
forestparkconservancy.org
Facebook: facebook.com/forestpark
conservancy
Twitter: @pdxforestpark

FRIENDS OF THE COLUMBIA GORGE

522 SW Fifth Ave., Ste. 720
Portland, OR 97204
503-241-3762
gorgefriends.org
Facebook: facebook.com/gorgefriends
Twitter: @gorgefriends

MAZAMAS

527 SE 43rd Ave., Portland, OR 97215
503-227-2345
mazamas.org
Facebook: facebook.com/mazamaspdx
Twitter: @mazamas

PORTLAND PARKS & RECREATION

503-823-play (7529)
portlandoregon.gov/parks
Facebook: facebook.com/portlandparks
Twitter: @pdxparksandrec

SIERRA CLUB, OREGON CHAPTER

1821 SE Ankeny St., Portland, OR 97214
503-238-0442
oregon2.sierraclub.org/chapter
Hikes scheduled at meetup.com
/the-portland-vancouver-sierra-club
-outings
Facebook: facebook.com/orsierraclub
Twitter: @orsierraclub

TRAILS CLUB OF OREGON

503-233-2740
trailsclub.org
Hikes scheduled at meetup.com
/trails-club-of-oregon
Facebook: tinyurl.com/ortrailsclub

APPENDIX D: Online Resources

My website, paulgerald.com, features my blog, regular hike reviews, information on trail conditions, public appearances, and guided hiking trips. You can also find me at facebook.com/hikerpaul and twitter.com/60hikesportland.

Here are more excellent online resources:

➤ **Green Trails Maps** (greentrailsmaps.com) sells terrific recreation maps.

➤ **Meetup.com** hosts a dozen or so local groups related to hiking and outdoor adventures (see opposite page for a few examples).

➤ **Northwest Hiker** (nwhiker.com) is an excellent guide to Pacific Northwest hikes, with photos.

➤ **Find searchable listings of all Oregon State Parks** at oregonstateparks.org (Facebook: facebook.com/oregonstateparks, Twitter: @orstateparks).

➤ **On the nwhikers.net discussion boards,** thousands of members post trip reports and trail conditions from all over the Pacific Northwest.

➤ **Oregon Hikers** (oregonhikers.org) is an invaluable resource for finding up-to-date conditions, trail descriptions, and people to go hiking with in the Portland area. (Say hello to OneSpeed there—he wrote this book.)

➤ **Trailkeepers of Oregon** (trailkeepersoforegon.org, Facebook: facebook.com/trail keepersoregon) is a nonprofit dedicated to protecting and enhancing the Oregon hiking experience through advocacy, stewardship, outreach, and education. If you've ever wanted to do some work on an Oregon trail to keep it in shape—and that would be a fine thing to do—get in touch with these folks.

➤ **The massive summitpost.org message boards** discuss mountain ranges all over the world, from the Absarokas in Wyoming to the Zlatibor Massif in Serbia. Seriously.

➤ **The U.S. Forest Service** operates the following websites for national forests that are within the scope of this book: Columbia River Gorge National Scenic Area, www.fs.usda.gov/crgnsa; Gifford Pinchot National Forest, www.fs.usda .gov/giffordpinchot; Mount Hood National Forest, www.fs.usda.gov/mthood; Siuslaw National Forest, www.fs.usda.gov/siuslaw; and Willamette National Forest, www.fs.usda.gov/willamette.

➤ **Find information on Washington State Parks** at parks.wa.gov (Facebook: facebook.com/washingtonstateparks).

➤ **The nonprofit Washington Trails Association** (wta.org, Facebook: facebook .com/washingtontrails, Twitter: @wta_hikers) promotes hiking, leads trips, and coordinates trail maintenance.

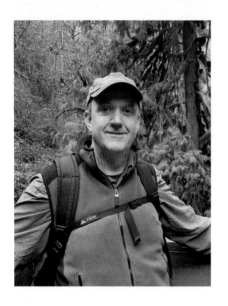

Paul Gerald has written professionally for newspapers, magazines and websites for more than 30 years. After growing up in Memphis, Tennessee, and graduating from Southern Methodist University in Dallas, he moved to Portland in 1996 to be closer to the mountains and ocean. Since then, he has written hundreds of freelance articles and four books in addition to this one: *Peaceful Places: Portland, Day and Section Hikes Pacific Crest Trail: Oregon, Best Tent Camping: Oregon,* and *Breakfast in Bridgetown: The Definitive Guide to Portland's Favorite Meal.*

Paul's hiking life started at the age of 12, when he went to a summer camp in the Absaroka Mountains of Wyoming. He's hiked in the Rocky Mountains from New Mexico to Montana and in Appalachia, Alaska, Argentina, Italy, the UK, and Nepal. He has led hikes, outings, and tours, both domestic and international, for Evergreen Escapes of Portland, Embark Exploration Co. (a Portland-based adventure-travel company), and the Mazamas mountaineering club. He is also on the board of Trailkeepers of Oregon and has worked as a driver for Radio Cab Company.

His latest passion is English soccer; he's writing and publishing a travel and cultural guide called *An American's Guide to Soccer in England,* which is great fun except when the research conflicts with seeing his beloved Portland Timbers.

Paul enjoys meeting people who use his books out on the trails; he's also grateful that none of them have appeared to be lost or angry. He does hope, however, that any feedback will be directed to him, care of the publisher, or to paulgerald.com, facebook.com/hikerpaul, or twitter.com/60hikesportland. And he hopes people will continue to enjoy and benefit from the fruits of his labor—if hiking and writing can truly be called labor.